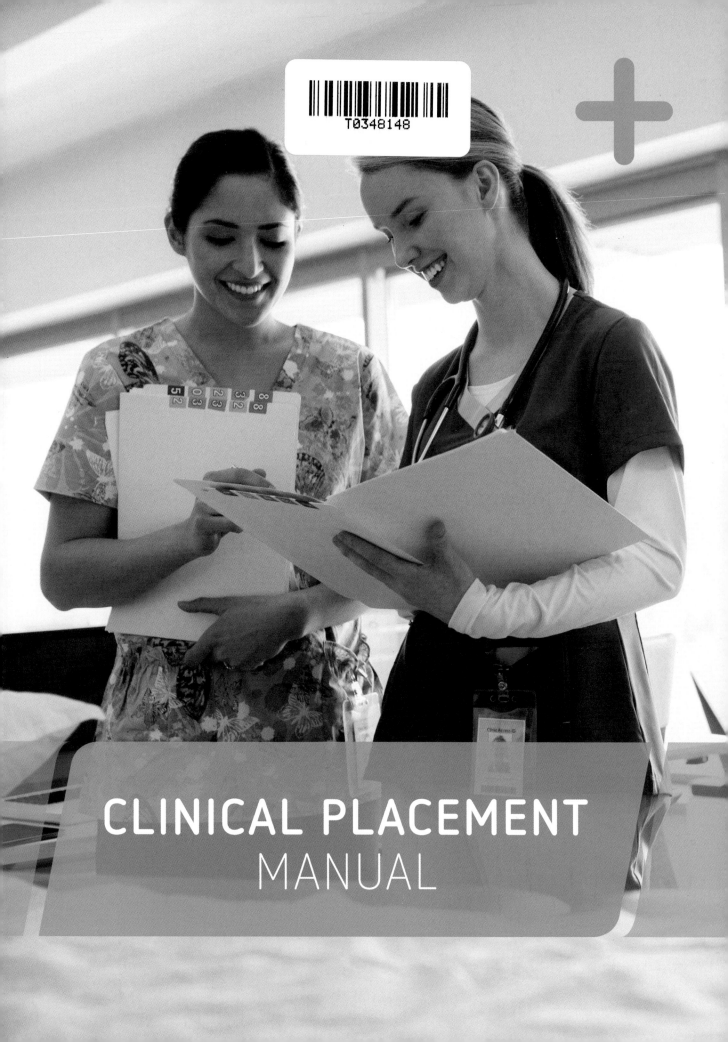

CLINICAL PLACEMENT
MANUAL

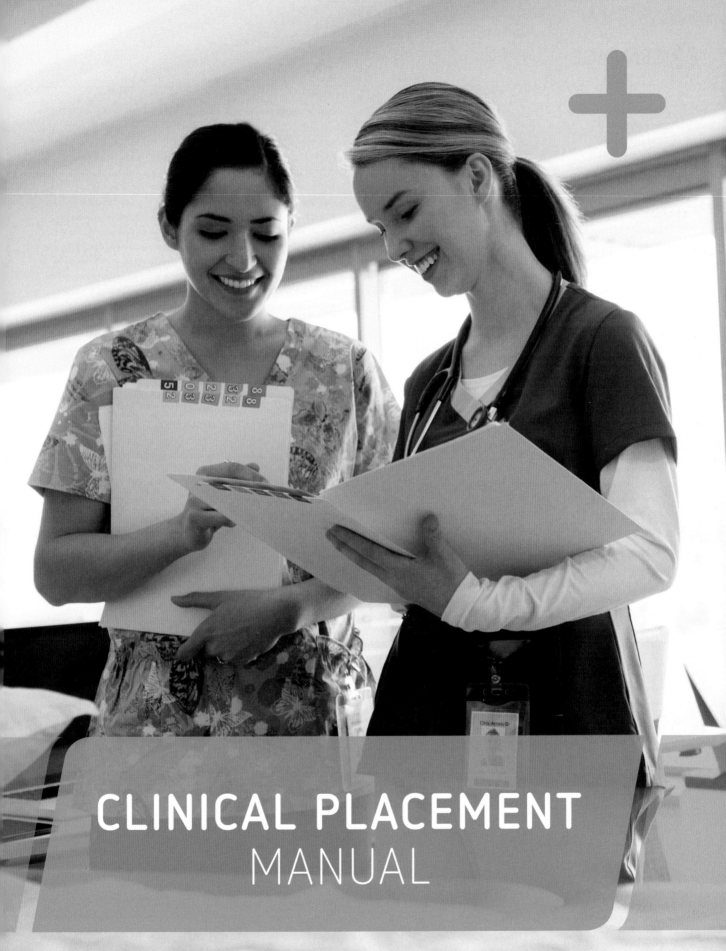

CLINICAL PLACEMENT
MANUAL

Catherine JOUSTRA, Ali MOLONEY

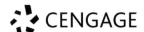

Clinical Placement Manual
1st Edition
Catherine Joustra
Ali Moloney

Head of content management: Dorothy Chiu
Content manager: Sophie Kalienicki
Content development manager: Jessica Brennan
Project editor: Sutha Surenddar
Editor: Craig MacKenzie
Proofreader: Jade Jakovcic
Permissions/Photo researcher: Jessica Boland (Boland Consulting)
Text designer: Rina Gargano (Alba Design)
Project designer: James Steer
Cover: Getty Images/Hero Images
MPS Limited

Any URLs contained in this publication were checked for currency during the production process. Note, however, that the publisher cannot vouch for the ongoing currency of URLs.

Acknowledgements
Part opener images
Part 1: Shutterstock.com/Photographee.eu; Part 2: Shutterstock.com/Photographee.eu; Part 3: Shutterstock.com/Photographee.eu; Part 4: iStock.com/Steve Debenport; Part 5: iStock.com/Ridofranz; Part 6: Shutterstock.com/Photographee.eu; Part 7: iStock.com/FatCamera

Notice to the Reader: Publisher does not warrant or guarantee any of the products described herein or perform any independent analysis in connection with any of the product information contained herein. Publisher does not assume, and expressly disclaims, any obligation to obtain and include information other than that provided to it by the manufacturer. The reader is expressly warned to consider and adopt all safety precautions that might be indicated by the activities described herein and to avoid all potential hazards. By following the instructions contained herein, the reader willingly assumes all risks in connection with such instructions. The publisher makes no representations or warranties of any kind, including but not limited to, the warranties of fitness for particular purpose or merchantability, nor are any such representations implied with respect to the material set forth herein, and the publisher takes no responsibility with respect to such material. The publisher shall not be liable for any special, consequential, or exemplary damages resulting, in whole or part, from the readers' use of, or reliance upon, this material.

For product information and technology assistance,
in Australia call **1300 790 853**;
in New Zealand call **0800 449 725**

For permission to use material from this text or product, please email **aust.permissions@cengage.com**

National Library of Australia Cataloguing-in-Publication Data

Creator:	Catherine Joustra, author
Title:	Clinical Placement Manual/Catherine Joustra/Ali Moloney (author).
Edition:	1st
ISBN:	9780170407021 (paperback)
Notes:	Includes index.
Other Creators/Contributors:	
	Ali Moloney (author).

Cengage Learning Australia
Level 7, 80 Dorcas Street
South Melbourne, Victoria Australia 3205

Cengage Learning New Zealand
Unit 4B Rosedale Office Park
331 Rosedale Road, Albany, North Shore 0632, NZ

For learning solutions, visit **cengage.com.au**

Printed in China by China Translation & Printing Services.
1 2 3 4 5 6 7 22 21 20 19 18

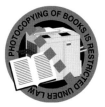

Brief contents

PART 1   CLINICAL PLACEMENT AGED CARE   1

Chapter 1   Safe work practices for direct client care   3

Chapter 2   Infection prevention and control   16

Chapter 3   Care of the older person   31

Chapter 4   Legal and ethical parameters for nursing practice   54

Chapter 5   Clinical assessment and planning nursing care   68

Chapter 6   Communication skills in nursing practice   80

Chapter 7   Physical health status   90

Chapter 8   Nursing within the Australian health-care system   106

Chapter 9   Working with diverse people   124

PART 2   CLINICAL PLACEMENT PALLIATIVE   136

Chapter 10   A palliative approach to nursing practice   139

PART 3   CLINICAL PLACEMENT REHABILITATION/SUBACUTE   157

Chapter 11   Client health information   159

Chapter 12   Nursing care for a person with complex needs   174

Chapter 13   Principles of wound management   188

Chapter 14   Nursing care plans   201

Chapter 15   Improving professional practice   215

Chapter 16   Care for a person with chronic health problems   224

Chapter 17   Researching and applying evidence to practice   239

Chapter 18   Care for a person with diabetes   253

PART 4   CLINICAL PLACEMENT MENTAL HEALTH   272

Chapter 19   Care for a person with mental health conditions   275

PART 5   CLINICAL PLACEMENT ACUTE   290

Chapter 20   Medicines and intravenous therapy   293

Chapter 21   Care for a person with acute health problems   319

PART 6   CLINICAL PLACEMENT COMMUNITY   331

Chapter 22   Nursing practice in the primary health-care setting   333

Chapter 23   Aboriginal and/or Torres Strait Islander health care   352

Chapter 24   Maternal and infant health care   366

PART 7   CLINICAL PLACEMENT MATERNITY   379

Chapter 25   Improving clinical practice   381

Contents

Guide to the text   xv
Guide to the online resources   xviii
Preface   xix
About the authors   xx
Acknowledgements   xxi
Introduction to clinical
placement   xxii

PART 1 CLINICAL PLACEMENT AGED CARE

Chapter 1 Safe work practices for direct
client care   3
1.1 Safe work practices for direct client care   4
    Workplace policies and procedures   4
    Hazards in the workplace   6
    Working safely with clients   7
    Reducing risk in the workplace   8
    Incidents and injuries   9
1.2 Safe work practices for manual handling   9
1.3 Safe work practices for managing infection
    control   11
1.4 Working as a team to ensure a safe working
    environment   13
1.5 Reflecting on your own safe work
    practices   13
    Summary   14
    Self-test questions   15
    Bibliography   15

Chapter 2 Infection prevention and control   16
2.1 Standard and additional precautions
    for infection prevention and control   17
    Standard precautions   17
2.2 Identifying infection hazards and
    assessing risks   26
    Infection hazards associated with your
    own role and work environment   26
    Areas of responsibility in relation
    to infection prevention and control   27
    Assessing risk   27
    Documenting and reporting activities
    and tasks that put you, clients, visitors
    and/or other workers at risk   27
    Control measures to minimise risk in
    accordance with organisation's
    procedures   28

2.3 Managing risks associated with
    specific hazards   28
    Protocols for care after exposure to blood
    and other bodily fluids   29
    Contamination considerations   29
    Minimising contamination   30
    Summary   30
    Self-test questions   30
    Bibliography   30

Chapter 3 Care of the older person   31
3.1 Health requirements of an older person   32
    Age-related physical changes and psychosocial
    needs of a person, their family or carer   32
    Age-related effects of drugs and medications   34
    Age-related pathophysiological disorders
    and preventative care   35
    Communicating effectively and making
    adjustments for people who have sensory
    impairments   36
    Preventative health assessment   36
    Theories of ageing   36
    Companionship and social inclusion   37
    Oral health problems   37
    Identify and respond to signs of distress   38
3.2 Care planning for the older person   38
    Aged care assessment tools   38
    Documentation and reporting   39
    Identifying abilities and limitations for
    self-care   40
    Contribute to the development of
    nursing care plans   41
    Understanding the implications of
    the admission   41
    Impacts of age-related disorders on ADLs
    and nursing interventions   41
3.3 Applying nursing practice in the aged care
    environment   42
    Stereotypes, attitudes, values and beliefs
    associated with ageing   42
    Impact of complex issues on family and carers   42
    Promoting health maintenance   43
    Community services   43
3.4 Aged care requirements and issues   44
    Identify legal requirements and ethical
    issues, and ensure work practice supports
    person's rights   44
    Elder abuse   45

Advocate for the person — 45
Responding to signs of stress — 46
Providing care for a deceased person — 46
Providing support in grief and death — 47
3.5 Strategies for dementia — 47
Types of dementia — 47
3.6 Strategies to minimise the impact of challenging behaviours — 49
Determining triggers contributing to challenging behaviours — 49
Impact of behaviours on person and others — 50
Best practice strategies to minimise impact — 50
Summary — 52
Self-test questions — 52
Bibliography — 52

Chapter 4 Legal and ethical parameters for nursing practice — 54
4.1 The scope of professional nursing practice — 55
Acts, guidelines, codes and nursing practice — 55
Scope of practice — 56
Responding to complaints — 57
Requests for information — 57
Documentation — 57
Monitoring your own compliance — 58
4.2 Applying knowledge of the legal framework to nursing practice — 59
Negligence, duty of care and vicarious liability — 59
Consent — 60
Restraint — 60
Common legal terms — 61
Writing reports — 61
Mandatory reporting processes — 61
Privacy and confidentiality — 62
Interpret referrals or requests for tests on receipt — 62
4.3 Ethics — 62
Demonstrating ethical practice — 63
Contemporary ethical issues — 63
Reporting potential ethical issues — 63
Resolving ethical issues — 63
4.4 Supporting the rights, interests and needs of patients and their families — 64
Duty of care — 64
Supporting the person's rights and interests, and encouraging decisions — 64
Advocating for the person — 65
4.5 Open disclosure processes — 66
Other health-care workers in relation to open disclosure — 66

Summary — 67
Self-test questions — 67
Bibliography — 67

Chapter 5 Clinical assessment and planning nursing care — 68
5.1 Collecting and interpreting health data — 69
Introduction and explanations — 69
Gathering information — 69
What to include in the primary health assessment — 69
Vital signs — 70
Developmental stages — 70
Other data to collect — 71
Families and carers — 72
Critical thinking — 73
Communication when a person's condition deteriorates — 74
5.2 Admission and discharge procedures — 74
Data for admission and discharge — 74
Issues that may impact on discharge — 74
Community supports — 75
Requirements for discharge — 76
5.3 Planning nursing care for clients — 76
Identifying risks and the health care that is required — 76
5.4 Ongoing development of nursing care plans — 77
Analysis of rationale behind decisions — 77
Confirming that nursing interventions are meeting client's needs — 78
Conflicts between the nursing care plan and the already prescribed plan of care — 79
Summary — 79
Self-test questions — 79
Bibliography — 79

Chapter 6 Communication skills in nursing practice — 80
6.1 Effective communication in complex situations — 81
Listening skills — 83
6.2 Identifying and addressing constraints to communication — 84
6.3 Using information technology to support communication in nursing practice — 85
6.4 Leading small group discussions — 85
6.5 Giving and receiving feedback for performance improvement — 86
Performance review — 86
Self-evaluation — 87
Reflecting on feedback — 88

6.6 Evaluating effectiveness of
     communication in complex situations   88
     Summary   *89*
     Self-test questions   *89*
     Bibliography   *89*

Chapter 7 Physical health status   90

7.1 Obtaining accurate information
     about physical health   91
     Interpreting information based on the
     structure and functioning of body systems   91
     Using information obtained to identify
     actual or potential health problems   96
     Factors that can impact on
     physical conditions   97

7.2 Checking the physical health status of clients   99
     Importance of checking client's physical
     health status before delivery of interventions   99
     Job role and organisation requirements
     for interventions   99
     Clarification of client's physical health status   100

7.3 Identifying variations from normal
     physical health status   100
     Identifying variations from normal health
     status using standard methods and protocols   100
     Potential factors responsible for variations
     in health status   103
     Risk factors associated with variations
     from normal health status   104
     When to refer issues   104
     Summary   *105*
     Self-test questions   *105*
     Bibliography   *105*

**Chapter 8 Nursing within the Australian
health-care system   106**

8.1 Principles and knowledge required of
     nurses in a health-care system   107
     Principles of primary health and wellness   107
     Agencies that facilitate positive
     health outcomes   107
     Sociocultural and social influences
     that affect health   108
     Political and economic impacts on health   109
     Non-Western approaches to health
     care and nursing practice   110
     Strategies the nurse can use to maintain
     standards of care   111
     Current health issues for health-care delivery   112

8.2 Funding sources for health care in Australia   113
     Awareness of appropriate sources of funding   113
     Discussing health-care services   113

8.3 Identifying and responding to factors
     and issues affecting health in Australia   114
     Factors affecting health   114
     Risk factors for health   115
     Existing health services   115
     Effectiveness of community
     health promotion   116
     Emotional and social wellbeing   117

8.4 Working in the context of professional
     nursing practice   118
     Historical development and current
     perspectives of nursing   118
     Nursing theorists   118
     Professional nursing bodies   119
     The principles and parameters of
     nursing practice   119
     Audits and accreditation processes   120
     Scope of practice framework   120
     Role of the nurse   120

8.5 Contributing to a professional
     work team   121
     Collaborative relationships   121
     How reflective practice impacts
     nursing practice   121
     Effective teamwork   121
     Summary   *122*
     Self-test questions   *122*
     Bibliography   *123*

Chapter 9 Working with diverse people   124

9.1 Reflecting on your own perspectives   125
     Social and cultural perspectives
     and biases   125
     Improving self and social awareness   126

9.2 The benefits of diversity and
     inclusiveness   127
     Professional relationships   128
     Work practices for a safe environment 129

9.3 Communicating with people from diverse
     backgrounds and situations   129
     Using verbal and non-verbal
     communication constructively   130
     Effective strategies to manage
     language barriers   131
     Seeking assistance according to
     communication needs   131

9.4 Promoting understanding across diverse
     groups   133
     Issues that may cause communication
     misunderstandings   133
     The impact of social and cultural diversity   133

Resolving differences 134
Summary 135
Self-test questions 135
Bibliography 135

PART 2 CLINICAL PLACEMENT PALLIATIVE

Chapter 10 A palliative approach
to nursing practice 139

10.1 The needs of a person requiring
a palliative approach to care 140
Principles of palliative care
and the palliative approach 140
Pathophysiological changes 141
Pain management 141
Social, emotional and spiritual needs 143
Working with the interdisciplinary team 144
Psychosocial impact of palliative care
on family and carers 144

10.2 Supporting the person, family or
carers using the palliative approach 146
Discussing spiritual and cultural issues
in an open and non-judgemental manner 146
Communication techniques and
support services 146
Monitoring the patient's condition
and respecting their wishes 147
Advance care planning and directives 147

10.3 Signs of deterioration and the stages
of dying 148
Physiology of dying 148
Management of respiratory and
swallowing difficulties 149
Malignant wound management 149
Signs of deterioration or
imminent death 150
Dignity in death 150
Ethical issues and concerns 151
Signs of clinical death 151

10.4 Caring for the person's body after death and
providing support for the family and others 152
Legislation (and policy and procedures) 152
Autopsy 152
Organ donation 152
Care of the body after death 153
Support needs and resources
for bereavement care 154
Emotional support relating to grief,
loss and bereavement 154

10.5 Self-care in the palliative care role 155
Self-care and supporting wellbeing 155
Support and professional debriefing 155
Summary 156
Self-test questions 156
Bibliography 156

PART 3 CLINICAL PLACEMENT REHABILITATION/SUBACUTE

Chapter 11 Client health information 159

11.1 Assessing clients' health status 160
Planning services to meet a client's needs 160
Recognising normal readings for vital
signs, tests and observations 161
Identifying pathophysiology through
observation, physical assessment and analysis 161
The impact of specific interventions 162
Disease 162
Health status 163
Homeostasis 163

11.2 Planning to address identified health status 170
Documentation 173
Summary 173
Self-test questions 173
Bibliography 173

Chapter 12 Nursing care for a person
with complex needs 174

12.1 Nursing interventions to assist a person
with complex needs 175
Nursing interventions based on
predetermined care plans 176
Nursing interventions demonstrating
respect for dignity and cultural diversity 176
Encouraging patient involvement
during care interventions 178
Physical, emotional and psychosocial
needs to consider 179
The importance of reporting
and recording 179

12.2 Nursing care of people with common
disorders and conditions 180
Nursing care for complex conditions 181

12.3 Critical thinking to improve care quality 185
Identifying nursing interventions 185
Quality improvement processes 186
Summary 187
Self-test questions 187
Bibliography 187

Chapter 13 Principles of wound management   188

13.1 Applying protocols for wound assessment   189
Client cooperation and consent   190
Maintaining client dignity and privacy   190
Documentation and reporting   190
Non-disturbance of wounds   190
Strategies to minimise cross-contamination and spread of infection   192
13.2 Assessing the impact of wounds   193
13.3 Planning care   194
13.4 Clinical nursing care of wounds   196
13.5 Complex or challenging wounds   197
13.6 Evaluating outcomes of nursing action in wound care   198
Wound review and reassessment   199
Documentation   199
Summary   199
Self-test questions   200
Bibliography   200

Chapter 14 Nursing care plans   201

14.1 Preparing a person for care procedures   202
Consent   202
Documentation   202
Dignity   204
14.2 Implementing care procedures to meet identified needs   205
Personal hygiene   206
Skin integrity   206
Nutritional needs   207
Respiratory function   207
Encouraging the person to contribute to their own independence and mobility   208
Comfort, rest and sleep   208
Dealing with emergencies   209
14.3 Monitoring a person's identified care needs   210
Ongoing assessment through observation, monitoring equipment and devices   210
Risks associated with hospitalisation   210
Reporting and recording changes   211
14.4 Evaluating outcomes of care provided   211
Consulting and collaborating with the interdisciplinary health-care team   211
Evaluating outcomes and changing care plans   211
Discharge planning   213
Summary   214
Self-test questions   214
Bibliography   214

Chapter 15 Improving professional practice   215

15.1 Reflecting on your own practice   216
Barriers to reflective practice   217
Models of reflective practice   217
Actively seeking feedback from others   218
15.2 Enhancing your own practice   219
Support networks   219
Self-care and support   220
Recognising the need for self-development   220
15.3 Facilitating ongoing professional development   221
Professional development   221
Confirming own practice against ethical and legal requirements   221
Performance review   222
Review processes   222
Summary   223
Self-test questions   223
Bibliography   223

Chapter 16 Care for a person with chronic health problems   224

16.1 Identifying the impacts of chronic health conditions   225
Chronic health problems and possible impacts   225
The person's and their carer's understanding of the disease process   229
Current treatments   232
Community-based care services   234
Involving the person   234
16.2 Contributing to a coordinated service approach   235
Other supports available   235
Support of the family or carer   235
Role and responsibilities for communication and reporting   236
Variations in the person's needs and the response of the health-care team   237
Health education and the role of the health-care team   237
Summary   238
Self-test questions   238
Bibliography   238

Chapter 17 Researching and applying evidence to practice   239

17.1 Planning information-gathering activities   240
How research can support and improve work practice   240
Current trends   241

Research objectives 241
Credible sources of data
and evidence 243
Cultural and ethical considerations
for research 243
17.2 Gathering information 244
Selecting and evaluating information 244
A systematic approach 245
Relevance of research 245
Organising information 246
17.3 Analysing information 247
Prioritising information 247
Comparing and contrasting information 247
Strength, relevance, reliability and currency 248
Feasibility, benefits and risks 248
Conclusions 249
17.4 Using information in practice 250
Identifying potential areas for change
and further research 250
Actions to address outcomes of research 250
Summary 252
Self-test questions 252
Bibliography 252

Chapter 18 Care for a person with diabetes 253
18.1 Diabetes care services 254
Information on diabetes care and
sources of funding for related services 254
Specialist services and complementary
roles of organisations 255
Liaising with referring agencies and
community organisations 256
18.2 Assessing the needs of a person
with diabetes 256
Pathophysiology of diabetes 256
Holistic nursing assessment 259
Determining the person's understanding
of their condition, self-management
strategies and medications 260
Possible factors impacting the person's
health 260
The family or carer's understanding of and
involvement in the person's diabetes care 261
18.3 Complex nursing interventions to achieve
and maintain optimal diabetes health 262
Managing nursing workload and re-
prioritising care activities for the person 262
Complex care needs of a person
with diabetes 262
Ongoing management of the
person's condition 264

Administering prescribed emergency
medication 264
Evaluating and interpreting blood
and urine test results related to diabetic
conditions 265
Alterations in the person's condition 266
18.4 Evaluating the care plan for a person with
diabetes, and supporting self-management 267
Reviewing and modifying the care plan 267
Considering outcomes against evidence-
based best practice 267
The person's understanding of their diabetes
condition, medications, therapeutic regimes
and self-management 268
Promoting the person's self-
management of their condition 269
Specific health promotion initiatives
to support self-management 269
Summary 271
Self-test questions 271
Bibliography 271

PART 4 CLINICAL PLACEMENT MENTAL HEALTH

Chapter 19 Care for a person with
mental health conditions 275
19.1 State/territory mental health legislation
requirements 276
Key features of mental health legislation 277
The values and philosophies that apply
to mental health care 277
The rights of the person 278
Legal issues in nursing 279
19.2 Responding appropriately to signs
of mental illness 279
Conditions and behaviours 280
Signs and symptoms 281
Biopsychosocial effects 281
Stereotyping and stigma 281
Using negotiation skills 282
19.3 Contributing to care planning and conducting
initial clinical observations for a person
with a mental health condition 282
Risk assessment 282
The interdisciplinary health-care team 284
Observing the person's behaviour
and physical health 285
Health promotion and educational
strategies 286

Interdisciplinary team meetings and service providers   286

Recovery principles with support from interdisciplinary team   286

19.4 Contributing to the recovery of a person with a mental health condition   286

Planning, prioritising and implementing nursing interventions   287

Respect for the person's dignity and uniqueness   287

Assisting the client, carer or family in appropriate therapeutic interventions   287

Medication   287

Community resources and opportunities   288

Supporting and valuing the person with a mental health illness   288

Summary   289

Self-test questions   289

Bibliography   289

PART 5 CLINICAL PLACEMENT ACUTE

Chapter 20 Medicines and intravenous therapy   293

20.1 Minimising potential risk to ensure safe administration of medications   294

Drugs and poisons schedules and classifications   294

Purpose and function of prescribed medicine and intravenous (IV) therapy   296

Pharmacology and substance incompatibilities when administering medication, blood and blood products   296

20.2 Preparing for medication administration and infusion of IV fluids   297

Explaining the processes of medication administration or IV fluid infusion   297

Identifying correct administration route or site for each medication or IV fluid   298

Considering the medication's effect on the body   299

Calculating accurate dosages and IV infusion rates   299

Legislative and organisational requirements   301

Techniques and precautions specific to the person's situation   301

Preparing blood and blood products for blood transfusions   304

20.3 Administering and storing medication   305

Applying the 'rights of medication administration'   306

Securing medications in a safe manner   308

Applying quality practices and undertaking risk assessment   308

Reporting refusal of medication or IV therapy or suspected incomplete medication ingestion   308

Handling and storing of medications and blood products   309

20.4 Monitoring and evaluating a person's response to administered medication, IV fluids, blood and blood products   309

Documenting and monitoring the person's response   310

Acute and delayed adverse reactions   310

Fluid and electrolyte imbalances   311

Removing the IV cannula   311

Educating the person, their family or carer on administration of medicines   314

20.5 Assessing the effectiveness of pain-relieving therapy   314

Identifying signs of pain or discomfort   314

Clarify the location and nature of pain   315

Interpreting observations and evaluating the person's pain   315

Prescribed medications and complementary strategies that may alleviate pain and discomfort   316

Assessing effectiveness of pain-relieving medication and non-medication therapies   316

Recording observations of the effectiveness of pain management strategies   316

Summary   317

Self-test questions   318

Bibliography   318

Chapter 21 Care for a person with acute health problems   319

21.1 Impact of acute health problems on the person, family or carer   320

Preliminary health assessment and the health-care team   320

Physical and psychological impacts of acute problems on the client and the family or carer   321

Pathophysiology   322

21.2 Planning care for a person with acute health problems   323

Health-care team and care planning   323

Gather information, document and report changes to health-care team members   323

21.3 Performing nursing interventions to support health care   324

Compromised airway   324

Prioritising and modifying nursing interventions to reflect changes in the person's condition   325

Observe and identify the need for
psychological support and care   325
21.4 Pre- and post-operative nursing care   **326**
Promoting post-operative comfort using
pain management strategies   327
21.5 Emergency response in the acute care
environment   **328**
Medical Emergency Team   328
Identifying emergency situations and
responding to first-aid requests   329
Summary   *329*
Self-test questions   *330*
Bibliography   *330*

PART 6 CLINICAL PLACEMENT COMMUNITY

Chapter 22 Nursing practice in the primary
health-care setting   **333**
22.1 The interdisciplinary health-care team in
a primary health-care environment   **334**
Primary health-care principles and
philosophical framework   334
Service model and the roles of the
interdisciplinary health-care team   334
Your role in community
health-care service   335
Effective decision making in primary
health care   335
22.2 Impact of health problems on a
person in the primary health-care
environment   **336**
Health issues affecting the Australian
community   336
Clinical manifestations of health
conditions   340
Priorities and potential areas of risk   342
Sharing information   343
Physical, psychological and social
impacts on activities of daily living   343
Actual or potential environmental
health issues   344
22.3 Providing health education and health
promotion for illness prevention   **344**
Strategies to support the person   345
Health promotion programs   345
22.4 Performing nursing interventions that
support a person's health-care needs   **346**
Nursing practice to support dignity
and privacy   347
Families and carers   347

Adjusting nursing interventions   348
Prioritising nursing interventions
according to the person's needs   349
Emergency treatment   349
22.5 Evaluating outcomes of planned
primary health care and
suitable resources   **349**
Evaluating care and how to access
resources   350
Community supports   350
Summary   *350*
Self-test questions   *351*
Bibliography   *351*

Chapter 23 Aboriginal and/or Torres
Strait Islander health care   **352**
23.1 Identifying cultural safety issues in
the workplace   **353**
Critical issues that influence
relationships and communication   353
Cultural safety guidelines   355
23.2 Modelling cultural safety in your
own work   **355**
Communication techniques   356
23.3 Developing strategies for improved
cultural safety   **356**
Health strategies   359
23.4 Evaluating cultural safety strategies   **362**
Self-determination   362
Collaboration   363
Evaluation   363
In conclusion   363
Summary   *364*
Self-test questions   *364*
Bibliography   *364*

Chapter 24 Maternal and infant
health care   **366**
24.1 Caring for a mother and newborn infant as
part of the health-care team   **367**
Pregnancy and foetal development   367
Labour and birth   370
Nursing care – assisting the midwife   370
Using correct terminology   373
Assisting with lactation   373
Assisting the mother with safe practices
in infant care   374
Ongoing care of mother   374
Documenting and recording
observations of the mother and
newborn infant   375
Providing holistic care   375

24.2 Supporting mother and newborn infant
       towards identified goals   376
       Outcomes of care   376
       Planning care and care goals   377
       Education   377
       Summary   *378*
       Self-test questions   *378*
       Bibliography   *378*

PART 7 CLINICAL PLACEMENT MATERNITY

Chapter 25 Improving clinical practice   381
   25.1 Modelling high standards of performance   382
        Organisational vision   382
        Supporting colleagues   382
        Respectful and positive communication   383
        Continuous improvement   383
   25.2 Reflecting on clinical work practices
        and potential improvements   385
        Reflection   386
        Systemic improvements   386
        Discussing and exploring challenges   387
        Sourcing information   387

25.3 Participating in processes for systemic
     improvement   388
     Organisation forums   388
     Recognising opportunities for systemic
     improvements to clinical guidelines
     for nursing practice   389
     Presenting and arguing ideas for improving
     clinical practice   389
     Identifying and articulating issues and
     practical processes for implementing
     change   390
     Responding to questions with confidence
     and relevant information   390
     Engaging with others using professional
     terminology   390
     Feedback   390
     Summary   *391*
     Self-test questions   *391*
     Bibliography   *392*

Glossary   393
Index   397

Guide to the text

As you read this text you will find a number of features in every chapter to assist you in your work placement and to help you understand how the theory is applied in the real world.

PART OPENING FEATURES

Gain an insight into arenas of placement in each **Part opening section**. This is a real-world reflection, a nurse experience with an outline of the types of people you will encounter, the objectives of this work placement and a discussion of how work is allocated.

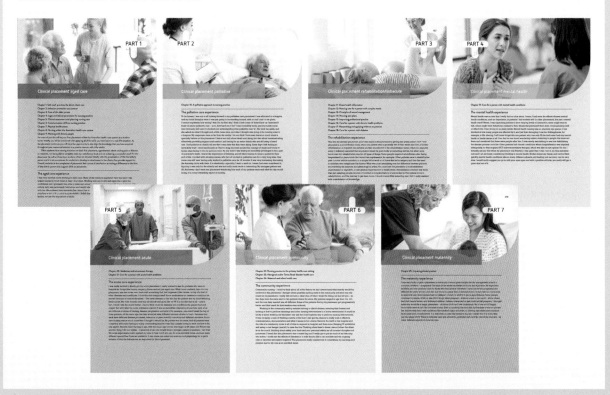

CHAPTER OPENING FEATURES

Identify the key concepts that the chapter will cover with the **Learning outcomes** at the start of each chapter.

Gain an insight into the placement experience in the **vignette** at the beginning of each chapter.

Care for a person with mental health conditions

CHAPTER
19

LEARNING OUTCOMES

After reading this chapter, you should have an understanding of:

19.1 State/territory mental health legislation requirements

19.2 Responding appropriately to signs of mental illness

19.3 Contributing to care planning and conducting initial clinical observations for a person with a mental health condition.

A dignified death

I was very apprehensive when I was told that my next clinical placement would be on the palliative care ward. I had never seen a person die and the only funerals I had attended had been for my grandfather who was elderly and had been ill for a long time.

On the first day I tiptoed quietly after my buddy and was very nervous even touching one of the clients in case I caused them to die. One of the clients I was involved with was Eileen.

Eileen was an elderly person in the palliative care ward. During her final weeks she required oxygen for breathing difficulties and medication for pain relief and anxiety. The nurses were all aware of Eileen's advance care plan and accepted her refusal of any lifesaving treatment to allow her to die a dignified death. They provided comfort care to Eileen and her family and she died surrounded by her loved ones.

The nursing staff had all got to know Eileen during her stay and at the debrief session they exchanged many tearful hugs and talked about their feelings. Although Eileen's death was upsetting, in Eileen's case she appeared comfortable and did not die alone. This helped everyone cope with the experience. I felt privileged to care for Eileen and her family.

FEATURES WITHIN CHAPTERS

Analyse **Case studies** that present issues in context, encouraging you to integrate and apply the concepts discussed in the chapter in preparation for your clinical placement.

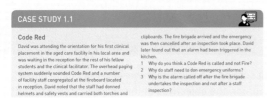

Engage actively and personally with the material by completing the practical activities in the **Reflective practice** boxes. These help you to assess your own knowledge, beliefs, traits and attitudes.

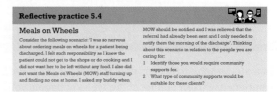

Practice the skills and knowledge required for placement with the **Activities**.

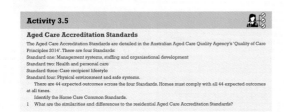

Be prepared for clinical placement by reviewing the **Tips** included throughout on the different situations you will encounter.

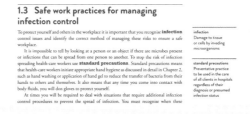

Important **Key terms** are marked in bold in the text when they are used in the text for the first time, with definitions included in the margin.

1.3 Safe work practices for managing infection control

To protect yourself and others in the workplace it is important that you recognise **infection** control issues and identify the correct method of managing these risks to ensure a safe workplace.

It is impossible to tell by looking at a person or an object if there are microbes present or infections that can be spread from one person to another. To stop the risk of infection spreading health-care workers use **standard precautions**. Standard precautions means that health-care workers initiate appropriate hand hygiene as discussed in detail in Chapter 2, such as hand washing or application of hand gel to reduce the transfer of bacteria from their hands to others and themselves. It also means that any time you come into contact with body fluids, you will don gloves to protect yourself.

At times you will be required to deal with situations that require additional infection control procedures to prevent the spread of infection. You must recognise when these

infection
Damage to tissue or cells by invading microorganisms

standard precautions
Preventative practice to be used in the care of all clients in hospitals regardless of their diagnosis or presumed infection status

ICONS

Link to skills and knowledge required for clinical placement with the

Review the skill in Tollefson *Essential Clinical*

- **Clinical Skills** icon that shows you where to find a detailed outline of the relevant skill in *Essential Clinical Skills*, 4th edition textbook by Joanne Tollefson, Gayle Watson, Eugenie Jelly, and Karen Tambree.

Explore the theory in *Foundations of Nursing*, Chapter 20: Infection control/asepsis

- **Theory** icon that shows you where to find an indepth discussion of relevant theory in *Foundations of Nursing*, 2nd edition textbook by Lois Elaine White, Gena Duncan, Wendy Baumle, Susie Gray and Leanne Ferris.

Collaboration

Feel confident that you are developing the foundational skills and abilities required to successfully complete your qualification by reviewing the content or completing the activities marked with a **Foundation Skills** icon.

END-OF-CHAPTER FEATURES

At the end of each chapter you will find several tools to help you to review, practise and extend your knowledge of the key learning outcomes.

- Review your understanding of the key chapter topics with the **Summary**.

- Test your knowledge and consolidate your learning through the **Self-test questions**.

- Take your study further by reviewing the source material in the **Bibliography**.

SUMMARY

- When providing nursing care to clients it is important for the health and safety of both client and nurse to follow safe work practices by identifying hazards, minimising risk, reporting issues, and following workplace policies and procedures.
- Manual handling is an activity that can pose a hazard in the workplace. Nurses need to identify risk and apply risk controls when undertaking these activities.

SELF-TEST QUESTIONS

1. What is the role of the enrolled nurse as part of the health-care team?
2. How can the enrolled nurse ensure that nursing interventions meet the needs of the individual?
3. What actions can the enrolled nurse take to ensure health promotion and health education is appropriate for individual clients?

BIBLIOGRAPHY

Advance Care Planning Australia, © Austin Health (2017). *The legal implications.* Retrieved from https://www.advancecareplanning.org. au/for-health-and-care-workers/legal-implications.

ANMC (2016). *National Competency Standard for Enrolled Nurse.* Retrieved from http://www.nursingmidwiferyboard.gov.au/Codes-Guidelines-Statements/Professional-standards.aspx.

Australian Commission on Safety and Quality in Health Care (2015). *National Consensus Statement, Essential Elements for Safe and High-Quality End-of-Life Care.* ACSQHC: Sydney.

Australian Government Department of Health (2010). *National Palliative Care Strategy 2010 – Supporting Australians to Live Well at the End of Life.* Retrieved from http://www.health.gov.au/internet/main/publishing.nsf/Content/EF57056BDB047E2FCA257BF000206168/$File/NationalPalliativeCareStrategy.pdf.

Australian Government Organ and Tissue Authority (n.d.). *Donate Life.* Retrieved from https://register.donatelife.gov.au/decide. Accessed 22 March 2018.

Guide to the online resources

FOR THE INSTRUCTOR

Cengage is pleased to provide you with a selection of resources that will help you prepare your students with pre-placement activities. These teaching tools are accessible via cengage.com.au/instructors for Australia or cengage.co.nz/instructors for New Zealand.

THE WORK EXPERIENCE TOOL AND LOGBOOK

Available in Word as a separate one-time institutional license to allow you to edit and customise the templates, these tools are designed to support your unique institution's clinical placement experience and assessment strategy for Diploma of Nursing. The **Work Experience Tool** section provides all the information regarding what is required for placement: what to expect, what to do in case of emergency or injury, what the students responsibilities are, what the facilitators responsibilities are. Later sections of this document can also be downloaded and provided to students for use as a **Logbook** to record their experience on each placement.

MAPPING GRID

The **Mapping grid** is a simple grid that shows how the content of this book relates to the units of competency needed to complete the Diploma of Nursing HLT54115.

INSTRUCTOR'S MANUAL

The **Instructor's manual** includes:
- chapter summary
- case question solutions
- answers to self-test questions
- additional material, such as additional content or activities.

TEST BANK

This bank of questions has been developed in conjunction with the text for creating quizzes, tests and exams for your students. Deliver these through your LMS and in your classroom.

POWERPOINT™ PRESENTATIONS

Use the chapter-by-chapter **PowerPoint slides** to enhance your lecture presentations and handouts by reinforcing the key principles of your subject.

ARTWORK FROM THE TEXT

Add the digital files of graphs, tables, pictures and flow charts into your course management system, use them in student handouts, or copy them into your lecture presentations.

Preface

Increasing demand and an ageing population continue to shape the changing context for the health workforce in Australia. This has resulted in the need for enrolled nurses who can provide a high standard of personal and clinical care for patients as well as meeting more complex needs. This will result in high-quality care for every patient and efficient use of health-care services, both within the health-care facilities and the community.

This text supports the beginning learner by describing the knowledge and skills required to work towards a Diploma of Nursing. This nationally recognised qualification reflects the role of a variety of workers who use a range of factual, technical and procedural knowledge to provide support to clients within a broad range of environments.

The enrolled nurse works collaboratively and under the supervision of registered nursing staff, and each chapter in the text identifies the scope of practice and range of activities that can be undertaken. The skills and knowledge required for effective delivery of care, with examples, are detailed throughout the text, with the capacity for the learner to self-assess, further discuss or extend their knowledge through activities, reflective practice sections and case studies throughout the chapter, as well as self-test questions at the end of each chapter.

Foundation knowledge and skills are developed throughout the initial chapters on work health and safety (WHS), infection control, anatomy and physiology, and terminology and communication, with an emphasis on their practical application. This underpinning knowledge can then be applied to gain a greater understanding of the specialist care chapters that follow. These discuss nursing in a variety of environments, complex and acute needs, and behaviours of concern. Additional chapters identify nursing care for people from culturally and linguistically diverse (CALD) backgrounds, and people with mental health and palliative care needs. This highlights the ever-expanding role of the enrolled nurse.

Using this text will enable students to meet high standards of patient-focused care and provide teachers and facilitators with tools to support students throughout their learning journey, with an application to the work environment.

Resources for Students, Educators and Institutions

The **Clinical Placement Manual** was built to assist students, educators and institutions preparing for placement. The resource consists of three parts:

Text: This book was designed as a student reference manual, to review key theory and skills and to explain what they will experience during their field placement. Organised by parts corresponding to commonly organised placements the chapters open with a vignette detailing real world experience and contain cases and activities that anchor the student in the work environment – the linking of theory to practice. Also, within each chapter there are reference points to skills and theory, that encourage the student to research and revise learning. Icons indicate the development of foundation skills.

Ancillary material: To support nurse educators in preparing students for the placement – instructor's guide with answers to in-text case studies, questions and activities, a mapping grid to performance criteria level, testbank of additional questions for in class or assignment and PowerPoint slides – part based for pre-placement teaching.

Work Experience Tool: Available in Word as a separate one-time institutional license to allow educators to edit and customise the templates, these tools are designed to support your unique institution's clinical placement experience and assessment strategy for Diploma of Nursing. The **Work Experience** Tool section provides the information required for placement: what to expect, what to do in case of emergency or injury, what the students responsibilities are, what the facilitators responsibilities are. Later sections of this document can also be downloaded and provided to students for use as a **Logbook** to record their experience on each placement.

About the authors

Catherine Joustra M Ed, Grad Dip Ed Psych, Grad Dip Ed, BA, Cert IV TAE, Div. 1 RN is an educator with over 10 years' experience fostering cohesive student learning atmospheres. She is currently a curriculum developer with Healthcareers. Catherine worked for over 20 years in the clinical environment in acute and rehabilitation areas before focusing on education and curriculum design. Catherine has also previously created support materials for the *Disability Support Worker* 2e and for *The Experienced Carer* 2e.

Ali Moloney BN, GCert CardiacN GCert AdvN, GCert FlightN, Cert IV TAE graduated from Griffith University in 1995 and has advanced qualifications and extensive experience in critical care nursing, with over 20 years as a clinical registered nurse. She has developed curriculum for the Diploma of Nursing at TAFE Queensland, and other registered training organisations. Ali has over 10 years' experience in vocational education and the delivery of the Diploma of Nursing and continues to work in the delivery of nurse education. Ali has also previously created support materials for the *Foundations of Nursing* 1e and contributed to *Foundations of Nursing* 2e.

Kathryn Austin Dip AppSc Nursing, CIV TAE, Grad Dip VET, MEd, MBA has been working in the Community Services and Health Faculty of TAFE NSW as a manager, head teacher and facilitator for over 20 years. Other roles have included capability development with a focus on leadership and culture and how they can impact on effective workplace teams.

Kathryn is a principled advocate for health and aged-care services and has presented at conferences on the changing needs of the health-care sector and current vocational education and training issues. She is an industry representative on accreditation and advisory groups for health-care training and is committed to improving educational standards and promoting a culture of mentoring and performance awareness among health-care and educational professionals.

Acknowledgements

Catherine

To my family for their support and time spent completing this work. Thank you to Ali for being ready to listen and assist when needed. A thank you to Cengage for providing this wonderful opportunity and supporting us through the process.

Ali

To Mags, a kabillion thanks! To my tiny humans Hayden, Brendan, Emma & Caitlyn, Mum did it, sorry for being cranky sometimes. To Mum and Dad, thank you for always believing in me, I know Dad would be proud. Thank you also to Catherine, it has been a journey for sure! And finally, thank you to Cengage, your patience, support and guidance is truly appreciated.

The authors and Cengage Learning would like to thank the following reviewers for their incisive and helpful feedback:

- Christine Baker, Eastern Health
- Ann Bolton, Charles Darwin University
- Kim Congues, Southern Cross Education Institute
- Ingrid Devlin, Health Skills Australia
- Leanne Ferris, Mater Hospital – Brisbane
- Annelize Grech, RDNS Training South Australia
- Michelle Hall, Holmesglen Institute of TAFE
- Isabella Hastings, Estia Health
- Hellene Heron, TAFE SA
- Helen Hilton, TAFE NSW
- Narelle Howell, TasTAFE
- Suzanne Howlett, TAFE Queensland – Gold Coast
- Leonie Kelly, South West Institute of TAFE
- Vivian Lindsay, Consultant
- Musa Masenda, Institute of Health and Nursing
- Louise Posa, TAFE Western
- Emma Sheppard, TAFE QLD
- Lara Tramacco, TAFE NSW – Shellharbour
- Nygell Topp, North Regional TAFE

Introduction to clinical placement

How placement fits into your course

Placement is the opportunity for you to put your newly acquired knowledge and skills to the test. It not only allows you to showcase your nursing skills but also your interpersonal and emotional readiness to undertake nursing in the Australian health-care environment.

The opportunity to undertake placement will occur at set points throughout the course. Most students will attend placement at set intervals after mastering specific knowledge and skills. The majority of students will undertake placement in aged care, rehabilitation or subacute care, mental health, acute care and in community centres. Before attending placement, you will have undergone rigorous testing of knowledge and skills. It is vital that you have the fundamental skills and knowledge in order to gain from and give the most to the clinical placement experience.

Competency is assessed through classroom-based learning, practical laboratory skills and in real life situations that occur on placement.

Why it is important

Clinical placement is important. Often when undertaking the acquisition of theoretical and laboratory skills, learning can appear disjointed, carefully separated into sections or topics. Clinical placement allows you to draw on all of your learning experiences, including previous clinical placement, to make sense of nursing in today's health-care environment. After placement you will be able to relate new learning and skills to those that you have already encountered and practiced in the workplace.

Being part of the team and fostering professional relationships between clients, peers and other professionals can enrich the clinical placement experience. It enables you to better understand the health-care environment and the role and contribution of the nurse.

How this book will assist you on placement

This book can assist you in several ways. The book has been divided into topics that encompass the core units of the Diploma of Nursing and some additional units that may be chosen as part of the nursing course. This book will be an excellent reference point for both theory and practical components, while also offering insight and some real life examples from nursing students and nurses.

Pre-placement

The book can be viewed before placement to assist the student to understand how the topic relates to clinical placement.

A variety of case studies have been included to assist the student before placement to identify key knowledge elements that are applied to a practical setting.

There are also a variety of reflective exercises that are designed primarily for use by the student on placement but can also be used as a guide for the student to use to analyse scenarios and situations that can arise in the clinical setting.

On placement

The book contains activities that the student can undertake on placement to enrich the learning experience. These activities will assist the student to make the best use of the clinical placement by ensuring they research key learning areas in the workplace.

There are many tips to assist the student in their new roles on placement and ensure their preparedness for the clinical situations they encounter. The book summarises some of the key knowledge areas. It provides a useful tool linking both theory and practical skills in a way that allows the student to refresh and consolidate their learning while in the clinical setting. Hopefully it will assist the student to gain a greater understanding of the role and responsibilities of the nurse in the clinical environment.

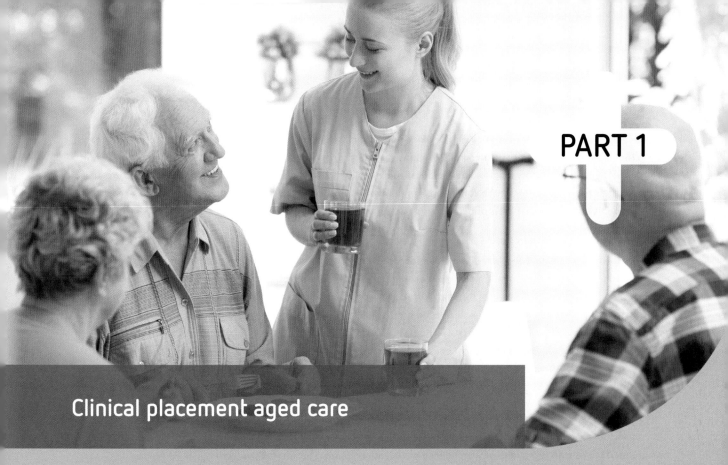

PART 1

Clinical placement aged care

Chapter 1: Safe work practices for direct client care

Chapter 2: Infection prevention and control

Chapter 3: Care of the older person

Chapter 4: Legal and ethical parameters for nursing practice

Chapter 5: Clinical assessment and planning nursing care

Chapter 6: Communication skills in nursing practice

Chapter 7: Physical health status

Chapter 8: Nursing within the Australian health-care system

Chapter 9: Working with diverse people

For most of you this will be your first placement within the Australian health-care system as a student nurse. Initially you will be concerned with applying all of the skills you have learnt in a real-life situation. As the placement continues you will have the opportunity to also align the knowledge that you have acquired throughout your course and interact in a positive manner with older adults.

Often students have varying emotions on their first placement, apprehension about causing pain or distress to residents, not being able to complete tasks to a satisfactory level and not achieving a successful result for the placement. As well as these fears students often are shocked initially with the presentation of the frail elderly person and it is not uncommon for students to develop an attachment to the clients they provide support to. Overall, students at the completion of placement feel a sense of satisfaction at making a difference to the lives of the elderly person they support while on placement.

The aged care experience

I was very nervous about working in aged care. Many of the residents appeared very frail and I was initially scared to touch them in case I hurt them. Working with my buddy and supervisor gave me confidence and I gradually was able to relax and actually enjoy my interaction with these residents. One elderly lady was particularly fond of me and would often want me just to hold her hand and spend time with her. She suffered from dementia but I found her to be extremely loving and I was very sad to say goodbye to her at the end of my placement. I found that I gained a lot from my experience in the aged care facility, not just the acquisition of skills.

Aged care is a specialised area where you will be able to put into practice all of the skills that you have learnt at school to date.

What is aged care? Aged care encompasses many different forms of care from community-based care to residential aged care. Society classes older adults as individuals who are aged over 65 years. The Australian Bureau of Statistics has analysed results of the statistics taken in 2011 and found that older Australians account for 14% of the population. It also found that 94% of people aged 65 and over lived in their own dwelling.

Who lives in residential care?

The number of individuals living in residential homes rose with increased age. Individuals aged between 65–74 years accounted for 2% while those aged 75–85 years accounted for 6% and this rose to 26% when people were aged 85 years or older. For older adults still living at home it was found that most required assistance with activities of daily living.

In this placement you will be based in an aged care residential facility. This is a community home for older adults who require increased assistance to maintain their activities of daily living. The majority of individuals who live in this type of accommodation have a long-term health condition, a disability or old age. The majority of elderly individuals that you will encounter are those we refer to as 'frail'. There will also be individuals who belong to a younger age group who reside in aged care due to supportive care needs.

Common experiences of student nurses in aged care

It can be confronting for students to see elderly people in aged care. Perhaps the hardest part to come to terms with is the level of dependence of the older person. This can include feeding, toileting and mobilisation. Students find that one of the hardest changes to accept is the loss of continence that may be present in older individuals along with the effects of age on the human body and mind. For some students it may be the first time that they have seen a naked person and the appearance of an older adult's body is very different to that of a younger adult due to the ageing process.

FS

Explore the theory in *Foundations of Nursing* 2e, Gray et al., Page 150, Chapter 7: Arenas of care

It is important to remember that this is the older person's home. While on placement you have been invited into their home and you need to balance the respect for this environment with the need to provide supportive care. The focus of this placement is to apply and consolidate foundation skills of nursing care, including assisting with all activities of daily living according to the care plan of the resident.

Objectives

The objectives that are to be set for this placement need to be contextualised to the aged care setting. Here are some examples of objectives:

*   Assist in supporting the resident in a home-like environment.
*   Provide care in line with resident's choices.
*   Manage the environment for residents with chronic illnesses including dementia or cognitive deficits.
*   Assess the physical state, including level of pain, for residents.
*   Assess palliative care requirements.

Work allocation

How work is undertaken in aged care will vary according to each facility. Some facilities use a team approach where a group works together for its allocated residents. Other facilities may allocate your own residents to be cared for under supervision or with a buddy. Medications may be administered by either a team leader of each section or by individual support workers who have been deemed competent by the facility. For more complex management there will be a registered nurse who will undertake these activities. All enrolled nurses and support staff work under the supervision of a registered Division 1 nurse.

Enjoy your placement and ensure you make good use of the valuable time you have with this cohort of people for whom you will provide supportive care.

Safe work practices for direct client care

LEARNING OUTCOMES

After reading this chapter, you should have an understanding of:

1.1   How to follow safe work practices for direct client care

1.2   How to follow safe work practices for manual handling

1.3   How to follow safe work practices for managing infection control

1.4   How to contribute to safe work practices in the workplace

1.5   How to reflect on your own safe work practices

Moving people safely

I was looking forward to my aged care placement but I was unsure if I would be able to complete all the physical requirements of moving people. I was aware that many of the elderly clients I would be caring for had limited movement.

In the class we learnt about safe work practices and had the opportunity to practice our manual handling skills in the nursing laboratory. I was relieved to learn that two people were required to assist with lifting machines. It was fun having a turn in the machines but I could imagine that some people would be very nervous when placed in the lifting machine. Some of my classmates were a little scared.

At the placement I was instructed on how to use the lifting machines; they were a little different from those in the classroom. I was glad that my supervisor watched and prompted me the first time I needed to use the machine.

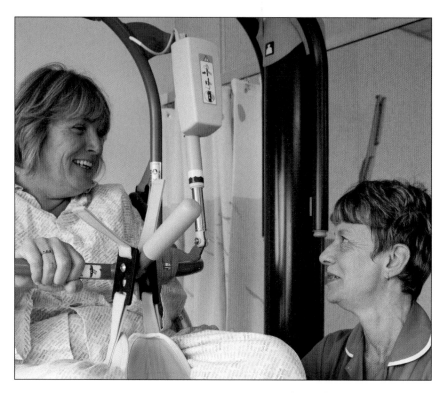

Science Photo Library/Life In View.

1.1 Safe work practices for direct client care

One of the main work health and safety (WHS) responsibilities of a registered nurse is to maintain a safe working environment, which needs to be safe for everyone including yourself.

On your clinical placement you will need to demonstrate safe methods of work, safe use of equipment and practices, and a thorough assessment of tasks.

Workplace policies and procedures

In Australia there is federal government legislation in place to protect the health and safety of people within the workplace. These Acts apply to all people, employees and those who access the workplace. As a student nurse on clinical placement you have an obligation to maintain a safe working environment.

There are a number of workplace policies and procedures that you must be familiar with to ensure safe working practices and maintain a safe environment. On orientation to the workplace, you will be required to locate and read the policies and procedures of the organisation. Often workplaces require you to sign that you have read and understood your obligations and responsibilities before undertaking work in the health-care facility. Policies and procedures are provided to all staff in either hardcopy or on a computer that staff are able to easily access.

Reading skills

Activity 1.1

Policies and procedures

On the first day of orientation locate the workplace policies and procedures.

1   List three policies that you locate and give a brief overview of how they relate to your work practice as a student nurse.

An area that you will need to familiarise yourself with during orientation is the workplace's **emergency procedures**. The workplace will have specific instructions on what to do in the case of emergencies. The Australian codes for emergencies are shown in **Figure 1.1**.

emergency procedure
Outlines an organisation's policies and procedures in response to emergency situations

Red	Code Red – Fire/Smoke R – Remove from immediate danger A – Alert C – Contain: close doors and windows E – Evacuate or extinguish if safe to do so
Orange	Code Orange – Evacuate Move laterally behind the next fire door and await instructions from fire warden Evacuate to evacuation point – Try to take list of clients
Blue	Code Blue – Medical/first aid emergencies Criteria for this code will vary from work place to work place
Yellow	Code Yellow – Failure or threat of failure to essential services
Brown	Code Brown – External emergencies
Purple	Code Purple – Bomb threat Obtain as much information as possible when call comes in Do immediate search of area for unusual packages Do not touch package but notify police Do not panic
Black	Code Black – Personal threat to others or self Press duress button if available Do not enter area where a Code Black is taking place
Green	Code Green – Correctional Health Services Emergency
Grey	Code Grey – Unarmed threat

FIGURE 1.1 Australian codes for emergencies

Source: Standards Australia

CASE STUDY 1.1

Code Red

David was attending the orientation for his first clinical placement in the aged care facility in his local area and was waiting in the reception for the rest of his fellow students and the clinical facilitator. The overhead paging system suddenly sounded Code Red and a number of facility staff congregated at the fireboard located in reception. David noted that the staff had donned helmets and safety vests and carried both torches and clipboards. The fire brigade arrived and the emergency was then cancelled after an inspection took place. David later found out that an alarm had been triggered in the kitchen.

1   Why do you think a Code Red is called and not Fire?
2   Why do staff need to don emergency uniforms?
3   Why is the alarm called off after the fire brigade undertakes the inspection and not after a staff inspection?

Activity 1.2

Emergency procedures

It is important to know the workplace emergency procedure for fire and evacuation. Answer the following questions:

1   What is your role in an emergency?
2   Where should you evacuate to in the health-care facility? What does 'RACE' stand for? What is the emergency number?

Hazards in the workplace

hazard
Anything that has the potential to harm the health and safety of a person

While you are on placement as a student nurse you may become aware of situations that pose a risk to the health and safety of people in the workplace. These are also known as hazards. A **hazard** is anything that could cause harm to a person or the environment, for example, exposure to certain chemicals, the potential for sharps injuries, aggressive behaviour or incorrect manual handling.

Safe Work Australia, the government agency that monitors the health and safety of workplaces on a national basis, requires all members of the workplace to identify and address any hazards that arise in their workplace. The identification of hazards is the first step in making the workplace safe. For example, all staff may be required to undertake regular housekeeping audits of the environment to identify potential hazards, such as faulty equipment, or specific procedures to deal with specific concerns addressed within that environment.

risk assessment
Analysis of a hazard in terms of the likelihood of it creating a workplace injury or illness

Once a hazard has been identified you will need to conduct a **risk assessment** and implement the appropriate controls to address the safety issues. It is vital to be familiar with the procedures that are in place to deal with specific hazards. These procedures that the workplace has implemented have arisen after the risk of the hazard has been assessed and the risk control methods have been identified. Risk is a mathematical means of assessing the likelihood of a person being adversely affected by the hazard and multiplied by the severity of the outcome. Risk control methods need to be introduced according to NIOSH's **hierarchy of risk control**, as shown in **Figure 1.2**. The hierarchy of risk control is constructed in a manner that attempts to address hazards, as you go down the hierarchy of risk control there is more risk and less control of the hazard. The type of control is determined by how often people encounter the hazard and what injury could result from the hazard.

hierarchy of risk control
The process for minimising or controlling risk

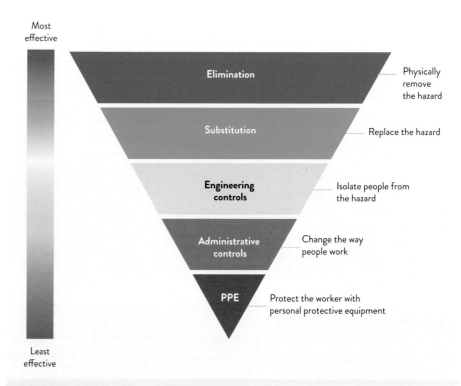

FIGURE 1.2 Hierarchy of risk control

National Institute for Occupational Safety and Health (NIOSH).

Everyone should identify hazards and report them. For the student nurse this may involve reporting verbally to the nurse manager, documenting the hazard using the workplace form or filling in the maintenance book. How you report the hazard will depend on the workplace policies and procedures.

You should be familiar and competent with the use of lifting machines and slide sheets as moving and repositioning people is a major hazard identified in nursing.

Technology

Review the skill in Tollefson *Essential Clinical Skills* 3.3 Assisting the patient to ambulate

---

Activity 1.3

Hazardous manual handling

Part of safe manual handling includes the ability to identify risk control methods used in the health-care facility. Read the following list of manual handling tasks that a nurse will encounter as part of her job role:

- moving patients on bed
- moving patients from bed to chair – **non-ambulant**, **non-weight bearing** and those that can stand but not work
- transporting patients in wheelchairs or on trolleys
- feeding patients
- applying **TED stockings**.

Where do these activities fit into the hierarchy of risk controls? Consider the policies and procedures of the health-care facility that you are completing your placement in when addressing the following questions:

1   How does the facility identify hazards that might be encountered in performing tasks such as those listed above?
2   What documentation is used? Complete a hazard form for one of your clients who requires manual handling.

CASE STUDY 1.2

Using lifting machines safely

David and his buddy Amelia had been allocated their residents for the morning shift. During handover and from reading the care plans David and Amelia planned how they would undertake the morning tasks of personal hygiene for their residents. One of their residents, Mr Crisp, was an elderly man of 78 who was unable to weight bear due to chronic arthritis that had seen his mobility deteriorate over the last 25 years. Mr Crisp also suffered from dementia and was assessed as being suitable for

full mobility assistance with two staff using the lifting hoist. On inspection of the hoist sling David and Amelia noted that there was some fraying around the straps. They decided that it would be safer to offer Mr Crisp a sponge bath, document the faulty equipment and report it according to workplace policies and procedures. David and Amelia also took care to label the faulty piece of equipment to prevent anybody else from using it.

1   Why is it important to follow the steps David and Amelia took with reporting faulty equipment?

Working safely with clients

Working with people, both clients and co-workers, can also pose hazards to the health and safety of others. Clients may have behaviours of concern; these can be aggression, anxiety, refusal to follow safety instructions, or other behaviours that pose a direct threat to other clients, co-workers and yourself. The workplace will have specific methods to capture and document these behaviours. At times specific instructions on how to care for the person may be documented in the client's case file, on a handover sheet or verbally handed over. All staff should document this information accurately and in a timely manner.

non-ambulant
Unable to walk

non-weight bearing
Unable to support themselves

TED stockings
Elastic stockings that apply pressure to limbs to return fluid back into the circulation system

incident report
A risk management tool used to describe and report any adverse event that occurs to a client, visitor or staff member

If a client exhibits a behaviour that does cause harm, an **incident report** will need to be completed and entered into the organisation's incident management system. In some facilities this is a paper-based system, while in others it can be a computer system such as 'Riskman'.

It is also important for the student nurse to recognise behaviour of co-workers that is inappropriate or not best practice and report the behaviour to the appropriate person. This could involve inappropriate manual handling techniques, verbal abuse or other behaviours that could cause harm to another individual in the environment.

Reflective practice 1.1

Caring for clients safely

A national report *Quality of Residential Care: The Consumer Perspective*, undertaken for Alzheimer's Australia, found that a number of people living in aged care are being shackled, assaulted and sedated against their wishes. This type of substandard care is abuse of the elderly. The report called for a collaborative approach by government, providers, unions and consumers as well as strategies to achieve cultural change in the attitudes towards older people. Some of the strategies outlined included:

- better funding for support and education of staff members and specialists
- extended mandatory reporting of physical and sexual assault
- giving approved volunteers a role in quality monitoring and accreditation
- ensuring complaints are dealt with properly and within set timeframes.

The report included a number of case studies provided by family members of aged care residents outlining specific incidences of elder abuse that had occurred in aged care institutions in Australia.

The full report can be accessed at https://www.dementia.org.au/sites/default/files/NATIONAL/documents/Alzheimers-Australia-Numbered-Publication-37.pdf.

Consider the following questions in relation to this report:

1   Are these behaviours appropriate in caring for people in an aged care facility?
2   What risks may occur to the person as a result of these strategies?

Source: Alzheimer's Australia, 2013, *Quality of Residential Aged Care: The consumer perspective*, Paper 37, https://www.dementia.org.au/sites/default/files/NATIONAL/documents/Alzheimers-Australia-Numbered-Publication-37.pdf.

Reducing risk in the workplace

One of the ways to reduce the risk of harm in the workplace is to follow workplace policies and procedures. In your workplace orientation you will be shown how to access the policies and procedures, given instruction on how to use safety equipment and shown how to report hazards in the workplace and where to find safety information. Each workplace is individual and the physical environment will have specific risks that you need to be aware of. You should be well prepared for your clinical placement by completing all of the theoretical components and by practising best practice techniques in the simulated environment before undertaking the task in the workplace. At times the workplaces may have specific situations that you may not have encountered in your learning environment. In such instances you should notify your clinical supervisor or the person in charge of the workplace so that individual coaching can be put into place to ensure safe practice.

Reflective practice 1.2

Unfamiliar tasks

Choose one of the nursing activities that you have undertaken for the first time on your placement. This could include using a lifting machine for a non-weight bearing person or feeding a client.

1   How did you feel doing this task?
2   What information or support did you need to complete the task?

Activity 1.4

Hazard documentation

Using the information from the hazardous manual handling activity complete a report for another task that you have undertaken. This could include assessment of a new patient to ascertain their mobility and completing the hazard form if they require assistance. Alternatively you could assess your posture when undertaking a task such as feeding or washing the lower legs or feet of a client who requires assistance with activities of daily living (ADLs).

1   Locate the hazard report used in the facility and complete this form with the activity you did in the reflective practice exercise above. Place a copy of the form in your file.

Incidents and injuries

When undertaking clinical placement, at times you may be involved in situations where it is necessary to report incidents. Incidents can be any occurrence where a person has been exposed to harm such as a fall or other **adverse event**. An adverse event is anything that occurs that causes harm. As noted above, it is important that documentation is completed according to the policies and procedures of the organisation. All incident reports are analysed and the information can be used to identify areas or hazards that may result in an incident and to implement strategies to prevent this from occurring.

Review the skill in Tollefson *Essential Clinical Skills* 7.1 Documentation

Numeracy, writing

Activity 1.5

Incident report documentation

Read the Ausmed article at http://www.ausmed.com.au/blog/entry/how-to-write-an-incident-report on 'How to write an incident report' and answer the following questions:

1   What are the two components of the incident report?
2   What should be included on the incident report?

1.2   Safe work practices for manual handling

As a nurse you will encounter many clients or types of work where **manual handling** is required. Safe Work has identified that nurses are particularly at risk of manual handling injuries due to the need to move heavy loads that can be unpredictable. Examples of manual handling situations are when dependent clients rely on nursing staff for their

Adverse event
An incident in which harm was done to a person receiving health care, for example from infections, falls resulting in injuries, or problems with medication and medical devices

See next page, Definitions *Continued*

>>

manual handling
Any activity that requires a person to use force to move, hold or restrain another person or thing

mobility needs or the nurse needs to assist the person into a particular position within the operating theatre.

Each organisation will have specific policies and procedures in place to address this issue and increase safety. There are a variety of different types of manual handling procedures such as 'No lift', 'Back safe' but they all rely on you following the procedures correctly.

The first step in identifying manual handling hazards is completing a risk assessment of the activity. This is completed for each client on their admission to the facility or after a significant change in their condition. Nurses need to assess the needs of the person on an ongoing basis and before any nursing interventions requiring mobility assistance. Facilities will have specific instructions on how to assess the person's mobility, from completing risk assessment forms, such as specific mobility assessment forms, to having a physiotherapy assessment before mobilising a person.

Information regarding the person's mobility may come from a variety of sources, such as the person themselves, a doctor's referral letter, a nursing letter, previous admissions or next of kin. You should document any type of mobility issue the person exhibits, such as holding onto furniture when walking, using a particular mobility aid or if the person's mobility changes due to other factors such as pain.

Other manual handling issues that affect nursing practice will depend on the type of equipment or task that is required. An example of a manual handling task that can cause injury is repetitive movements, bending or stretching the body to complete a task, such as feeding a person sitting in a chair. All activities that are part of the normal work practice need to be assessed and risk control measures put into place. In the example of feeding a person who is sitting in a chair the nurse also should sit to avoid bending. This creates a more social environment for the person who requires assistance. As with any hazard identified the risk control method is chosen from the hierarchy of risk controls.

CASE STUDY 1.3

Changes in a person's mobility

Mrs Fraser, a 76-year-old woman, was admitted to the medical ward with dizziness for investigation. Mrs Fraser had no other symptoms and was able to weight bear and mobilise independently. The next morning Susan, Mrs Fraser's nurse, came in and was preparing to assist

Mrs Fraser to have her shower. Mrs Fraser stated that she felt unwell and dizzy. Susan took a set of vital signs and decided to allow Mrs Fraser to rest in bed and assisted her with a sponge bath.

1 What could have occurred if Susan had attempted to mobilise Mrs Fraser at this time?

2 What other actions does Susan have to complete?

Activity 1.6

Moving people safely

Choose one of the clients that you are caring for and complete a risk assessment using the documentation from WorkSafe or the health-care facility (https://www.worksafe.vic.gov.au/__data/assets/pdf_file/0016/211273/ISBN-Transferring-people-safely-handbook-2009-07.pdf).

Activity 1.7

Mobility equipment

Complete the activities listed in **Table 1.1**:

TABLE 1.1 Activities undertaken with mobility equipment

Type of activity	Tollefson Clinical Skill
Demonstrates correct use of a hoist	None
Demonstrates correct use of a stand up lifter	None
Demonstrates correct use of slide sheets	3.12 Positioning of a dependent patient
Demonstrates correct use of bed mechanics to assist with mobility	3.12 Positioning of a dependent patient
Demonstrates correct use of body mechanics to assist mobility	3.12 Positioning of a dependent patient
Demonstrates correct use of a commode chair or wheelchair	None
Demonstrates correct use of mobility aids such as a pick-up frame, wheelie frame and single point stick	3.3 Assisting the patient to ambulate

1.3 Safe work practices for managing infection control

To protect yourself and others in the workplace it is important that you recognise **infection** control issues and identify the correct method of managing these risks to ensure a safe workplace.

It is impossible to tell by looking at a person or an object if there are microbes present or infections that can be spread from one person to another. To stop the risk of infection spreading health-care workers use **standard precautions**. Standard precautions means that health-care workers initiate appropriate hand hygiene as discussed in detail in Chapter 2, such as hand washing or application of hand gel to reduce the transfer of bacteria from their hands to others and themselves. It also means that any time you come into contact with body fluids, you will don gloves to protect yourself.

At times you will be required to deal with situations that require additional infection control procedures to prevent the spread of infection. You must recognise when these situations occur. You may get information from different sources such as handover, lab results and through observation of the patient. If additional precautions are required you need to know where to access the information, how to access resources and the required documentation and reporting that needs to be completed. This information will be in the policies and procedures document kept in the area, through documentation in the handover or case files, or through handover from infection control departments. An example of when this could occur would be in the event that a person starts vomiting and having loose bowel motions. These could indicate gastroenteritis that could easily be transmitted from one person to another if the implementation of additional precautions is not taken.

infection
Damage to tissue or cells by invading microorganisms

standard precautions
Preventative practice to be used in the care of all clients in hospitals regardless of their diagnosis or presumed infection status

Review the skill in Tollefson *Essential Clinical Skills* 1.1 Hand hygiene

Examples of additional precautions that may be required are:

- wearing of gloves when undertaking wound care
- placing a person into isolation within a ward environment
- wearing gloves and eye shields when emptying a catheter bag to prevent splash contamination
- wearing a special mask to protect against airborne infections.

Signs of infection are redness, swelling of local areas, odours, increased temperatures and lethargy. Other ways to identify infections may be from pathology reports that identify a pathogen or bacteria in a body fluid.

Reading

CASE STUDY 1.4

Managing infection control hazards in the workplace

Access the VicHealth web page 'A guide for the management and control of gastroenteritis outbreak in aged care, special case, health care and residential care facilities' at https://www2.health.vic.gov.au/about/publications/researchandreports/guide-for-management-and-control-of-gastroenteritis-outbreaks and answer the following questions:

1. When is the outbreak of gastroenteritis considered over?
2. What is the most important measure that health-care staff can perform to prevent the spread of infection?
3. List two additional infection control measures that should be implemented.

Activity 1.8

Preventing the spread of infection

Complete the activities listed in **Table 1.2**:

TABLE 1.2 Activities undertaken to prevent the spread of infection

Type of activity	Tollefson Clinical Skill
Demonstrates correct hand-washing techniques	*1.1 Hand hygiene*
Demonstrates correct disposal of body fluids	*3.7 Assisting the patient with elimination – urinary and bowel elimination*
Demonstrates correct use of gloves	*1.1 Hand hygiene*
Demonstrates correct use of masks if required	*8.13 Infection control – standard and transmission-based precautions*
Demonstrates correct technique for managing clients in isolation	*8.13 Infection control – standard and transmission-based precautions*

1.4 Working as a team to ensure a safe working environment

You must work together as a team to ensure a safe working environment. Ways that you can contribute to the team are:

- always follow workplace policies and procedures
- ensure equipment is in good order
- maintain a clean and tidy environment
- maintain currency in safe work practices
- complete safety documentation such as housekeeping inspections, equipment audits or the completion of hazard and incident reports
- participate in safe work practices and education.

If there is an issue with safety in the workplace it needs to be documented correctly and reported to the person in charge of the area. Each workplace will have a formal forum to discuss workplace safety issues. Everybody should be aware of the WHS meetings and either attend the meeting or read the minutes of the meeting.

TIP 1.1

Gloves

You should always wear gloves if you are coming in contact with body fluids. Always change gloves at the end of any procedure with the client. Always perform hand hygiene in between procedures and dispose of the gloves when leaving the client's bedside.

CASE STUDY 1.5

A team approach to safety in the workplace

John was a nursing student on his aged care placement. He was feeling overwhelmed by the large amount of skills and knowledge required for the placement to be successful. Everything felt new and alien to him. When he had to assist with the showering of an immobile patient using a hoist sling John was very nervous and determined to do everything by the book. After showering the client John dressed him appropriately and placed him in a fall out chair with his call bell within reach. John

was glad that he had managed this difficult task with the supervision of his buddy. His buddy left the room and John was also ready to leave when he noticed that he had not cleaned up the bathroom floor. John attended to this while his buddy returned, went into the bathroom to refill the client's water jug and did so safely.

1   Who is responsible for safety in the health-care facility?
2   What does John need to do at the end of the procedure, with the equipment he has used?
3   What could happen if the equipment is not attended to?

1.5 Reflecting on your own safe work practices

Each person needs to assume responsibility for their own health and safety, as well as others they work with or care for. For the student nurse this means being prepared, and the ways in which you can prepare are:

- reviewing theoretical areas relating to WHS
- ensuring that practical skills are revisited before placement
- attending to orientation
- reading the policies and procedures relating to WHS in the workplace
- asking questions if unsure before undertaking an activity.

Clinical placement can be tiring and you should take adequate measures to protect your own health. General areas to look at are:

- diet
- exercise
- sleep.

At times placement can cause stress and fatigue and it is important to recognise these if they occur and let your clinical facilitator know of any issues that arise.

As part of the clinical placement experience there will be times set aside for you to participate in clinical debriefing opportunities. These are ideal times to raise issues on which you require further clarification or instruction. They can also be valuable to review activities or incidents within a supportive environment.

CASE STUDY 1.6

Reflecting on safe working strategies

Justin was in Sundeep aged care facility for his clinical placement. Justin found that one of the residents, David, was very difficult to manage. David had been involved in a car accident five years ago and had an acquired brain injury and was confined to a wheelchair. David was 38 years old and before the accident held a job as a builder. David was married and had two young children. They often came to visit, but when they left David would become distressed. David was verbally aggressive when he did not want to do something and would fly into rages if his routine was altered. David had at times hit staff when agitated and would also hit and punch himself.

Justin was assigned to care for David with his buddy, Angela, who told Justin that David was being taken out of the facility to attend a family function and they would need to get him ready early. When they entered David's room, he was still sleepy and not wanting to get up. Angela told him that he was going out that day and needed to be ready. David just huddled under his doona. Angela told Justin that she would try again in 30 minutes

because it was important not to agitate David and they could assist another resident while they waited for David to fully wake up. Angela also told Justin that with David it was important not to rush him. Justin was glad that he did not have to attend to David by himself as he did not have enough experience with individuals with this type of behaviour.

Justin found that he was exhausted by the end of the shift and on returning home sat on the couch and just watched television till bedtime. Justin could not even be bothered to get himself a meal and just opened a packet of chips and a can of Coke.

Justin had a disturbed sleep and woke early thinking about what this day would bring and hoped that he would not have to attend to David on his own.

1   What strategies could Justin use to improve his knowledge in caring for David?
2   Describe some of the strategies that Justin could use to reduce his stress?
3   Explain how debriefing can assist the nurse in this situation?

Learning

SUMMARY

- When providing nursing care to clients it is important for the health and safety of both client and nurse to follow safe work practices by identifying hazards, minimising risk, reporting issues, and following workplace policies and procedures.
- Manual handling is an activity that can pose a hazard in the workplace. Nurses need to identify risk and apply risk controls when undertaking these activities.
- Direct client contact involves exposure to infection for both the nurse and the client. Infection risks need to be identified and risk control measures put in place to address these risks. Standard precautions are used at all times and additional precautions may be required if standard precautions are not sufficient to control the spread of infection.
- You should notify the appropriate person with regard to WHS issues in line with organisational policy. Participation in the WHS program at the workplace will assist in making the workplace safe for all who access it.
- Thinking about your own performance and maintaining currency of safe work practices will assist in maintaining your own wellbeing.

SELF-TEST QUESTIONS

1 What steps do I need to take to ensure safe work practices for direct client care?
2 How do I ensure safe practice when undertaking manual handling activities?
3 What measures can I employ to stop the transmission of infection?
4 How can I contribute to the safe working environment of the workplace?
5 What processes can I employ to ensure my own wellbeing in the workplace?

BIBLIOGRAPHY

Alzheimer's Australia (2013). *Quality of Residential Aged Care: The consumer perspective*, Paper 37, https://www.dementia.org.au/sites/default/files/NATIONAL/documents/Alzheimers-Australia-Numbered-Publication-37.pdf.

Australian Bureau of Statistics (2013). *Where and how do Australia's older people live?* http://www.abs.gov.au/ausstats/abs@.nsf/products/422C56F1DD0DE073CA257B50001D0EED?OpenDocument.

Australian Institute of Health and Welfare (2017). *How to write an incident report*, http://www.aihw.gov.au/haag11-12/adverse-events/.

Crouch, B. (2013). 'Residential aged care report says people are being shackled, assaulted and turned into "zombies"', *The Advertiser*, 12 November, http://www.news.com.au/national/residential-aged-care-report-says-people-are-being-shackled-assaulted-and-turned-into-zombies/story-fncynjr2-1226758258945.

O'Connell, B. (2014). 'Violent nursing home resident creates staffing headache', *Herald Sun*, 28 September, http://www.heraldsun.com.au/news/victoria/violent-nursing-home-resident-creates-staffing-headache/news-story/e641cf952e81e23d9f91ad06aea09d1d.

Tollefson, J., Watson, G., Jelly, E. & Tambree, K. (2016). *Essential Clinical Skills: Enrolled Division 2 Nurses* (3rd edition). Cengage Learning: South Melbourne.

VicHealth (2013). *A guide for the management and control of gastroenteritis outbreaks in aged care, special care, health care and residential aged care facilities*, https://www2.health.vic.gov.au/getfile/?sc_itemid=%7B13535B5B-D5C4-421D-9425-0CA9501C811D%7D&title=A%20guide%20for%20the%20management%20and%20control%20of%20gastroenteritis%20outbreaks%20in%20aged%20care,%20special%20care,%20health%20care%20and%20residential%20care%20facilities.

WorkSafe Victoria (2009). *Transferring people safely*, https://www.worksafe.vic.gov.au/__data/assets/pdf_file/0011/12224/Transferring_People_Safely_-_Web.pdf.

Infection prevention and control

LEARNING OUTCOMES

After reading this chapter, you should have an understanding of:

2.1 Following standard and additional precautions for infection prevention and control

2.2 Identifying infection hazards and assess risks

2.3 Following procedures for managing risks associated with specific hazards

Hand hygiene

As a student I was horrified to learn how many bugs were present on my skin. In class we had a solution applied and we were told to wash our hands thoroughly. The teacher then ran a UV light over our hands and we could see the areas that we had missed.

Reading about some of the complications that patients could get, such as MRSA in their operative site, I was determined to ensure good hand hygiene procedures. It was constantly reinforced during all practice sessions, I gradually took on the five moments of hand hygiene and it became something that I did automatically.

I was surprised at how often I was required to wash my hands and was glad that the teacher reinforced the need to apply moisturiser as my hands were not used to such frequent washing.

The most surprising thing I learnt was that gloves had minute holes and were not a substitute for hand washing.

2.1 Standard and additional precautions for infection prevention and control

As discussed in Chapter 1, all health-care facilities must implement policies, regulations and guidelines in accordance to federal, state and territory regulations, policies and Acts that relate to the control of infectious diseases and their transmission. Health-care facilities strive to provide an environment in which the health-care worker, patients/clients and visitors have minimal exposure to infectious diseases. The policies and procedures of infection control implemented are based on the research and recommendations of the National Health and Medical Research Council (NHMRC, https://www.nhmrc.gov.au/).

It is estimated that the length of stay due to surgical site infection is between 3.5 and 23 days, depending upon the nature of the infection. This is, obviously, a significant impact on the client and on the health-care budget. Furthermore, it is estimated that around 200 000 health-care-associated infections occur within Australia annually – that is, an infection acquired in hospital by the patient. At least half of these are preventable (NHMRC, 2010, p. 6).

Health-care workers of all disciplines have a responsibility to minimise the risk of all infections including **health-care acquired infections (HCAIs)**. In your clinical placement you will need to demonstrate your understanding of what constitutes an infection and infection risk as well as demonstrating the following standard precautions. Refer to Clarke et al. (2016), Chapter 20 'Infection control' for a detailed discussion of infection, the chain of infection and risk.

Standard precautions

In your placement you will need to demonstrate your ability to perform a range of standard precautions to help prevent the spread of infection (see **Figure 2.1**) and HAIs. These procedures include aseptic techniques, hand washing, the use of personal protective equipment, appropriate reprocessing of instruments and equipment, and ensuring environmental controls. They also incorporate the safe systems for handling of blood and other body fluids as well as non-intact skin and mucous membranes.

Universal precautions or standard precautions were originally developed to protect the health-care worker from the risk of transmission of blood-borne pathogens from a client. However, standard precautions expanded to also prevent staff-to-client transmission as well as client-to-staff transmission. The current Australian guidelines cover all pathogens that are likely to be present in any type of bodily fluid or substance.

Standard precautions should always be used when there is contact (or potential for contact) with blood or bodily fluids (for example, urine, faeces, vomit) and should also be considered when there is a break in skin integrity or if airborne pathogens are present (influenza) or if a client is immunosuppressed.

These guidelines apply to:
- blood
- all bodily fluids, secretions or excretions
- non-intact skin
- mucous membranes.

These guidelines include specific recommendations for the use of all personal protective equipment when contact with blood or body secretions is possible or probable.

Standard precautions are intended to supplement rather than replace routine infection control mechanisms such as hand washing, and using gloves to prevent the contamination of hands, especially when handling sharps.

Explore the theory in *Foundations of Nursing*, Chapter 20: Infection control/asepsis

health-care acquired infections (HCAIs)
Infections acquired in health-care facilities, or infections that occur as a result of an intervention in a health-care facility

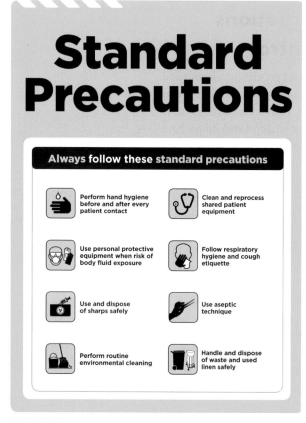

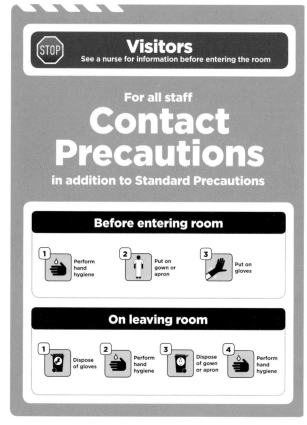

FIGURE 2.1 Standard precautions for infection control

Source: Australian Commission on Safety and Quality in Health Care.

Health-care facilities must provide all equipment for standard and additional precautions. A component of your role ties infection control in with work health and safety, whereby you are responsible for keeping your work area free from blood or other bodily fluid splatters or spills. You are responsible for wearing the appropriate protective equipment and protecting both yourself and your patients from the possibility of infection.

Hand washing

Hand washing is one of the most important and most basic techniques in preventing and controlling the spread of infection. Contaminated hands are a prime cause of cross infection.

You may have seen the phrase 'Clean hands save lives' in a hospital or health-care facility. So important is this notion that the World Health Organization (WHO) has established an annual campaign to highlight the importance of hand hygiene in health care to reduce antibiotic resistance.

The Australian organisation is 'Hand Hygiene Australia' and can be found at https://www.hha.org.au.

Hand washing should be undertaken for 10–15 seconds to remove the most transient organisms from the skin. If the hands are visibly soiled then more time may be needed. Routine hand washing may be performed with plain soap. Antimicrobial soap solutions are generally used in all acute care facilities, so this is what nurses predominantly use. When hands are not visibly soiled, alcohol-based hand rubs (in lieu of washing hands) can be used in the clinical setting.

There are different types of hand washing:

- The **social hand wash** comprises of a 10–15 second hand wash using plain soap. It is used for daily activities in the clinical ward and after going to the toilet.
- The **clinical hand wash** is used prior to aseptic procedures and involves one minute with antimicrobial soap or skin cleanser. It is used before any non-surgical procedures, which require aseptic technique, for example, wound dressings.
- The **surgical hand wash** is used before any invasive surgical procedure (in theatre) and is undertaken for at least five minutes.

Health-care acquired infections are still incredibly high in Australia, and a very big preventative measure is hand hygiene. The five moments for hand hygiene, as shown in **Figure 2.2**, will assist in preventing the spread of infection.

social hand wash
A 10–15 second plain soap hand wash used for daily activities

clinical hand wash
A one-minute hand wash using antimicrobial soap or skin cleanser performed prior to non-surgical procedures requiring aseptic technique

surgical hand wash
A five-minute hand scrub using antimicrobial soap performed before any invasive surgical procedure

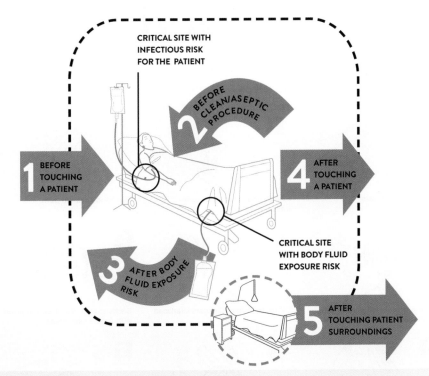

FIGURE 2.2 Five moments of hand hygiene

Your 5 Moments for Hand Hygiene from Hand Hygiene: How, Why & When?, World Health Organization, revised August 2009, © World Health Organization, http://www.who.int/gpsc/5may/Hand_Hygiene_Why_How_and_When_Brochure.pdf?ua=1, accessed 13 September 2018.

The principles of hand washing include:

- no jewellery – including wrist watch and rings
- short nails, inspect length of nails regularly (no false nails)
- no cuffs of sleeves
- no breaks in skin or cuts on hands
- cover lesions on own skin before providing patient care
- keep hands and uniform away from sink surface and do not stand against it
- use elbow taps to turn on water
- avoid splashing water against uniform
- use warm water and wet hands and wrists thoroughly under running water before applying soap
- keep hands and forearms lower than elbows during washing
- wash hands using soap, lather and friction for at least 10–15 seconds
- rinse hands thoroughly under running water and pat dry with paper towel from fingertips to wrists.

Review the skill in Tollefson *Essential Clinical Skills* 1.1 Hand hygiene

Activity 2.1

Review hand-washing facilities

Do a review of the different hand-washing facilities in the clinical area. You may find that there are a variety of different types, for example, long handled taps or automatic taps. Practise doing both the standard hand wash and the hand wash for clinical procedures.

Did you have any difficulty in completing the steps as outlined in **Figure 2.2** or according to the practice that you were taught in the lab?

TIP 2.2

Hand washing frequency

Nurses wash their hands many times in a single shift. Routinely inspect your hands for signs of cuts, infections, dermatitis, or dry, cracked skin. Application of a suitable moisturising cream is highly recommended.

Use of a moisturising hand cream will assist in maintaining the integrity of your own skin. Check hospital policy regarding available moisturisers in your place of employment.

The essential components of a good hand washing technique are outlined in **Figure 2.3**.

How to Handwash?

WASH HANDS WHEN VISIBLY SOILED! OTHERWISE, USE HANDRUB

Duration of the handwash (steps 2-7): 15-20 seconds

Duration of the entire procedure: 40-60 seconds

0
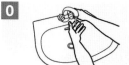
Wet hands with water

1

Apply enough soap to cover all hand surfaces

2
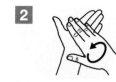
Rub hands palm to palm

3
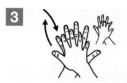
Right palm over left dorsum with interlaced fingers and vice versa

4
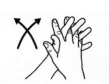
Palm to palm with fingers interlaced

5
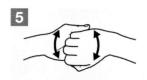
Backs of fingers to opposing palms with fingers interlocked

6
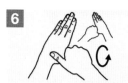
Rotational rubbing of left thumb clasped in right palm and vice versa

7
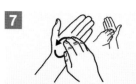
Rotational rubbing, backwards and forwards with clasped fingers of right hand in left palm and vice versa

8
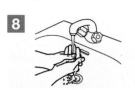
Rinse hands with water

9
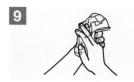
Dry hands thoroughly with a single use towel

10
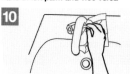
Use towel to turn off faucet

11
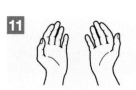
Your hands are now safe.

World Health Organization | **Patient Safety** A World Alliance for Safer Health Care | **SAVE LIVES** Clean **Your** Hands

FIGURE 2.3 How to handwash with alcohol-based hand rub

How to Handwash? poster, World Health Organization, May 2009, © World Health Organization, http://www.who.int/gpsc/5may/How_To_HandWash_Poster.pdf?ua=1, accessed 13 September 2018.

Personal protective equipment

All health-care facilities must provide their workers with appropriate *personal protective equipment* (PPE), which meets the Australian Standards (see some examples in **Figure 2.4**). PPE is to protect you, so you should be well informed about application, removal and appropriate use of PPE.

You have a responsibility to yourself, your clients, fellow workers, visitors and your employer to use PPE correctly and, importantly, at the appropriate times. PPE is an important measure to ensure that you do not come into contact with blood or other body substances, chemicals and all types of waste. The type of PPE required will vary depending on the task or procedure that you are undertaking, and you should always wear the PPE specified in the policies and procedures manual.

In health care, PPE will be required for using certain equipment or machinery; some examples would be lead aprons for x-ray, and certain types of gloves for cleaning of surgical equipment. PPE must work to ensure that you are not injured or infected whilst undertaking your nursing duties.

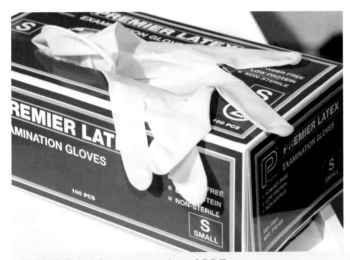
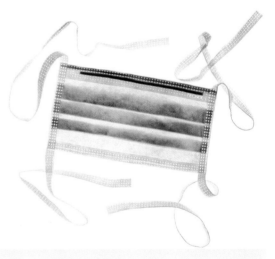

FIGURE 2.4 Some examples of PPE

Science Photo Library/Life in View;
Science Photo Library/Kevin Curtis.

Activity 2.2

Types of PPE

Locate the different types of PPE that are available in the clinical area. Find out what activities require the use of PPE.

- How do you access these items if they are not present in the steri-room?

- How do you dispose of the PPE at the end of the intervention? Check the requirements for removal of gloves and masks.

Aprons and gowns

Aprons and gowns should be used when there is a likelihood of splashes or contamination of clothing or skin with blood or body substances.

- Use impermeable or fluid-resistant aprons or gowns where possible as they prevent fluids seeping through to your underlying skin.
- Dispose of used aprons and gowns immediately
- Do not ever reuse without washing at a later time – this increases the risk of cross infection and contamination of yourself.
- If aprons or gowns are laundered and reused they should be placed in the appropriate linen container immediately after use to minimise the risk of transmission of infection (for example, in the operating room).

Most aprons and gowns are unsterile, the exception being for operating room gowns which are sterilised prior to use.

Eye shields/safety glasses and face protection

Eye shields or safety glasses are often referred to as 'goggles'. These should be used when there is a likelihood of splashing or spattering of blood or body substances. This includes when cleaning up blood or other body fluids.

- Eye and face protective equipment should be close fitting and protect the side of the face as well.
- When non-disposable equipment is supplied it must be thoroughly cleaned as per the manufacturer's instructions after each use.
- Many hospitals supply a pair of goggles for each staff member and it becomes your responsibility to keep your pair clean and operational.
- Eye and face protection should be available in both clean and dirty utility rooms as well as laundry areas.

TIP 2.3

Goggles or safety glasses
It is important that fluids do not enter the eye. You can apply the goggles over your personal glasses if required. Goggles provide more coverage of the eye area.

Masks

Masks must be worn when there is a risk of contamination from airborne droplets such as when caring for a client with a productive cough or an airborne transmissible disease. Care should be taken to ensure that the mask is applied correctly – there are suppliers' instructions on the side of every box stipulating what the mask is to be used for and how to apply, remove and dispose of it.

Masks limit the dispersal of droplets, but are not a total protection from droplet infection. Masks must be:

- worn for aseptic procedures
- not touched with hands or gloves once in place
- removed by touching the ties or loops only – not the actual maskpiece
- used once then disposed of correctly
- never left hanging around the neck
- fluid repellent
- work as per manufacturers guidelines – some masks in certain clinical situations are only effective for 4–6 hours and require replacement.

Gloves

Latex gloves, both sterile and non-sterile, have been provided for many years for health-care workers. However, some health-care workers have developed latex allergies, as have patients. Most states and territories in Australia have ceased supply of latex gloves, and now supply latex-free gloves for staff at their health-care facilities. Gloves are worn as a barrier to protect the wearer's hands from contamination and also prevent cross infection from organisms already on the health-care worker's hands (normal epidermal flora).

Gloves must be worn when handling blood and body substances, waste, or when there is a risk of coming into contact with blood or other body substances. Disposable gloves are worn for:

- clinical procedures such as venepuncture and finger or heel sticks/pricks
- where there is risk from contamination from blood, other body substances or infectious material
- when a health-care worker has broken skin, wounds on their hands or has a skin condition (dermatitis etc.)
- plastic or vinyl gloves should be used in all food preparation areas
- sterile gloves must be worn for all sterile procedures
- rubber utility gloves must be used for housekeeping and waste handling tasks
- hands must be washed after removing gloves.

Figure 2.5 outlines the guidelines that should be adhered to for the use of gloves.

Activity 2.3

Application and removal of sterile gloves

It is important to apply sterile gloves correctly. This is to ensure you do not contaminate them with your own skin. Read the policy about application and removal of sterile gloves and do this activity following the steps given.

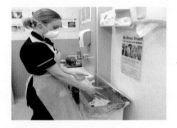
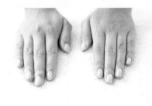

Hand hygiene is required with glove use	
The need to wash your hands still exists when wearing gloves	
When should gloves been worn?	• when handling blood, body substances, waste • when there is a risk of coming into contact with blood or body substances • when staff have skin breaks or lesions on their hands
When should gloves be changed?	• must be changed and discarded when torn or punctured or damaged in any way
How should gloves be handled and disposed?	• should be disposed of in general waste unless they are heavily contaminated, then they must be disposed of in the clinical waste bin • clean or used gloves should never be carried in pockets • remove jewellery when wearing gloves as sharp edges will puncture the gloves allowing contamination • long fingernails can puncture or tear gloves and nail polish can chip or flake and cause contamination • most health-care facilities have strict policies concerning both jewellery and long nails – neither is generally tolerated in the clinical setting

FIGURE 2.5 Gloving guidelines

Respiratory hygiene and cough etiquette are further infection control principles that need to be followed at all times. The NHMRC guidelines are shown in **Figure 2.6**.

Anyone with signs and symptoms of a respiratory infection, regardless of the cause, should follow or be instructed to follow respiratory hygiene and cough etiquette as follows:

- Cover the nose/mouth with disposable single-use tissues when coughing, sneezing, wiping and blowing noses.
- Use tissues to contain respiratory secretions.
- Dispose of tissues in the nearest waste receptacle or bin after use.
- If no tissues are available, cough or sneeze into the inner elbow rather than the hand.
- Practise hand hygiene after contact with respiratory secretions and contaminated objects/materials.
- Keep contaminated hands away from the mucous membranes of the eyes and nose.

FIGURE 2.6 Steps in respiratory hygiene and cough etiquette

Source: NHMRC (2011), Table B1.15: Steps in respiratory hygiene and cough etiquette, https://www.nhmrc.gov.au/book/australian-guidelines-prevention-and-control-infection-healthcare-2010/b1-6-respiratory-hygiene. Creative Commons BY 3.0 AU licence. https://creativecommons.org/licenses/by/3.0/au/.

Environmental cleaning

Infection control is the responsibility of all health-care workers. Cleaning is a very large component of infection control. We will now look at what is required in the health-care setting with respect to environmental cleaning.

Cleanliness and hygiene are interdependent. Unwanted microbes and 'soils' are generally located together and must be considered together. A sound working knowledge of methods of cleaning and correct use of chemicals is therefore an essential requirement in understanding the role of cleaning in a health-care facility. The actual methods and chemicals to be used on equipment must be understood to achieve the required standard of hygiene.

Cleaning is the removal of 'soil' or other unwanted matter. 'Soil' is defined as 'matter in the wrong place'. A high standard of cleanliness is absolutely essential for clients' welfare as well as the health of the staff. Soils fall into two main groups: those which comprise visible dirt, spills or stains, and those which comprise or contain dangerous microorganisms. Visible soils cause untidy and unappealing appearance.

Microbial or bacterial soils are capable of being moved from one part of a building area to another. This will cause cross infection. Both types of soils must be removed constantly to achieve the necessary level of hygiene and for the efficient operation of the health-care facility.

Activity 2.4

Using trolleys and equipment

In the clinical area, you will need to use clean trolleys for performing certain nursing interventions. Examples include dressings, catheterisation or using equipment such as the bladder assessment trolley, hoists and monitoring equipment.

1 What are the requirements for cleaning the equipment?
2 Why should you clean from top down?
3 Do you need to use a special type of cleaning solution?

Waste management

Safe disposal of wastes in correct containers is essential not only for protecting yourself, but other workers in the clinical setting. In the hospital environment, it is likely that a wider and more hazardous type of waste will be encountered. However, as with any waste management, if the correct precautions and procedures are followed, the risk of contamination is minimal. Think for one minute about what constitutes waste in a hospital and then think about the possibilities for contamination. They are large if the correct procedures are not followed by everyone associated with waste disposal and management.

All health-care facilities have protocols and procedures in place to ensure effective waste management. In most health service inductions, you will receive a lecture or information session concerning the correct waste segregation in your health-care facility. These policies are formulated in line with federal and state or territory government legislation – management of poisons, cytotoxic waste, disposal of sharps etc.

Health-care facilities are responsible for all waste generated within the hospital until its final disposal. All staff working within the facility have an obligation to abide by the policies and procedures and regulatory requirements to protect the safety of clients, visitors and co-workers as well as their own safety.

When waste is not handled correctly and safely it poses a risk to everyone. Inappropriate handling of waste can also lead to significant financial burdens – clinical waste is incinerated at extremely high temperatures and is incredibly expensive and detrimental to the environment in its disposal.

CASE STUDY 2.1

Unexpected guests

You are completing clinical placement on a general medical ward. Your patient Flynn Grahams requires an IV antibiotic. You are observing your buddy nurse give the medication, and as she is preparing to administer the medication she touches the patient's wound dressing that is soiled and falling off. She then administers the IV medication without washing her hands.

1   What are the moments of hand hygiene here that were missed?
2   Potentially, what has the nurse exposed this patient to?
3   Is this practising within infection control standards?

The environment protection authority (EPA) in each state and territory must license waste-disposal contractors. The responsibility of the health-care facility's management for waste generated onsite continues until, and including, the actual disposal. Management and staff must also include the following waste disposal points in their infection control strategy.

Bins must be:
- weather safe, and secure against animals and vermin
- emptied on a needs basis, but at least weekly
- secured from public access.

Waste bags must:
- never be braced against the body or dragged across the floor
- not be compacted with the hands or the feet
- be inspected regularly to ensure contents are appropriate to the type of the bag.

Incontinence pads, colostomy bags and urinary drainage bags can be disposed of in the general waste for landfill after the contents have been drained into the sewerage.

Figure 2.7 gives a general overview of the colours of bags for waste in health care.

Type of waste	Colour of bags / containers	Colour of letters	Symbols
Clinical	Yellow	**Black**	
Cytotoxic	Lilac	Violet	
Radioactive	Scarlet	**Black**	
General Waste	opaque white	**no colour**	no symbol

FIGURE 2.7 The colours of bags for waste in health care

Activity 2.5

Managing clinical waste

Do a workplace inspection on the clinical area.
* What types of waste are present? For each type of waste locate the policy and procedure.
* What are the requirements for disposal of each type of waste?

2.2 Identifying infection hazards and assessing risks

You are responsible for taking reasonable care to protect your own health and the safety of others. Occupational exposure is direct contact with blood and bodily fluids during the course of your normal duties.

Infection hazards associated with your own role and work environment

The first step in protecting yourself is identification of a hazard. When providing nursing care for a client there are a number of times that physical contact occurs. Any person with an infection that is identified on admission needs to have a risk assessment of all care tasks. Can the infection be transmitted? How is it transmitted?

If the person does not have a documented infection on admission, the nurse will assess them and a full assessment of all of the body systems is undertaken. Examples of assessment taken on admission are:
* if the person has a temperature, the cause is investigated
* if there is a wound, a wound swab is taken
* routine urinalysis is conducted.

Areas of responsibility in relation to infection prevention and control

As a nurse you must be aware of your own responsibilities to prevent the spread of infection. The best way of ensuring this is by following the facility's policies and procedures, maintaining hand hygiene and caring for all clients using standard precautions.

If you have an illness such as a cold or cold sore, you need to follow the policies and procedures relating to staff illness and report to the supervisor. One way that nurses demonstrate their responsibilities in the prevention of infections is by ensuring that they have undertaken the required immunisations before attending placement. This protects them from contacting an infection and also prevents them from transmitting infections to vulnerable groups of people they come in contact with.

Assessing risk

A risk assessment of the identified hazard then needs to be undertaken. This will determine how likely the hazard is to cause harm and what could occur. For infection control there are a number of infection hazards present in the hospital. Examples are used needles, dirty linen and equipment, and body fluids and waste.

Other infection hazards that nurses need to be aware of relate more to the infectious diseases that people may have when they are admitted. A person who has vomiting and diarrhoea may have gastroenteritis that could spread quickly and cause the health-care facility to close down, and in some vulnerable groups may cause severe illness or even death.

Activity 2.6

Infectious diseases

Locate the policy and procedures relating to infectious diseases. Find the policy that relates to:

- gastroenteritis
- influenza
- measles.
  Identify the precautions the facility has put in place when these situations occur.

Documenting and reporting activities and tasks that put you, clients, visitors and/or other workers at risk

If you note an area of concern regarding infection you need to document this and report to the supervisor of the area. Ensure that other clients are not exposed to the infection by proper hand hygiene and required nursing actions to prevent the spread of infections.

Health-care facilities commonly use an infection control consultant or nurse to assist in the management of infection. You may be required to also complete additional nursing actions to notify this department.

TIP 2.6
Required immunisations
Locate the staff policies and procedures that relate to staff immunisations. Have you had all of the immunisations listed?

Activity 2.7

Prevention of infection

Locate the policy and procedures relating to preventing the spread of infection. Find the policy that relates to:
- management of linen and equipment
- sharps and needle sticks
- body fluids.

Identify the precautions the facility has put in place when these situations occur.

Control measures to minimise risk in accordance with organisation's procedures

As a health-care facility's business is the provision of support to all people who access their services, special procedures have been implemented to control the spread of infection that could occur as a result of daily activities when undertaking nursing care of clients. Often the procedures do not eliminate the infection risk but control it using a variety of measures. These are implemented by ranking the risk of the hazard and addressing the most serious risks first, then applying measures such as isolation, engineering, PPE or administrative controls.

Reflective practice 2.1

Germs, germs everywhere!

I can recall one of my first clinical placements in an acute care facility. It was on a respiratory ward. I would go home and hear coughing in my sleep. Sputum was a daily experience, and there was all sorts of sputum that is for sure. I never realised just how projectile coughing can be! Sputum and saliva sure can move at speed, and it was in this placement that I learnt the value of PPE. I would carry goggles on me, and would always ensure I had gloves and an apron on when performing care. I never realised just how simply infection could be spread until I could 'see' it in action on a respiratory ward. Prior to this placement I was not always using goggles, as they got hot and annoying at times. I soon learnt to adjust to working with them on!

Joanne, 24, Enrolled Nurse

1 How can you undertake work in a manner that prevents the spread of infection?
2 What resources could you use if you are unsure about the actions that you need to take to prevent the spread of infection?

2.3 Managing risks associated with specific hazards

All facilities will have protocols and procedures in place for any exposure. After hours exposure often has a slightly different management plan due to decreased staff working. In any case, you should always ensure you familiarise yourself with the policies so you can assist or ensure you are following correct procedure.

Activity 2.8

Spill management

Locate the policy and procedure for spill management.
    Find the spill kit and investigate the contents.
- Is all equipment in the kit?
- If you have to use it, where or how is the equipment replenished?

Protocols for care after exposure to blood and other bodily fluids

In the event of exposure to blood or other bodily fluids or substances, your immediate steps should be:
- Flush the area with copious amounts of running water.
- Pat dry and cover with a sterile adhesive dressing.
- If eyes are affected, flush them thoroughly and gently several times while open with water or normal saline.
- If clothing is contaminated, remove and shower.
- Report exposure to an appropriate person (follow organisational policies and procedures) to ensure that necessary follow up action can be taken.
- Complete appropriate work injury paperwork (WorkSafe, workers' compensation etc.)

All incidents of exposure to blood or other bodily fluids must be reported and a risk assessment of the significance of the exposure can then occur. The significance of the exposure will depend on the nature and extent of the injury, the item that caused the injury or exposure and the body substance involved, and the amount of substance involved.

Activity 2.9

Exposure to blood or body fluids

Locate the facility's policy and procedure for exposure to blood.
    Imagine you have had a needle stick injury after giving an injection of insulin. Complete an incident report on this injury. You can make up the patient details – do not use real details.

Contamination considerations

Effective infection control requires that you understand how infection is spread and ensure you abide by infection control policies in place at your place of employment. In any health-care setting, a client should have their own set of personal care items such as toothbrush, comb and linen.

Because microorganisms travel easily through the air, you should not shake bed linen (clean or dirty) or bedclothes. To prevent the transmission of microorganisms through indirect contact, do not allow soiled items and equipment to touch your clothing – a common error is to carry dirty linen against the uniform or to drop on the floor rather than dispose directly into the appropriate containers.

TIP 2.7

Equipment

When using a stethoscope, it is desirable to wash off the bell or diaphragm with a neutral detergent prior to proceeding to your next patient. This will stop the spread of infection from one client to another. For your own protection you should also wipe the ear pieces with an alcohol wipe before inserting into your own ear canals.

Minimising contamination

In each ward or health-care facility there are designated clean and dirty areas. This is also a consideration for minimising the risk of cross infection/contamination. There are often 'glove free' or 'non-clinical' areas, which are usually common areas where computers and phones are kept. Think about the contamination that could occur if you were to use the computer to contact someone with contaminated gloves or dirty hands – those germs would be left on the equipment to be passed on to the next user, and so begins the chain of infection!

Infection control is a major component of our everyday roles as nurses. Linked with WHS (workplace health and safety), it underpins every procedure we undertake. With this in mind it is imperative that we adhere to clean work areas. Dirty utilities must be clearly signed and the area responsibly kept clean. If you take a dirty bed pan into the room, you clean it! It is unsafe to leave this lying around for other workers to potentially spill, and it can cause harm or cross infection. Infection control requires you to be aware of the risks of contamination and limit them as much as possible. The health-care facility you are attending will have a detailed infection control policy that will outline your responsibilities and the facility's procedures for containment etc. Ensure that you read this policy and that you abide by it – for your safety and that of your patients and colleagues.

SUMMARY

- When performing nursing interventions the nurse needs to use the appropriate standard or additional precautions to prevent and control infection. Responding appropriately to situations where additional precautions are needed will reduce the risk of the spread of infection.
- To prevent the spread of infection nurses need to identify infection hazards, assess the risk and implement control measures as part of their professional responsibilities.
- Policies and procedures of health-care facilities need to be followed to ensure infection is not spread through exposure or contamination.

SELF-TEST QUESTIONS

1 What is the difference between standard and additional precautions for managing infection?
2 What actions do I need to take if there is an infectious hazard that requires additional precautions?
3 How can I identify infection hazards and control the spread of infections?
4 Where do I locate the additional equipment required to manage infections that require additional precautions?
5 What documentation and action is required if I suffer an exposure to blood in the workplace?

BIBLIOGRAPHY

Clarke, L., Gray, S., White, L., Duncan, G. & Baumle, W. (2016). *Foundations of Nursing: Enrolled Division 2 Nurses* (ANZ edition). Cengage Learning: South Melbourne.

DeLaune, S.C., Ladner, P.K., McTier, L., Tollefson, J. & Lawrence, J. (2016). *Australian and New Zealand Fundamentals of Nursing* (revised edition). Cengage Learning: South Melbourne.

Hand Hygiene Australia (2018). *5 moments for hand hygiene*, http://www.hha.org.au/home/5-moments-for-hand-hygiene.aspx.

National Health and Medical Research Council (NHMRC) (2010). *Australian Guidelines for the Prevention & Control of Infection in Healthcare*. Retrieved from http://www.nhmrc.gov.au/_files_nhmrc/publications/attachments/cd33_complete.pdf.

Tollefson, J., Watson, G., Jelly, E. & Tambree, K. (2016). *Essential Clinical Skills: Enrolled Division 2 Nurses* (3rd edn). Cengage Learning: South Melbourne.

World Health Organization (2009). *My 5 moments for hand hygiene*, http://www.who.int/gpsc/5may/background/5moments/en/index.html.

Care of the older person

LEARNING OUTCOMES

After reading this chapter, you should have an understanding of:

3.1 Responding to the health requirements of an older person

3.2 Contributing to the care plan for an older person

3.3 Applying nursing practice in the aged care environment

3.4 Identifying requirements and addressing issues in aged care nursing practice

3.5 Using strategies that relate to the progressive and variable nature of dementia

3.6 Developing and implementing strategies to minimise the impact of challenging behaviours

Working in aged care

I was really excited to be going on my first clinical nursing placement. I was going along with seven other classmates to the local aged care facility. I was looking forward to putting into place all the techniques that we had learnt about in class.

On the first morning we assembled in the corridor of the aged care facility. The first thing I noticed was the smell. It was not unpleasant, but very strong. The clinical educator told us that it was due to the chemicals that were used to clean the facility.

I was assigned to look after eight residents with a buddy. I was shocked at how frail some of the residents were. Some were so incapacitated they could not move or even feed themselves. Showering the residents also provided some shocks. It was hard to relate to their bodies, they were so wrinkled, and some of the female residents even had whiskers that needed to be removed.

At debrief I was close to tears, and told my clinical educator that I did not think I could do this work. The clinical educator encouraged me to come back the next day. Over the next few days, I got to know more details about the lives that the residents had had and why they had come to the facility. One of the residents had been a musician and I was amazed to see a photograph of him playing in the Royal Symphonic Orchestra when he was a young man. He had been very handsome.

Gradually I became used to the care requirements and felt pleased that I could provide care for the residents.

At the end of the placement, I felt sad that I would not see some of the residents I had cared for. One resident kissed me and told me that she would miss me greatly. I gained a lot from the placement and was glad that I had seen it through.

3.1 Health requirements of an older person

When you work with aged people, you have to know it all. It is so comprehensive because the patients have multiple issues. In order to provide holistic care you have to know about all the body systems and how ageing affects their function, as well as insight into allied areas – occupational therapy, physiotherapy, speech therapy, dietetics, social work and counselling.

By working with older people you can make a tremendous difference to their quality of life and achieve real personal satisfaction through your work.

The ageing process affects us all in different ways with some older people ageing faster than others. Factors which may contribute to the ageing process include heredity, nutrition, environmental and social factors, with both the person and their family or carers being affected. It is important to recognise these changes and respond appropriately so that the quality of life in an older person is optimised.

Age-related physical changes and psychosocial needs of a person, their family or carer

Normal ageing involves physical and mental changes which may impact on sight, hearing, memory, motor sensory skills, mobility and balance. The rate of ageing varies between individuals with many older people remaining healthy and others experiencing increasing levels of ill health, including chronic diseases and other age-related disorders such as cancer. This diversity can also be influenced by socioeconomic disadvantage, which can increase the incidence of disease or disability later in life. **Table 3.1** outlines the main physical changes associated with ageing.

TABLE 3.1 Physical changes associated with ageing

System	Physical changes
Cardiovascular	• valves thicker and more rigid • stroke volume decreases by 1% per year • vessels lose elasticity • oxygen utilisation decreases • decreased cardiac output
Respiratory	• reflexes become weaker • alveoli become larger resulting in less surface area for oxygen to diffuse across • chest muscles become more rigid • lungs unable to fully inflate • ciliary action decreases leading to more mucous buildup
Musculoskeletal	• bones become weaker and tendons less flexible • loss of muscle tissue • decline in reflexes
Integumentary	• skin becomes dry and less elastic • skin becomes thinner • wrinkles and spots/lesions appear
Gastrointestinal	• taste sensation diminished • dry mouth due to decrease in saliva production • decreased absorption occurs in the gut • more time required to move food through the gut

>>

System	Physical changes
Genitourinary	• pelvic floor muscles weaken • bladder capacity decreases Female: • decreased oestrogen and vaginal secretions • urgency and stress incontinence Male: • decreased testosterone, sperm count and testicular size • increased prostate size causing retention • urinary frequency
Neurological	• neuron function decreases • neurotransmitter function is diminished • brain mass reduces
Special senses	Vision: • close focus diminished • thickness of the lens occurs • decreased tear production causing dry eyes Hearing: • tympanic membrane atrophy • decreased high frequency hearing • cerumen is more likely to become impacted due to increased keratin Taste: • reduced saliva production causing dry mouth • ability to perceive bitter, salt and sour tastes diminishes Smell: • diminished smell sensation due to reduced sensory cells
Endocrine	• thyroid gland atrophies • hormonal secretion decreases • lower basal metabolic rate • decreased release of insulin and metabolism of glucose

Source: TAFE NSW (2012), HLTEN515B Implement and monitor nursing care for clients, http://www.vetres.net.au/product_files/HLTEN515B_5573_PROMO.pdf.

Activity 3.1

Assessment of the older person

Choose one of the clients you are providing care for and complete an assessment of the systems of the body. In aged care environments a resident is usually assessed each month. This is called 'the resident of the day'.

Are they exhibiting the changes as described above? Remember that everyone is individual and ageing occurs differently for each person. If you noticed some differences try to find out why they occurred. An example may be the skin. One person may have less wrinkles and spots than another or require a different dietary intake.

Psychosocial needs

Growing older means confronting many psychological, emotional and social issues that come with entering the last phase of life. These can include:

• **Dementia** – the irreversible deterioration of intellectual ability accompanied by emotional disturbance.

dementia
The irreversible deterioration of intellectual ability accompanied by emotional disturbance

Alzheimer's disease
A progressive disease that leaves a person unable to form new memories and is marked by the loss of other mental functions

- **Alzheimer's disease** – a progressive disease that leaves a person unable to form new memories and is marked by the loss of other mental functions.
- Sleep problems – as people age, deep sleep is decreased and their sleep becomes lighter with frequent waking. This results in daytime fatigue.
- Dependency – as people age, they become more dependent on others. They may also struggle with feelings of guilt, shame or depression because of their increased dependency, especially in societies where the elderly are viewed as a burden.
- Loneliness and isolation – many older people contend with these feelings as their loved ones pass away, which can negatively impact their health and wellbeing.
- Rejection – a feeling of rejection and loss of purpose in life may also be felt by the older person which can lead to decreased self esteem.

Activity 3.2

Enhancing self-esteem

Complete the table by giving examples of how a nurse can enhance self-esteem for the aged person.

Strategy	Example
Develop a trusting relationship	
Treat the person with dignity and respect	
Give positive reinforcement for progress	
Encourage verbalisation	
Practise active listening	
Include the person in decision making	
Use verbal and non-verbal communication	
Encourage socialisation	

Age-related effects of drugs and medications

Older people tend to take more drugs than younger people because they are more likely to have more than one chronic medical disorder. Consideration needs to be made when caring for the elderly who are taking multiple medications:

- The use of multiple medications increases the potential for **adverse drug reactions (ADRs)** and drug interactions.
- Age-related pharmacokinetic changes can alter drug absorption, distribution, metabolism and excretion.
- As the person ages, the body systems become less effective and this can cause the effects of medications to change. This is due to poor absorption, distribution thoughout the body, metabolism of the medication and excretion of the medication. This can lead to a change in the effect of the medication on the older person.
- Elderly individuals who have challenging behaviours may refuse to take prescribed medication due to cognitive changes.
- Loss of hearing, vision and manual dexterity may make it difficult for the elderly person to take medication as prescribed.

adverse drug reactions (ADRs)
Any medication effect other than what is therapeutically intended

TIP 3.1

Medication effects in the elderly

The metabolism and excretion of many drugs decrease in the elderly and this can lead to adverse effects or over dosage. The elderly often take many drugs (polypharmacy) which can lead to drug–drug interaction. Make sure to check all medications prior to dispensing and report any concerns to the RN or pharmacist.

Activity 3.3

Medication and the elderly

Choose one of the clients for whom you are providing care. Make a list of the medications that the person is taking. List the side effects of the medication. Why have they been prescribed this medication?

Try to find another person who exhibits challenging behaviours or a dementia and complete the medication activity for this person.

Age-related pathophysiological disorders and preventative care

As people age, their body systems also change and the chances of developing chronic disease increases. **Table 3.2** lists common pathophysiological disorders associated with ageing and the preventative care measures that can be implemented to meet the person's needs.

Learning

TABLE 3.2 Pathophysiological disorders and monitoring

System	Disorder	Preventative care
Central nervous system	Dementia and changes to brain function e.g. impaired judgement, difficulty understanding, stroke	Risk assess – increased likelihood of falling, mental health deterioration
Cardiovascular system	Blood pressure abnormalities e.g. hypertension and orthostatic hypotension	Monitoring medications
Integumentary system	Decreased elasticity of body tissue and thin skin causing tears and pressure sores	Monitoring wounds as they take longer to heal Pressure relieving devices
Respiratory system	Chronic lung disease	Do not over exert Deep breathing and coughing
Gastrointestinal and urinary system	Constipation Difficulty swallowing Incontinence Renal failure	Smaller, regular meals High fibre foods Regular toileting
Endocrine system	Diabetes Osteoporosis	Healthy diet Risk of falls – encourage exercise
Musculoskeletal system	Osteoarthritis Rheumatoid arthritis Fractures	Active and passive exercises Mobility aids and adaptive devices
Special senses	Cataracts, hearing decline	Adaptive equipment e.g. glasses, hearing aids
Immune system	Cancers	Regular monitoring

CASE STUDY 3.1

Pathophysiology and polypharmacy

Richard, aged 91, was admitted with dehydration and anaemia. He has a history of heart problems, incontinence, arthritis, hearing difficulties and early onset dementia. He takes antihypertensive and anticoagulant medication for arthritis, vitamin deficiency, pain relief and dementia. His wife is 89 years old and is having difficulties caring for him at home.

1. What are the key physical issues facing Richard?
2. What psychosocial issues need to be addressed?
3. Richard has been identified as a high risk for experiencing ADRs due to polypharmacy. What are some nursing strategies that can be implemented to reduce this risk?

Communicating effectively and making adjustments for people who have sensory impairments

Communication is integral to implementing effective nursing care for the older person. When the patient is able to see the reason behind planned care and the benefit to themselves, they are more likely to be compliant and cooperative.

As a nurse in aged care your communication skills are crucial in delivering quality care to your older clients. How effective you are as a communicator will greatly influence your relationship with clients and work colleagues. **Table 3.3** identifies strategies for communicating effectively with people who have sensory impairments.

TABLE 3.3 Communication strategies for sensory impairment

Impairment	Communication strategy
Hearing impairment	• Sit on the side where the person can hear better. Ensure they can see your face as older people can pick up words from lip movements. • Ensure that there is no other noise present to compete with your voice. • Speak slowly and precisely.
Vision impairment	• Clear verbal communication is important. • It is important to provide a large written material or audio material for the person to refer to after verbal communication.

Speech impairment	• A speech therapist can assist to promote effective communication though the provision of communication aids such as:
	  – sign language
	  – communication boards
	  – artificial voice box for a person who has had a laryngectomy
	  – computer devices.
	It is important to allow enough time for the person to respond.

Preventative health assessment

Normal ageing changes and health problems frequently show themselves as declines in the functional status of older people. Assessment of functional ability becomes more important to nurses as well as other members of the interdisciplinary team.

Preventative health assessment tools are used as an aid to assess the emotional, psychological, mental, physical and functional abilities of the patient and allow the health-care team to plan care more effectively (Section 3.2 'Care planning for the older person', describes common assessment tools in aged care).

Theories of ageing

People are living longer now due to better medical interventions. Biological theories look to the effects living has on the person's cells (Physiopedia, n.d.). The structural-functional theory of ageing proposes that withdrawing from society the person is acknowledging the end of their life and as a result loses both mental and physical capabilities (Study.com, n.d.) **Table 3.4** outlines four theories of ageing.

TABLE 3.4 Theories of ageing

Theory	Description
Programmed theories	A person is born programmed to die and this is part of their genetic makeup.
Damage or error theories	The effect of the environment a person lives in causes damage to build up over their lifespan.
Disengagement theory	The person withdraws from society and society accepts this withdrawal.
Activity theory	Roles held by people in society are linked to physical and mental health. If a person stops these activities they lose the benefits of the previous activities.

Source: Physiopedia, *Theories of aging*, https://www.physio-pedia.com/Theories_of_Aging.

Companionship and social inclusion

Companionship and social inclusion is important for both mental and physical wellbeing.
Mental benefits include:
- increased sense of purpose
- prevention of loneliness
- maintenance of social skills
- feeling of value.
  Physical benefits include:
- participation in physical activities together
- maintaining healthy habits
- supporting each other in achieving goals.

A person's social interaction provides the individual with a life that is enriched through interaction with others in society. Section 3.3 'Applying nursing practice in the aged care environment' identifies social networks and organisations that the older person can use.

Oral health problems

A common problem with elderly people is poor oral health. Studies have shown that there is a link between oral health and illness. Reasons given for this are:
- a healthy mouth is one of the body's defence mechanisms
- pain can lead to poor nutrition
- appearance can lead to low self-esteem and isolation
- difficulty in communicating verbally (Victorian Government Department of Human Service, 2002).

Table 3.5 outlines preventative care for oral and/or dental problems in the elderly.

TIP 3.3

Oral hygiene
As part of the care routine cleaning of the oral cavity and brushing of teeth/dentures should be undertaken twice a day. Regular fluid intake of water after meals should also be encouraged.

TABLE 3.5 Oral health preventative measures

Oral/dental problem	Prevention
Dental caries and tooth loss	Provide oral hygiene and dental care regularly to maintain teeth and gums in good condition Regular teeth brushing and flossing Oral care, mouth toilets, artificial saliva Dental checks and treatment
Gum disease: gingivitis and periodontitis	Good oral hygiene and oral inspection
Xerostomia (dry mouth)	Good hydration Artificial saliva
Oral infections and ulcerations	Antifungal/antibiotic treatment is effective Brushing of dentures after eating Removing dentures at night Dental checks to ensure dentures fit properly

Identify and respond to signs of distress

Because symptoms of distress can vary, you must become familiar with the causes of the person's behaviour through their care plan and current medical conditions in order to recognise the early warning signs. Once you have identified these signs, you and the health-care team can determine strategies to prevent the behaviour from escalating. **Table 3.6** lists common signs of distress with appropriate responses.

TABLE 3.6 Signs and responses to distress

Signs and symptoms	Responses
Restlessness	Identification of triggers that may cause distress
Impaired ability to make decisions	Do not become anxious as this may increase the patient's distress
Rapid heartbeat	Do not command or argue with the patient; be polite, tolerant and respectful
Nausea	Give the patient physical space
Sweating	Convey a message of empathy and reassurance to the person concerned

3.2 Care planning for the older person

Caring for the older person requires a diverse range of skills that require all members of the multidisciplinary team to address. Good assessment is the first step in planning care for individuals. There are a number of risk assessment tools that can be used when planning the care for the older person.

Aged care assessment tools

Preventative health assessment tools (see **Table 3.7**) are used to assess the emotional, psychological, mental, physical and functional abilities of the person, allowing the health worker to plan care more comprehensively.

TABLE 3.7 Assessment tools

Tool	Description
Mini mental status examination (MMSE)	Most commonly used instrument for screening global cognitive decline. Shows any decline in cognitive functioning, particularly in memory function.
Index of Independence in Activities of Daily Living (Katz ADL)	The Index assesses functional status by measuring the person's ability to perform ADLs. The six functions are: bathing, dressing, toileting, transferring, continence and feeding. Patients are scored yes/no for independence in each of the six functions. The lower the score, the greater the functional impairment.
Norton scale	This scale identifies the need for preventative pressure area care. Each of the five criteria – physical condition, mental condition, activity, mobility and incontinence – are scored from 1–4 with the lower score rating the person 'at risk' of developing pressure sores and requiring preventative care.
Braden scale	An assessment tool for predicting the risk of pressure ulcers, based on the total of scores given in the categories: sensory perception, moisture, activity, mobility, nutrition, and friction and shear.

TIP 3.4

Falls screening and risk assessment tools

Falls screening aims to identify people at increased risk of falls, whereby falls risk assessments aims to identify factors that increase falls risk, and that may be responsive to intervention.

Both these tools need to be linked to an action plan to address any modifiable falls risk factors they identify.

>>

Tool	Description
Waterlow scale	Gives an estimated risk for the development of a pressure sore. Areas are assessed for each patient and assigned a point value. High risk is a score >20: • build/weight for height • skin type/visual risk areas • sex and age • malnutrition screening tool • continence • mobility.
Geriatric depression Scale	A 30-item self-report assessment used to identify depression in the elderly.
Falls risk assessment tools	A process used to identify underlying risk factors for falling. Some falls risk assessments also classify people into low and high falls risk groups.

CASE STUDY 3.2

Risk assessment

Mrs Porter, aged 89, was admitted to the local hospital after falling down her front steps and suffering a fractured humerus. Falls risk assessments indicated high risk. Her past history indicated two falls in the past six months, impaired vision, frequency and incontinence.

On discharge a management program was implemented that included a community physiotherapist for ongoing strength and balance exercises.

1   What other referrals would be beneficial for Mrs Porter and why?
2   What physiological changes occur in the elderly to make them more prone to falls?

ACAT assessment

If an older person needs help at home or is considering moving into an aged care home, respite care or transition care, they may first need an assessment by an **Aged Care Assessment Team**. ACAT will ask questions about the person's activities of daily living and if they need help with all or some of them. They will also ask about the general state of the person's health and specific health conditions to help work out how much and what type of help is needed.

Aged Care Assessment Team
An interdisciplinary team made up of a doctor, a registered nurse, a social worker and an occupational therapist, assisting the elderly and their carers to determine the care level required to meet the client's needs

Activity 3.4

Assessment tools

Assessment tools are particularly beneficial because they can form part of routine clinical management and inform further assessment and care for all patients.

Identify the assessment tools used in your facility:

1   What risk management strategies are implemented for these tools?
2   Who are the members of the multidisciplinary team that contribute to the ongoing management for people at risk?

Documentation and reporting

Government funding for aged care is based on meeting standards and providing quality care. This means that correct documentation is essential to ensure that appropriate funding is allocated and that evidence of acceptable standards is reported.

Aged care standards/accreditation

Residential aged care in Australia is regulated by the *Aged Care Act 1997*. The Act specifies the standards that facilities must achieve. Part of the Act details the accreditation process to which federal government funded residential facilities must adhere. For facilities to receive government funding they must pass accreditation. Accreditation is usually for a specific time frame, for example, three or five years (see **Activity 3.5**).

Activity 3.5

Aged Care Accreditation Standards

The Aged Care Accreditation Standards are detailed in the Australian Aged Care Quality Agency's 'Quality of Care Principles 2014'. There are four Standards:

Standard one: Management systems, staffing and organisational development

Standard two: Health and personal care

Standard three: Care recipient lifestyle

Standard four: Physical environment and safe systems.

There are 44 expected outcomes across the four Standards. Homes must comply with all 44 expected outcomes at all times.

Identify the Home Care Common Standards.

1   What are the similarities and differences to the residential Aged Care Accreditation Standards?

Aged Care Funding

Aged Care Funding Instrument (ACFI)
A resource allocation instrument that assesses the needs of residents and enables allocation of government funding

The **Aged Care Funding Instrument (ACFI)** is a resource allocation instrument. The ACFI assesses core care needs as a basis for allocating funding. These needs are related to day to day, high frequency need for care (see **Activity 3.6**).

The ACFI is primarily intended to deliver funding to the organisation providing the care, which is the residential aged care home. When completed on all residents in the facility, the ACFI determines the overall care needs profile of the facility and the subsequent funding.

Activity 3.6

Aged Care Funding Instrument (ACFI)

The ACFI is in the form of 12 questions about individual aged care needs, divided into three broad domains: activities of daily living, behaviour and complex health care. Based on the answers/assessments, each of these areas is allocated funding according to the following needs: high, medium, low or nil.

1   List the categories in each of the three domains.

2   What is the role of the nursing staff in completing ACFI forms?

3   Describe in more detail the complex health-care domain.

Learning

Identifying abilities and limitations for self-care

Recognising and acknowledging that older people have abilities and limitations in self-care can reduce the feelings of distress in the person. Early detection of limitations can prevent more complex problems developing. This might require adaptive aids, therapies or medications that can be tailored to suit the individual.

Consideration must be made in regard to:

• monitoring of current health problems

• medication monitoring

- continence care
- mobility assessment
- ability to achieve activities of daily living
- ability to maintain sleep and rest
- ability to participate in regular activity and exercise
- monitoring of mental state.

Collaboration

Activity 3.7

Applying a holistic approach to aged care

Choose a client that you have been caring for in the aged care environment:

1   How are their physical needs being met?
2   How are their social, emotional and spiritual needs being met?
3   Are there any additional needs that need to be addressed?

Contribute to the development of nursing care plans

The purpose of a nursing care plan is to provide a detailed guide for individualised client care and to put client goals, priorities, deadlines and nursing actions in writing. The plan provides a line of communication for nursing team members and coordinates the work of the team. The older person and their family should be encouraged to participate in the planning to ensure that it meets all needs.

Understanding the implications of the admission

When an older person is admitted to hospital, their care needs can change from self-sufficiency to dependency due to their underlying condition. This can make care delivery and discharge planning challenging. The person may return home independently, may return home with a home care package, or may be admitted to nursing home care. The following section looks at the impacts of age-related disorders on activities of daily living and the associated nursing interventions to promote independence and wellbeing for the elderly patient.

Reflective practice 3.1

Reflection about aged care admissions

The Australian Institute of Health and Welfare (AIHW, 2013) notes that people are more likely to be admitted into residential care than return to the community after hospitalisation.

Reflect on your experiences with older people and consider what factors may contribute to this occurring.

Impacts of age-related disorders on ADLs and nursing interventions

Caring for older people requires a diverse range of skills that need to be provided by members of a multidisciplinary health-care team. Maintaining dignity, privacy and confidentiality, as well as infection control due to the increased susceptibility of the older person to infection are particularly important. Complete **Activity 3.8** to identify nursing interventions for each of the activities of daily living.

Activity 3.8

Nursing care of the older person

Choose a client that you have been caring for in an aged care environment and complete the activity below to identify age-related disorders and appropriate nursing interventions.

Activity of daily living	Age-related disorder	Nursing intervention
Mobility		
Hygiene		
Elimination		
Breathing		
Communication		
Rest and sleep		
Pain		

Problem solving

3.3 Applying nursing practice in the aged care environment

Much of the way we feel about growing older is based on attitudes that are prevalent in our society. The term *ageism* was first used in 1976 by Robert Butler to describe the process of stereotyping and discrimination against people who are old.

Stereotypes, attitudes, values and beliefs associated with ageing

Stereotypes of ageing include assumptions and generalisations about how people at or over a certain age should behave, and what they are likely to experience, without regard for individual differences or unique circumstances.

Activity 3.9

Myths about ageing

1   Why are negative attitudes about older persons prevalent in our society?
2   Research common myths about ageing and discuss the reality regarding these myths.

TIP 3.5

Are you stereotyping?

It is important to evaluate our own ideas about ageing.

We must be open to new ideas and eliminate our own judgements regarding growing older so that we can provide effective care to the older person.

Impact of complex issues on family and carers

Carers are usually family members or friends who provide support to an older person who has a disability, mental illness, chronic condition or is too frail to provide care for themselves.

Caring for someone can be a demanding job and most people need extra assistance to manage. In Australia, federal, state or territory and local governments have a number of services available to help carers and their family members.

Activity 3.10

Respite care

Respite care (or short-term care) is an option that carers can access to give them an opportunity to have a holiday or a break from caring.

Research the different types of respite services available through the Commonwealth Home Support Program.

1   What is transition care and how is it different to respite care?

Promoting health maintenance

The older person can be encouraged to adopt strategies to support health maintenance (see **Table 3.8**). This will promote their physical and emotional wellbeing.

respite care
Care and services that provides a break to caregivers and is used for a few hours a week, for an occasional weekend or for longer periods of time

TABLE 3.8 Healthy lifestyle practices

Healthy lifestyle practice	Implementation
Adequate nutrition	Include a variety of fresh fruit, vegetables, grains, dairy, meats. Avoid excess sugars and fats
Maintaining healthy weight	Regular exercise Refer to dietician if malnourished or overweight
Staying mentally active	Participation in social activities Refer to diversional therapist for opportunities for older people to stay mentally active
Regular sleep	Maintain regular sleep patterns Refer to GP if the person is having sleep difficulties
Moderation with alcohol	Monitor intake and educate about healthy alcohol limits
No smoking	Educate about dangers of smoking-related diseases Refer to GP for strategies to stop smoking

Community services

Community support services help older people by providing additional supports and services such as home and community care, Meals on Wheels, transportation and various recreational facilities. Other services include are discussed below.

Day Therapy Centres

Day Therapy Centres offer physiotherapy, occupational and speech therapy, podiatry and other therapy services to older people in a community setting. People can attend these centres on a needs basis. Some may have access to a community bus to allow easier access to the facility.

Transition Care Programs

The Transition Care Program provides goal-oriented, time-limited and therapy-focused care to provide support to older people at the conclusion of a hospital stay. This is a temporary arrangement with the person eventually returning home (Australian Government Department of Health, 2017b).

Aged care residential facilities

People enter aged care for different reasons. A person may only need to stay for a short time in order to recuperate or provide a solution for when their normal carer is not available. At other times, a decision is made that a permanent arrangement needs to be organised

TIP 3.6

People from CALD backgrounds

Many organisations now offer specific diets, activities, languages or spiritual needs, to cater for different cultural, linguistic or spiritual backgrounds.

There are organisations in each state and territory that work as part of the Partners in Culturally Appropriate Care (PICAC) program to support aged care providers to deliver culturally appropriate care to older people from culturally and linguistically diverse (CALD) communities.

Collaboration

to support the older person. Permanent care provides accommodation for people who are unable to continue living independently in their own homes. Both options are available to the older person who has been assessed and approved to receive it.

Home care packages

The Home Care Packages Program helps you live independently in your own home for as long as you can. The Australian Government provides a subsidy to an approved home care provider towards a package of care, services and case management to meet your individual needs. The older person will need an ACAT assessment to determine eligibility for these packages.

Additional support services

The following additional support services may be required:

- community nursing care
- allied health care
- meals and other food services
- domestic assistance
- personal care
- home modification and maintenance
- shopping
- transport
- respite care
- counselling, support, information and advocacy
- hospice care.

Activity 3.11

My Aged Care

My Aged Care is a website that serves as the main entry point to the aged care system in Australia. It provides information and tools to assist and support older people in their care.

Look up http://www.myagedcare.gov.au/ to answer the questions below:

1   Identify the services that support the older person to stay at home.
2   How can family members seek extra help and support when caring for someone at home?
3   What is the Community Visitors Scheme?
4   How can the older person access culturally appropriate aged care services?

3.4 Aged care requirements and issues

There are various legal and ethical issues that impact on aged care. This includes providing care for the deceased person and support for a grieving family. When working in aged care the nurse must ensure their own work practice complies with ethical and legal requirements and supports the rights and dignity of the older person and their family or carer at all times.

Identify legal requirements and ethical issues, and ensure work practice supports person's rights

All aged care facilities and staff must comply with legislation, standards, and policies and procedures. This ensures that a quality framework is provided and that older people have care that maximises their wellbeing. **Table 3.9** lists policies and procedures that are common in aged care.

TABLE 3.9 Policies and procedures

Policy and procedure	Description
Work health and safety	Hazard identification and reporting Risk minimisation
Documentation	Documentation that must be completed for compliance and safety within the organisation
Assessment	Which assessment tools are used in the facility and how they are used
Privacy and confidentiality	Information about the rights of the older person
Complaints	Information for residents on how to lodge a complaint against staff or others
Consent	To give permission for a procedure or activity, it is imperative that the person giving consent has decision-making capacity. Informed consent is made for specific interventions
Guardianship	Protects the rights of people who are unable to make their own decisions
Advanced care directive	Sometimes called a living will, this is when a person makes decisions about their future preferences for medical treatment in cases where they may become incapacitated
Power of attorney	A legal document which gives the person you choose the power to manage your financial and health affairs while you are alive

Elder abuse

This is the infliction of physical, emotional and/or psychological harm on an older, vulnerable person. Elder abuse can take the form of financial exploitation, intentional neglect of an older person by the carer, or unintentional abuse due to ignorance of care issues.

Signs and symptoms may include:
- poor personal hygiene; decayed teeth, overgrown nails
- weight loss
- missing personal aids such as hearing devices, dentures, etc.
- frequent injuries with implausible stories behind them
- old and new looking abrasions, bruises, welts or burns
- bleeding, bruising, pain or itching of the genital area
- behaviour changes such as withdrawal
- reluctance to be undressed/showered (to hide injuries)
- carer insists on being present during all conversations
- client seems fearful of upsetting the carer/relative
- lack of money
- being described as 'accident prone' or 'clumsy'.

Advocate for the person

Advocacy is the ability to stand up for or represent the interests or rights of another person (advocacy will be discussed in more detail in Chapter 4). The National Aged Care Advocacy Program (NACAP) is funded by the Australian Government under the *Aged Care Act 1997*. It provides free, confidential advocacy support and information to consumers of the Australian Government subsidised Home Care Packages and residential aged care services by:
- supporting consumers to find residential aged care services or Home Care Packages to be involved in decisions that affect their life and their care needs

advocacy
The ability to stand up for or represent the interests or rights of another person

TIP 3.7

Charter of rights and responsibilities
As an aged care worker you must be aware of the Charter of Resident Rights and Responsibilities (http://www.agedrights.asn.au/rights/rights_charter.html).

This charter recognises that residents of nursing homes or hostels have the responsibility to ensure that the exercising of their individual rights does not affect others' individual rights, including those providing care.

- providing consumers receiving, or who may receive, residential aged care services or Home Care Packages with information and advice about their rights and responsibilities
- assisting consumers of residential aged care services or Home Care Packages and/or their representatives to resolve problems or complaints in relation to aged care services, through the provision of advocacy
- promoting the rights of consumers receiving residential aged care services or Home Care Packages to aged care service providers (Australian Government Department of Health, 2017a.).

CASE STUDY 3.3

Being an advocate

Mrs Morris is 80 years old and lives alone in the family home. She has vision and mobility problems and shortness of breath. She confides in you that she uses taxi services for all her medical appointments and for shopping, because she is concerned about falling if she uses public transport. This leaves her minimal money for paying bills and supporting family occasions.

The nurse advocated successfully for Mrs Morris and it was arranged that she could use the community transport service in her area.

1   What other services could Mrs Morris be eligible for given her health issues?

Learning, speaking, listening

Responding to signs of stress

As the person ages, so do their cells. Heart fitness and lung capacity decline, which keeps the body from adequately accommodating the natural stress response. People with chronic disease have an additional burden on the body, which makes it even harder to bounce back physically from the toll the stress response takes.

Common sources of stress in the elderly include:
- changes of lifestyle and financial status after retirement
- caring for a sick spouse
- death of relatives, beloved or close friends
- deterioration of physical abilities and chronic illness
- worries about not being able to live independently.

FS

Listening

Stress management

- The elderly can share their difficulties and feelings in facing stress with those they can confide in to help ventilate emotions.
- An active social life, healthy lifestyle and relaxation exercises are all useful ways to handle stress.
- Positive thinking, such as appreciating one's achievements and strengths, can help to enhance self-confidence and to cope with stress.
- The elderly can seek help from professionals in case of need.

Providing care for a deceased person

When the patient dies, their body should be treated with the same respect as when they were alive. Depending on the cultural situation you may have to prepare the body for viewing by the family. You may have to warn family members about post-mortem changes to the body such as the cooling or mottling of the skin. Chapter 10 'A palliative approach to nursing practice', outlines the care of the body after death in more detail.

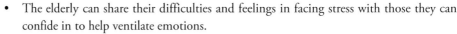

Providing support in grief and death

The older person, due to their age, often experiences situations of grief and death of friends and family. Strategies to support the person who is grieving include:

- Talk to the person about the loss. Sharing memories can help to identify the person's feelings and cope with the emotional distress.
- Give the person time. This shows respect and concern for their needs.
- Identify feelings to help the person become aware of their changes in behaviour.
- Spend time with the person so that they are not alone.
- Be alert for signs of depression so that referrals can be made if necessary.

Activity 3.12

Stages of grief

As a nurse it is important to understand the stages of grief so that you can support the person and encourage them to talk about their loss. Research further on the Internet to answer the following:

1 Describe the stages of grief as identified by Elizabeth Kübler-Ross.
2 What physical symptoms can accompany grief?
3 What organisations offer specialist services in grief support?

3.5 Strategies for dementia

Dementia is a broad term for a range of conditions that involves the progressive decline in a person's ability to function and can cause problems with memory, language, intellect, behaviour and normal emotional reactions.

Types of dementia

Although dementia mainly affects older people, it is not a normal part of ageing. **Table 3.10** lists the various types of dementia.

TABLE 3.10 Types of dementia

Reversible dementia	This is when the cause of the dementia can be treated and the patient makes a recovery from their symptoms. Causes can include ADRs, poisonings, psychological trauma, diabetes, physical disorders, dehydration, tumours, vitamin deficiency, post anaesthetic, infection.
Irreversible dementia	Dementia is irreversible when caused by degenerative disease or trauma. When the brain has been damaged through disease or trauma, mental functioning is unable to recover.
Alzheimer's disease	Alzheimer's disease is the most common form of dementia, affecting up to 70% of all people with dementia. It is distinguished by the buildup of amyloid plaques in the brain.
Lewy body disease	Lewy body disease is caused by the degeneration and death of nerve cells in the brain. This is due to abnormal proteins that somehow appear in nerve cells and impair functioning.
Vascular dementia	Blood supply to the brain is critical for healthy brain functioning. If the circulation is impaired parts of the tissue of the brain can be damaged. Depending on the area of the brain affected, the person will lose the functions associated with that area.
Frontotemporal dementia	The frontotemporal lobes of the brain control our thinking, personality, emotion and behaviour. The temporal region is responsible for language and recognising objects.
Alcohol-related dementia	Alcohol can cause brain damage that can lead to a decrease in mental functioning. (It may be referred to as Korsakoff's Syndrome.)
Other causes of dementia	People in the later stages of AIDS may develop HIV-related dementia. People with Parkinson's disease will often exhibit dementia in the later stages of their illness.

Source: healthdirect. *What causes dementia?* https://www.healthdirect.gov.au/what-causes-dementia.

Signs and symptoms of dementia

The progressive loss of mental function in people with dementia may include:

- loss of memory
- deterioration in intellect
- problems with learning
- inability to plan
- confusion or disorientation
- word finding
- lack of concentration
- deterioration in social skills
- abnormal emotional reactions
- hallucinations
- failure to recognise people
- gradual loss of ability to perform all tasks of daily living.

Activity 3.13

Is it dementia or depression?

There are many symptoms common to both dementia and depression that can lead to an incorrect diagnosis in an older person.

Depression is three to four times more common in people with dementia than in older people without dementia, but it can go unrecognised.

1   What symptoms are common for both dementia and depression?
2   What reasons could account for depression being unrecognised in a dementia patient?

Activities appropriate to the person with dementia

The aims of providing activities include increasing the self-esteem of the person with dementia, to maintain their existing skills and to provide fun and pleasure.

Physical mobility can be improved through range of motion exercises with joints, circulation, respiration and body sense being maintained or improved, allowing movement for pleasure. Social skills persist until death but they need to be supported and encouraged. To help a person feel as though they are part of society they need to experience a range of social activities that will help them fit in, while maintaining their own identity and individualism.

Strategies to relieve distress and agitation

Distress and agitation are common behaviours in dementia patients and can be expressed both physically and verbally. Patients with dementia can display agitation if they feel frustrated, frightened or threatened. The acute care environment can be frightening for patients who have difficulty coping with changed situations.

If you are confronted by a distressed or agitated person, remain calm and appease the person if possible. Try to find out what has triggered the distress and acknowledge the trigger.

Additional strategies include:

- Keep distance between yourself and the person and do not crowd them.
- Provide opportunities for the person to talk. This provides an outlet for their feelings.
- Try to listen and empathise with what they have to say. Do not argue.
- Do not turn your back on the person.

- Diversional activities can help to relax the distressed person. For example, change the focus of conversation, offer them a book to read or offer them a cup of tea.
- Do not argue with the person as this can turn to anger. Speak calmly and try to ease the mood.
- Ensure you have clear access to an exit should the situation get out of control.

If you are dealing with a grieving person, acknowledge their grief. It can be unhelpful to give personal examples of similar losses. The person's grief is unique to them, and should not be compared to that of others. Allow the person to grieve in their own way and use active listening. Let the person know that you will listen to them.

Listening, speaking

3.6 Strategies to minimise the impact of challenging behaviours

Challenging behaviours or behaviours of concern are any behaviours which causes stress, worry, and risk of or actual harm to the person, their carers, staff, family members or those around them. The person's background, needs and circumstances should be examined within the environment in which the behaviours of concern are occurring. Strategies and interventions are based on the patient's presentation and exhibition of behaviour. Examples of challenging behaviours include:

- verbal disruption
- physical aggression
- repetitive actions or questions
- resistance to personal care
- sexually inappropriate behaviour
- refusal to accept services
- problems associated with eating
- socially inappropriate behaviour
- wandering or intrusiveness
- sleep disturbance.

TIP 3.9

Considerations for behaviours of concern
Family and carers are a good source of information about the person with behaviours of concern, their history, personality and preferences.

Determining triggers contributing to challenging behaviours

To manage the behaviours of concern, the health-care team needs to examine the underlying causes or triggers (see **Table 3.11**). The triggers can be environmental, psychological or medical and should be noted in the care plan, patient history and progress notes, along with strategies to reduce their impact. Once the trigger is identified, the person can be referred to the appropriate health professional and management of the trigger commenced.

Problem solving

TABLE 3.11 Behaviours of concern – causes

Causes	Description
Environmental	A person may exhibit behaviours of concern when their needs are not met, for example, hunger, thirst, pain, fatigue, temperature, over/under stimulation, social engagement.
	Daily stress increases the susceptibility to environmental stressors such as noise, temperature, light.
Psychological	Pathological changes to the brain in dementia impair normal brain functions and cause behavioural symptoms.
	Confusion, grief, experience of abuse and mental illness can also cause challenging behaviours as the person may have limited ability to express themselves clearly.

>>

Causes	Description
Medical	Impaction (faecal impaction) Medications (sedatives, alcohol, polypharmacy) Systemic (dehydration, hypoglycaemia, vitamin B12 deficiency) Trauma (chronic pain, fractures) Infections (urinary tract infection, pneumonia, septicaemia) Metabolic (hypo/hyperthyroidism) Degenerative (chronic illness)

CASE STUDY 3.4

Managing behaviours of concern

Barbara is a 92-year-old lady with early stage dementia. She was admitted to hospital with dehydration, confusion and agitation. On the night shift she was found in another patient's room and when the nurse tried to take her back to her room she became aggressive and tried to hit the nurse. Barbara said that she was looking for her sister, who had passed away two years ago.

The nurse looked at triggers for her behaviour and noted:
- Barbara was in an unfamiliar environment.
- Barbara had not been sleeping well.
- Barbara was dehydrated.

The nurse used a calm tone when speaking to Barbara, while redirecting her back to bed. She respected her personal space. She made sure that Barbara's fluid intake was appropriate.

Barbara continued to wander, however, she can easily be redirected without expressing agitation.

1   What other strategies could the nurse use to minimise Barbara's behaviour?

Impact of behaviours on person and others

Behaviours of concern can be distressing not only for the person affected but also for the patient's family and friends and the health-care worker. This can be very confronting for families and carers to see the person's behaviour change in a negative way. Care also needs to be given to support the family/carer at this time. A detailed explanation of why the person is exhibiting these behaviours is required and it can be helpful to include the family/carer in the planning of interventions.

Best practice strategies to minimise impact

A number of approaches have been developed based on trust and support necessary to a person's wellbeing when they exhibit challenging behaviours.

All interventions should be based on:
- comprehensive assessment of the challenging behaviours
- strategies which alleviate or address the triggering factors
- evaluating the effectiveness of the strategy
- preventing recurrence of the behaviour.

Communication

It is vital that you convey a message of empathy and reassurance to the person concerned. By using both non-verbal communication and verbal communication, you can allay anxiety to minimise concerning behaviours. Techniques include:
- speaking slowly
- using simple sentences

- establishing eye contact
- getting down to their level
- using a warm tone of voice
- not using 'baby talk'
- paraphrasing what the client has said and asking for clarification if unsure
- not arguing unless it is an issue of safety
- using positive statements
- offering simple choices
- responding more to the emotion expressed rather than the words spoken
- ASKING if they would like to do something
- using appropriate touch
- observing for non-verbal cues.

Validation therapy

Validation therapy is used to make a connection with a person by acknowledging their reality and not forcing them to adopt the present reality. This prevents agitation and stress for the person (Dementia Australia, 2012).

Music therapy

Music used as a sensory and intellectual stimulation can help maintain a person's quality of life or even improve it by shifting mood, managing stress-induced agitation and stimulating positive interactions. It works by allowing the person to relive a past experience.

Reminiscence

This is a way of reviewing past events that have been meaningful for the patient. Looking back on the past may help to highlight lifelong accomplishments and can calm a confused or agitated person.

Reality orientation

Presenting orientating information, such as time, place, and person, gives the confused person information of where they are, what time it is, and who they are dealing with. A person may gain a sense of control and understanding by using this technique.
- Talk about orientation, including the time of day, the date and the season.
- Use the person's name frequently.
- Discuss current events.
- Refer to clocks and calendars.
- Place signs and labels on doors and cupboards.
- Ask questions about photos or other decorations.

Complementary therapies

Pet therapy, art therapy, massage and aromatherapy are used to promote wellbeing for people living with dementia.

Some of the therapies work by stimulating the person either physically or mentally while others, such as massage and aromatherapy, provide relaxation to ease stress on the individual.

TIP 3.10

Validation

Reality orientation can lead to anger, frustration and more confusion for some people with dementia. Use sensitivity and consider the person's emotional situation. It may be best to use validation therapy to acknowledge the person's feelings and their questions or try to engage them in a task.

Speaking, collaboration

CASE STUDY 3.5

Complementary therapies

Mrs Yee, an 85-year-old, could not be encouraged to eat. She had signs of early dementia and was confused. Her family was keen to provide her with food from their own culture but did not want it to interfere with her conventional medicine. A traditional practitioner suggested a combination of herbs, beans and meats that could be made into a soup. The health-care team reassured the family that this would not cause adverse medication effects and Mrs Yee was able to be nutritionally maintained.

The reassurance by both the health-care team and the traditional practitioner was extremely valuable in supporting the health-care needs of Mrs Yee and her family.

1   What other alternative therapies could be useful for patients from a Chinese culture?
2   What is the difference between complementary and alternative therapies?

SUMMARY

- Age-related changes – physical, psychological and social – require specialised health requirements for the older person.
- All members of the health-care team as well as the individual and their family and carers, are involved in the formation of the care plan.
- A non-judgemental attitude and a solid knowledge base for the ageing process are required to ensure appropriate nursing care for the older person.
- Legal and ethical issues are essential aspects of nursing care for the older person.
- A nurse needs to maintain current knowledge of best practice for interventions and strategies when caring for the older people with dementia.
- Challenging behaviours requires the nurse to determine triggers and implement best practice strategies to manage the behaviours to avoid harm to the person and others that are affected by the behaviour.

SELF-TEST QUESTIONS

1   What are the specialised health requirements of an older person?
2   How can the nurse contribute to the care planning for an older person?
3   What nursing practices are appropriate in the aged care environment?
4   How can the nurse address the legal and ethical issues when caring for a person in the aged care environment?
5   What strategies can be used to assist the person with dementia in the aged care environment?
6   What strategies can the nurse use to minimise the impact of challenging behaviours?

BIBLIOGRAPHY

Australian Aged Care Quality Agency (2014) *Quality of Care Principles 2014*. Retrieved from https://www.legislation.gov.au/Details/F2014L00830.

Australian Aged Care Quality Agency (2017). *Standards*. Retrieved from https://www.aacqa.gov.au/providers/accreditation-standards.

Australian Commission on Safety and Quality in Healthcare (ASQHC) (2009). *Preventing falls and harm from falls in older people - best practice guidelines for Australian hospitals*, Commonwealth of Australia.

Australian Government (2017a). *Find the help you need with My Age Care*. Retrieved from http://www.seniors.gov.au/. Accessed 21 October 2017.

Australian Government (2017b). *My Aged Care*. Retrieved from http://www.myagedcare.gov.au/.

Australian Government Department of Health (2017a). *Consultation on the draft National Aged Care Advocacy framework*. Retrieved from https://agedcare.health.gov.au/support-services/national-aged-care-advocacy-framework-consultation.

Australian Government Department of Health (2017b). *Transition care program*. Retrieved from https://agedcare.health.gov.au/programs-services/flexible-care/transition-care-programme.

Australian Institute of Health and Welfare (AIHW) (2013). *Movement between hospital and residential aged care*. Retrieved from http://www.aihw.gov.au/WorkArea/DownloadAsset.aspx?id=60129547766.

Cappo, D. (2002). *Social inclusion initiative. Social inclusion, participation and empowerment*. Address to Australian Council of Social Services National Congress 28–29 November 2002, Hobart.

Carers Australia, http://www.carersaustralia.com.au/. Accessed 21 October 2017.

Department of Health (2011). *Promoting older people's oral health*. Middlesex, UK: RCN Publishing Company.

Dementia Australia (2012). *Therapies and communication approaches*. Retrieved from https://www.dementia.org.au/sites/default/files/helpsheets/Helpsheet-CaringForSomeone02-TherapiesAndCommunicationApproaches_english.pdf

Devon Dementia (2017). *Complementary therapies*. Retrieved from http://www.devondementia.org/the-power-of-complimentary-or-alternative-therapies-in-the-treatment-of-dementia/. Accessed 21 October 2017.

Healthdirect (n.d.). *What causes dementia*? Retrieved from https://www.healthdirect.gov.au/what-causes-dementia.

Helguide.org. *Depression in older adults and the elderly*. Retrieved from http://www.helpguide.org/mental/depression_elderly.htm. Accessed 21 October 2017.

National Prescribing Service, http://www.nps.org.au. Accessed 21 October 2017.

NSW Department of Ageing, Disability and Home Care (DADHC). *Help at home*. Retrieved from http://www.adhc.nsw.gov.au/individuals/help_at_home. Accessed 21 October 2017.

NSW Department of Health, http://www.health.nsw.gov.au. Accessed 21 October 2017.

Nursing and Midwifery Board of Australia (2016). *Enrolled nurse standards for practice*. Retrieved from http://www.nursingmidwiferyboard.gov.au/Codes-Guidelines-Statements/Professional-standards/enrolled-nurse-standards-for-practice.aspx.

Physiopedia, *Theories of aging*. Retrieved from https://www.physio-pedia.com/Theories_of_Aging.

Queensland Government Department of Communities, Child Safety and Disability Services (2012). *Ageing Myth and Reality*. Retrieved from https://www.qld.gov.au/seniors/documents/retirement/ageing-myth-reality.pdf.

Study.com (n.d.). *Theories of Aging: Structural-Functional, Symbolic-Interaction & Social-Conflict*. Retrieved from https://study.com/academy/lesson/theories-of-aging-structural-functional-symbolic-interaction-social-conflict.html.

TAFE NSW (2012). *HLTEN515B Implement and monitor nursing care for clients*. Retrieved from http://www.vetres.net.au/product_files/HLTEN515B_5573_PROMO.pdf.

Victorian Government Department of Health (n.d.). *Older people in hospital*. Retrieved from https://www2.health.vic.gov.au/hospitals-and-health-services/patient-care/older-people. Accessed 13 March 2018.

Victorian Government Department of Human Services (2002). *Oral Health for Older People: A Practical Guide for Aged Care Services*. Retrieved from https://www.dhsv.org.au/__data/assets/pdf_file/0020/3269/oral-health-for-older-people.pdf.

Legal and ethical parameters for nursing practice

LEARNING OUTCOMES

After reading this chapter, you should have an understanding of:

4.1 The enrolled nurse's scope of professional practice

4.2 The legal framework applied to nursing practice

4.3 Ethical concepts underpinning clinical practice

4.4 How the enrolled nurse can support the rights, interests and needs of the patient and their family

4.5 The enrolled nurse's role in open disclosure

Legal and ethical responsibilities as a nurse

On one hand I was excited to undertake my first clinical placement as a student enrolled nurse but on the other I was nervous about meeting all the legal requirements.

I felt that I would not struggle much with the ethical requirements as I was a good person and wanted to do the best for my patients.

We had learnt about all the legislation that we needed to abide by and there seemed to be a lot. I hoped I could remember all the requirements in real practice.

I had been scouring the newspaper and television for current articles and reports on issues affecting nurses and I felt that I was on a roller coaster of emotions. I was shocked at some of the actions of the nurses that were reported because it seemed that they did not care for the person at all, and saddened by the plight of some of the frail, elderly people who had been badly cared for. At times the stories were positive and I felt proud that I was undertaking this work so that I could also contribute and make a difference.

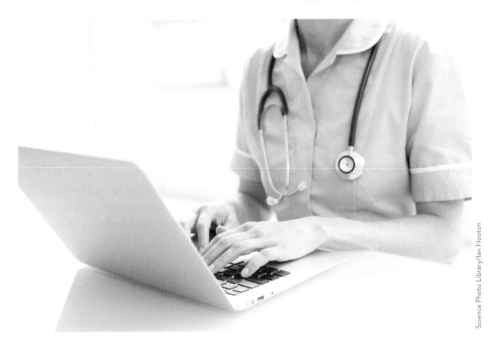

Science Photo Library/Ian Hooton

4.1 The scope of professional nursing practice

Nursing is undertaken in complex environments that combine many elements that must be performed at the same time. Legal and ethical requirements underpin all aspects of contemporary nursing practice.

Acts, guidelines, codes and nursing practice

As student nurses it is important to always use the codes of ethics, codes of conduct and the competency standards to guide your practice. The health-care environment is a dynamic one and there are constantly new procedures and equipment being developed for nurses to use.

Real nursing situations can become 'murky' in regards to right and wrong and the goalposts may change quickly. There is a lot to remember and when you are busy you are often focusing on what has to be achieved rather than thinking about legalities and ethics. This may happen later in the day when you spend time reflecting on the day and writing in your journal. So how do we know what to do and what not to do? The easiest way is to always follow the policies and procedures of the facility as these have been based on legal requirements and ethical principles. Always ask if you are unsure of an intervention or if you do not feel comfortable with an action that is required.

Ethics consist of personal values, attitudes and beliefs that a person holds towards others and actions. **Law** is a rule that exists and is enforced within a society. It is important to know the difference between legal obligations and ethical requirements.

For example, for a patient in pain the most effective pain relief may be an illegal substance, but while using this might be argued as the ethical choice it is not a legal one (Gray et al., 2018, p. 101).

ethics
Branch of philosophy concerned with determining right from wrong on the basis of a body of knowledge rather than on opinions

law
Decisions about conduct that guide the interactions of people. Laws are necessary, binding and enforceable so people can live and work together

Reading

professional misconduct
Poor conduct of a nurse outside their duty as a nurse such as being drunk and disorderly in a public place

unprofessional conduct
Poor conduct while undertaking the duties of a nurse. Not providing the agreed level of care

As nurses we fall under the *Health Practitioner Regulation National Law Act 2009* which defines and describes the scope of nursing practice. This has given the Nurse and Midwifery Board of Australia (NMBA) the right to determine standards and investigate and apply disciplinary action if required. The board has set codes and guidelines that govern nursing practice.

If a complaint against a nurse is made to the board it might find it was **professional misconduct** or **unprofessional conduct**. There are a number of actions that the board can impose on an individual nurse such as:

• a fine
• deregistration, either temporary or permanent
• direction to undertake further training
• limitation on areas of nursing practice
• reprimand or caution.

The reputation of the facility may be compromised if poor nursing standards are in place. The facility may also be fined if legal action is taken by the client, family or carer.

scope of practice
Outlines the procedures, tasks and care permitted under the criteria of the professional licence held by an individual

Explore the theory in *Foundations of Nursing*, Chapter 5: Legal and ethical responsibilities, Page 105

Scope of practice

As a nurse it is important that you undertake work duties within your **scope of practice**. What does this mean for the student nurse?

This means that you must first have the necessary knowledge, have practised the skill and have been supervised. For example, to give medications you must know the medication, the dosage that is usually prescribed, why it is prescribed, the side effects and the nursing actions that are required. If you are unsure you can refer to ANMAC's decision-making framework (http://www.nursingmidwiferyboard.gov.au/Codes-Guidelines-Statements/Frameworks.aspx) or check with the supervisor. Sometimes even though you have completed all the practice and skills there may be a person who is better qualified to complete the task.

Reflective practice 4.2

Determining competence

Thinking about the subjects and skills that you have practised at school, how ready are you to put these into practice?

1   Is the activity within your scope of practice?

2   Does this intervention follow ANMAC's decision-making framework?

3   Do you need to complete any further activity (acquisition of knowledge or skill practice) before undertaking the intervention?

Responding to complaints

Providing care to clients accessing a health-care facility is a complex task. At times it can result in a complaint being made either about the facility, the people who work there or yourself. At times the complaint is not a personal issue but may reflect other issues the client is experiencing, such as a person who is kept waiting while anxious about picking up the children from school.

Complaints are a useful means of improving health care and customer services. The planning of services from management or administration may not reflect the user experience and complaints from customers highlight areas that could be improved.

It is important to remember that clients who make complaints may feel vulnerable and it is important to always maintain a professional attitude when dealing with a person who has made a complaint.

Requests for information

It can sometimes be confusing as to what action to take in regard to providing information. The case file notes, while containing information about the person, belong to the health-care facility. This means that the file cannot leave the health-care premises. At times there will be requests for a person's information. This could come from family members/carers who want to know the person's progress or from another organisation in order to plan further care or investigations. As a nurse, personal and private information must be kept secure and falls under the privacy legislation. At times information does need to be shared with other health-care or allied health services and consent must be obtained from the person for this to occur (Gray et al., 2018, p. 106).

Documentation

Part of maintaining standards and incorporating legal and ethical requirements of nursing practice is to ensure documentation is completed accurately and in a timely manner.

TIP 4.1

Complaints

It is important not to react to the complaint but to listen, reflect, investigate and respond to the complaint. It can be difficult to maintain a professional attitude if your own emotions become involved. In this case your supervisor is the best person to assist you in handling the complaint.

TIP 4.2

Information

Your supervisor is the most appropriate person to refer requests for information. The privacy legislation imposes legal action if personal information is given out inappropriately. The registered nurse will seek the person's consent for sharing their personal information or will liaise with the person requesting the information to inform them that this is not possible if consent is not obtained.

TIP 4.3

Documentation

Always carry a blue, red and black pen as part of your nursing kit. There may be resources on the ward but some documentation is required to be completed at the time the nursing intervention is undertaken. For example, recording of blood glucose measurement. You may find that if you do not document this immediately you may forget or remember the level incorrectly. This will cause the client to have to undergo the procedure again, which will be a waste of time (which is a precious resource), give a poor impression of yourself as a professional and could lead to more serious consequences such as giving the wrong amount of insulin.

Review the skill in Tollefson *Essential Clinical Skills* 7.1 Documentation

Writing

Activity 4.3

Documentation

Read the legal rules for documentation and locate the guide on how the unit requires file notes to be written. Choose one of the clients you are caring for to write a progress note. You might want to write this on a scrap piece of paper first and have it checked by your supervisor.

Monitoring your own compliance

How do we know if we are working within our legal obligations and requirements? An example of this is a patient in palliative care who requires large amounts of morphine to control their pain. You may feel concerned that you are hastening the dying process and hold conflicting emotions about the nursing intervention. Discussion with the supervisor may assist in clarifying the issues with which you are concerned. You do not want the client to feel pain but are unsure that giving the amount of morphine is in the person's best interests.

CASE STUDY 4.1

Acting outside scope of practice

Navpreet was excited to be undertaking his first clinical placement as an enrolled nurse within the aged health-care environment. Navpreet felt very confident as all his theory and practical work had gone well and he felt that he had acquired a comprehensive knowledge and skill base. Navpreet was assigned to a large aged-care facility that provided support to a variety of clients with different needs. The facility had ageing in place and the residents ranged from very frail to only needing assistance with activities of daily living. Navpreet was buddied up with Angela who nine months earlier had completed her training as an enrolled nurse.

On the first day of placement Navpreet went through the handover chart with Angela and noted down the salient points of which residents required full assistance with mobility, any behavioural problems and those who required diabetic testing. Navpreet found that he worked well with the residents and Angela complimented him on his ability to engage the residents in conversation while providing personal care. After a couple of days Navpreet felt very comfortable with the routine and felt that he managed the workload well, better in fact than Angela who he felt was very slow when using the hoist machine and mobilising clients.

Navpreet asked Angela if he could be allowed to provide total support to two of the residents as he thought that this would improve his time management skills. Angela agreed to his suggestion and checked at morning tea and at lunch how Navpreet was managing. Navpreet

felt that everything was going well and he had managed to complete all of the nursing care that was documented on the care plan for his two clients. After lunch Napreet was filling in the fluid balance chart when the local GP entered the room. Navpreet went to get Angela but the resident Mr Davis asked Navpreet to stay. The GP examined Mr Davis and after consulting with him told Navpreet that he would order stronger pain medication as Mr Davis had chest pain due to cardiac problems. Mrs Davis entered the room as she always visited her husband at lunchtime and wanted to know what the doctor had said. Mr Davis told his wife that 'he was as fit as a fiddle'. Navpreet interrupted and told Mrs Davis what the doctor had told him.

Mr Davis asked Navpreet if he could have some pain killers as he felt uncomfortable and he had not had any pain medication since breakfast time. Mrs Davis was quite anxious and told Navpreet that nobody helps her husband as they would have noticed that he was in pain and would have done something about it sooner. Navpreet told Mr Davis that he would go and inform Angela that Mr Davis required some pain relief. Navpreet found Angela with Mrs Reynolds, a very frail resident who required full nursing care with all her ADLs including feeding. Navpreet passed on Mr Davis' request and told Angela what the doctor had told him about increasing the pain relief for Mr Davis. Angela, who had been giving Mrs Reynolds her midday lunch and tablets, agreed but was unable to do so immediately. Angela told Navpreet to take over the feeding for Mrs Reynolds while she went to obtain the medication from the drug trolley. When Angela

>>

came back she noticed that Mrs Reynolds was coughing and put the medication on the overbed table while she assisted Navpreet to reposition Mrs Reynolds. Angela told Navpreet to take the tablets to Mr Davis while she completed the feed for Mrs Reynolds. Navpreet was keen to get Mr Davis his pain medication as he did not want Mrs Davis to think he did not care.

Navpreet gave the medication to Mr Davis and completed the remainder of the lunchtime duties, removing trays and filling in food and fluid charts. Navpreet noticed that Mr Davis appeared pale, sweaty and when talking was slurring his words. Navpreet sponged Mr Davis and settled him for a sleep. Navpreet told Angela that he had given the medication.

Later as Angela and Navpreet were doing their round assisting residents to position themselves for afternoon tea they found they could hardly rouse Mr Davis. Angela went to get the registered nurse who came and took a set of observations. The nurse noticed the sweating and also took a BGL which was 2.7mmol. The nurse asked about the medication that Mr Davis had been given as he was not a diabetic and had never previously displayed the symptoms of hypoglycaemia before. Angela admitted that she had given Navpreet the medication to give Mr Davis while in Mrs Reynold's room. Mrs Reynolds was a non-insulin-dependent diabetes mellitus (NIDDM) patient who was on oral hypoglycaemic medication. The nurse rang for the ambulance and gave some oral glucose. The nurse told Navpreet and Angela to write up an incident report regarding the wrong administration of medication.

1. What legal and regulatory requirements govern Navpreet's practice as a student nurse?
2. What actions did Navpreet do that are non-compliant with current legislation?
3. Identify the codes of ethics, conduct and competency standards that were involved in this incident.
4. Explain how Napreet functioned outside the scope of enrolled nurse practice.
5. How should Navpreet handle the complaint the resident's wife has made about the nursing staff?
6. Should Navpreet give the patient's wife the information about the pain medication?
7. What documentation needs to be completed for the two patients that Navpreet was caring for?
8. What legal obligations and requirements should Navpreet have followed during his clinical placement?

4.2 Applying knowledge of the legal framework to nursing practice

As nurses we not only come under the nursing board but we are also held to account to the laws and penalties that operate within our state or territory and country.

See more detail on the different aspects of the law as relevant to you in Clarke et al. (2016), *Foundations of Nursing: Enrolled Division 2 Nurses*, Chapter 4.

Negligence, duty of care and vicarious liability

The most common areas that nurses may be held liable in a court of law are **negligence**, **duty of care** and **vicarious liability**. To be found negligent it must be proved that the person was owed a duty of care and that you did not fulfil this duty of care, either through an act or omission and as a result the person suffered either physical, mental or financial harm. If a nurse is found to be deliberately reckless the nurse may be found to be criminally negligent.

negligence
A general term referring to careless acts on the part of an individual who is not exercising reasonable prudent judgement

duty of care
An obligation both moral and legal to ensure the safety of others

vicarious liability
Where another person or the facility is held responsible for the actions of employees

Activity 4.4

Indemnity insurance

When working as a nurse you may be involved in an incident with legal consequences. What types of insurance are available for legal costs and how do you access them?

Consent

When we want to undertake a nursing intervention with a client it is necessary to obtain their **informed consent**. This is an integral part of the nursing process. Consent may be verbal, with the client saying 'yes go ahead', written if the client is having an invasive procedure such as surgery (this is then the doctor's responsibility to obtain) or implied consent where the person does an action that makes clear their agreement. An example of implied consent is where you need to administer an intramuscular injection into the upper arm and the client rolls up their sleeve and holds their arm for you.

There are three elements to a valid consent:

- It must be given voluntarily.
- The person giving consent must have the capacity and competence to understand what they are agreeing to.
- Enough information must be given to make a decision (Gray et al., 2018, p. 108).

CASE STUDY 4.2

Duty of care

Jonti was completing her first clinical placement in the aged-care facility attached to the local hospital. As well as the permanent residents there were also some residents who required ongoing support following their hospitalisation, and undertook physiotherapy while waiting for a place in the rehabilitation ward. Jonti was assigned with her buddy to care for six residents, one of whom was rehabilitating after having a hip replacement procedure. Jonti was confident at the end of the first week with personal hygiene needs and wound care and asked her clinical supervisor to assess her competence. The supervisor found that Jonti was proficient and complimented her on her ability to complete the tasks in a professional manner.

Jonti was not so happy the second week as she was assigned to Errol, who was to be her buddy for that week. Errol felt that he should do all the more technical tasks as he was qualified and Jonti was just a student. Jonti felt Errol was demeaning her and complained to the clinical supervisor, Rita, who spoke with Errol and he agreed to allow Jonti more scope to practise her skills.

The next morning Errol assigned Mr Hedgman to Jonti. Mr Hedgman was a 74-year-old who had been admitted for respite care following a total hip replacement and was also suffering from unstable diabetes. Jonti found Mr Hedgman had been incontinent of urine and was sweating profusely. Jonti decided to shower him before breakfast. Mr Hedgeman was reluctant and did not want to have a shower. Jonti ignored his protests and assisted him out of bed into the shower. Jonti noted that Mr Hedgman was unsteady on his feet and required assistance of one staff member and a four-wheelie frame to ambulate. In the shower, Mr Hedgman bumped the towels onto the wet floor. Jonti did not want to call Errol and told Mr Hedgman to sit still and she would pop out and get another towel. On returning to the shower Jonti found Mr Hedgman on the floor. The leg that had been operated on was shortened and rotated. Jonti called for assistance.

1. Has Jonti broken any laws or principles of nursing practice in this scenario? Why/why not?
2. What penalties might apply to Jonti as a result of her actions?
3. Has Jonti been negligent in her nursing care of this person? Discuss applying the concepts of duty of care and vicarious liability.
4. Why is it important to gain consent before undertaking nursing interventions?

Restraint

At times restraint is necessary to protect the person or others from harm or to promote a positive health outcome, for example:

- physical – application of straps, sheets or other devices used to restrict movement
- chemical – medication used to control behaviour
- aversive treatment – withholding of basic human rights or needs
- environmental – isolating a client.

In order to protect the person from harm while using restraints, there are a number of actions that need to be put into place. These are:

- introduction of self and explanation for restraints
- consultation with the family and doctor. The family does not have the legal power to consent to restraint as it is a clinical decision made by the health-care team (Australian Government Department of Health and Ageing, 2012)
- applying the restraints in a safe manner to avoid injury or harm to the person
- frequently checking the person when a restraining device has been applied
- reviewing the need for the restraints at frequent intervals
- removal of restraints when the need for such measures is no longer required.

Common legal terms

As well as using the correct medical terminology it is important to use the correct common legal terms associated with nursing practice when recording a refusal of treatment or a consent for an intervention. Documenting clearly and objectively is required. Client files are a legal document and the rules for documentation are clearly outlined in Clarke et al. (2016), *Foundations of Nursing: Enrolled Division 2 Nurses*, Chapter 4. All variations to the care plan are documented in the file note, 'If it is not documented it did not happen'. Most clinical areas will have examples of how to complete the documentation for clients (see Clarke et al., Chapter 9).

Writing reports

Case files are a legal document and there are strict rules that apply to nursing documentation. Consideration must be given to the following:

- date and time
- timing – frequency of reporting may be adjusted in line with client's condition
- all entries must be legible
- entries must be recorded in ink for permanency
- use of commonly accepted abbreviations
- correct spelling
- signature – includes name and title
- accuracy
- document in time line order
- only record information related to the health of the client
- the entries need to be complete and reflect the nursing process; this will also include care that is omitted
- the entry needs to be brief.

In some clinical areas report writing will follow the care plan documentation, or a brief summary of the person's progress is written that summarises the pathway that is used as the care plan tool.

Mandatory reporting processes

There is a legal obligation for nurses to report to the AHPRA if they believe a registered staff member is likely to cause harm to a member of the public. You should notify your supervisor if you are unsure about any incident or action in the workplace. A student may be reported if a staff member feels that the student has an impairment or condition that puts the public at risk of harm. Read the fact sheets from the NMBA on mandatory reporting for further information and decision flow charts at http://www.nursingmidwiferyboard.gov.au/Codes-Guidelines-Statements/Codes-Guidelines/Guidelines-for-mandatory-notifications.aspx.

TIP 4.4

Restraint

If you feel uncomfortable caring for a client who requires restraint you should ask your clinical supervisor to review the decision, the means of restraint and the policy and procedures for restraint. It is always helpful to discuss emotions and those of the client to avoid build-up of stress.

Privacy and confidentiality

privacy
The right to be left alone, to choose care based on personal beliefs, to govern body integrity, and to choose when and how sensitive information is shared

As a nursing student you have access to a person's private and confidential information. You have an obligation to protect that information and not disclose it unless the client has given consent to do so. To protect your patient's **privacy**:

- Access client files in an appropriate environment, usually at the nurses' station.
- Keep all other information, such as handover sheets, in the nursing area and do not remove them from there.
- Be mindful where you verbally discuss a client, to ensure that other people do not overhear personal details.
- Knock on doors before entering a room.
- In shared rooms, keep privacy curtains pulled around the bed area if the person is disrobing.

Where a client needs to disrobe for an examination, use blankets or towels to keep the client covered, exposing only the part of the body that needs to be examined. Another area to be mindful of is social media; once information is on the web it is there forever. Students are often inclined to want to take photographs of themselves or the people they are caring for. This is against privacy and confidentiality rules and a breach of legal and ethical boundaries. Taking photographs of documentation is also not permitted as these are legal documents and include sensitive data.

Interpret referrals or requests for tests on receipt

TIP 4.5

Debriefing

At times during clinical placement you may want to ask questions about a person's condition or discuss what has happened during your time in the clinical area. These discussions should be undertaken during debrief in a private area. Support from colleagues can assist and alleviate stress or confusion and your supervisor can give you additional support during this process.

During your placement in different clinical areas you will be required to organise tests for clients. These investigations can range from blood tests to invasive procedures in an effort to diagnose the health status of the person. It is important that the client is correctly prepared for any test that is ordered, for example, the client may need to give consent, be fasted or have transport organised.

When test results come back they need to be correctly interpreted and communicated to the appropriate member of the health-care team. All blood test results are transmitted back via computer or hard copy. The result's sheet will include a normal reference range to check the person's result against. All test results that are abnormal are also marked with an asterisk to alert staff to the abnormal reading and this will have an impact on treatment.

Even if the results are normal the doctor may need to be notified as this can have a direct impact on treatment. For example, the discontinuation of a medication, such as antibiotics, if test results are normal.

4.3 Ethics

bioethics
The application of general ethical principles to health care

Ethics refers to the branch of philosophy concerned with determining right from wrong on the basis of a body of knowledge.

Bioethics is ethics that are involved in health care or human life. The guiding principles of bioethics are:

- autonomy – to be self-determining
- non-maleficence – to do no harm
- beneficence – to do good
- justice – fairness
- fidelity – to be faithful to agreements
- veracity – to tell the truth.

At your placement you will need to demonstrate familiarity with the code of ethics for nurses in Australia. Go to http://www.nursingmidwiferyboard.gov.au/Codes-Guidelines-Statements/Professional-standards.aspx.

Review the skill in Tollefson *Essential Clinical Skills* 7.3 Clinical handover – change of shift

Demonstrating ethical practice

Every interaction you make with a person, family or colleague involves the use of ethical behaviour. Even interactions that you do not make may be an example of ethical behaviour. An example of this is referring nursing interventions to the most appropriate staff member.

Reflective practice 4.3

Ethical practice

Choose an interaction with a client that involved an emotional response from yourself.

1   Did the emotion colour the interaction?

2   Did the emotional response undermine your actions and ethics?

3   Does the policy and procedure follow the principles outlined for bioethics? Why? Why not?

Contemporary ethical issues

As a nurse you need to be aware of issues and potential conflicts of interest that may impact upon nursing practice. Cultural demographics are constantly changing in Australia and it is important that nursing practice supports the culture of the area in which it is based. Information regarding changes may be accessed through a variety of mediums, for example:

* newspapers and media
* Internet
* nurses' journals and communiqués
* research articles
* policies and procedures
* memos
* complaints
* incident reports.

FS

Reading, computer skills

Reporting potential ethical issues

With so many practices changing in health care it can be difficult to stay on top of new developments in managing the care of individuals. In some areas of nursing new approaches to caring for palliative patients can make you feel sad or uncomfortable. Researching areas that make you feel uncomfortable may give you additional knowledge that can assist in aligning new practice with nursing ethics.

At times there will be instances where ethical issues arise and it is important that these are fully documented and reported in line with the organisation's policies and procedures. This will alert staff to issues and it may need additional resources or interventions to manage the situation.

TIP 4.6

Talking about ethical issues

If you feel uncomfortable about any interventions it is important to raise it with your clinical supervisor. They may assist you to identify underlying ethical issues and help you manage your emotional response. Sometimes talking with someone else can assist in helping you manage difficult situations.

Resolving ethical issues

How do you resolve ethical issues that arise during clinical practice? Firstly, discuss the issue with your supervisor. Perhaps it is not an ethical issue but more an instance where further explanation or knowledge is required.

Secondly, refer to the policies and procedures of the organisation to ensure that nursing actions being undertaken are appropriate. Always follow the decision-making guidelines and codes of ethics for nursing for ensuring nursing interventions meet professional standards. Access the professional standards at http://www.nursingmidwiferyboard.gov.au/Codes-Guidelines-Statements/Professional-standards.aspx.

CASE STUDY 4.3

Ethical dilemmas

Mark, an 18-year old enrolled nursing student, was assigned to the Baringa unit providing care for residents who had brain injuries as a result of motor vehicle accidents that also resulted in both physical and mental health issues that could not be supported in the community. The residents in these units would stay till their condition stabilised and they could be transferred to an aged-care facility close to where their family lived. Mark had had no previous experience with clients with mental health issues other than what he had learnt in school.

At first Mark was overwhelmed with sadness when he saw the young men trying to regain their lives. Mark required a lot of support from his clinical facilitator to manage his emotional response to these clients. Eventually Mark felt more comfortable and looked forward to his days in the unit.

Mark had struck up a friendship with John, who was only a couple of years younger, and like him was a passionate Aussie Rules follower. Mark and John often spent time watching replays of recent matches and listening to talkback shows discussing a footballer's performance and umpiring decisions.

During Mark's second week he had accepted John's invitation to watch a football match on Friday. During the match Mark noticed that John appeared excited and agitated. Mark discovered that John had taken illegal substances and this had resulted in an euphoric mood. John asked Mark not to report it as he told Mark it made him feel better and he had not taken much, just enough to function properly.

1 What should Mark do in this situation?
2 What ethical issues are involved?
3 Who should be notified?

4.4 Supporting the rights, interests and needs of patients and their families

Providing care for the person also involves supporting carers, relatives or other people who provide support. Include carers and relatives of the person in the care planning process to ensure that their rights and needs are also addressed.

Duty of care

Duty of care is a legal term that underpins standards of care. You must only provide care for a person when the intervention is one that you have the required knowledge and skills to undertake. At times it may be in the person's interests that another member of the health-care team undertakes the required intervention. An example of this is the care for a specialised dressing technique. Even though you have completed the wound care module, you may not have the knowledge and skills for this specialised care intervention.

Supporting the person's rights, interests and encouraging decisions

At times the person you are caring for may choose not to accept the planned care or may want to try an alternative treatment. It is important to support the person through active listening, explanation of care and discussion. The enrolled nurse needs to document the client's preferences or decisions and report these to the supervisor or appropriate member of the health-care team.

However, it is important that the client is able to make informed decisions about their care. The enrolled nurse is able to contribute to this process through discussion and explanation of care activities. Information needs to include the positive and negative aspects of the intervention in order for the person to make an informed choice. For example, if a

Review the skill in Tollefson *Essential Clinical Skills* 7.3 Clinical handover - change of shift 7.1 Documentation

person refuses to have a particular medication, you provide information and education on why the medication has been ordered but ultimately the person needs to consent to have the medication. If they choose not to consent, you would document your actions on a drug chart, note the decisions made in the client file, and verbally report the actions and decisions to the supervisor and the doctor.

Activity 4.5

Care planning

Choose one of the clients you are caring for. Locate their case file and care plan.

1   How has the client been involved in the care planning process?

Advocating for the person

You can demonstrate respect and support the dignity of the client and family by ensuring that you practise in an inclusive manner, for example, by encouraging the person or their family to ask questions and give consent for all interactions and incorporating their wishes into the care plan.

For the enrolled nurse **advocating** for the person involves reporting and documenting the person's wishes clearly according to organisational policies and procedures. It may also involve suggesting referrals to other agencies or health-care professionals that can assist the person to achieve their goals.

advocating
To publicly safeguard a person's decisions, wishes and preferences; to ensure the person is treated with respect and that they have the necessary information and support to make an informed choice

CASE STUDY 4.4

Advocating for clients

Amandeep was undertaking her palliative care placement in the aged-care facility that offered this support to residents. Amandeep was assigned to Julie, an experienced enrolled nurse who told Amandeep that she was passionate about caring and providing support to residents who were dying. One of the residents Amandeep was caring for was Mrs Hedley who was 84 years old and was admitted to the facility following a right cerebrovascular accident (CVA). Mrs Hedley had been found by her carer after spending the night on the floor.

On admission to the facility after transfer from the local hospital Mrs Hedley was noted to have a large amount of skin tissue breakdown necessitating the need for very particular pressure area care. Mrs Hedley was also unable to speak and had refused to have a PEG tube inserted for nutrition when it was found that she was unable to swallow food safely. The doctors had documented that Mrs Hedley's condition was unlikely to improve. An advanced care directive had not been made

by Mrs Hedley before having the stroke and her daughter who had medical and legal power of attorney had agreed for her mother to enter the facility and be supported with palliative care. Mrs Hedley's daughter told Amandeep that her mother had dreaded this situation and had told her that is she was incapacitated and was unable to recover to previous health status she did not wish to have medical intervention to prolong her life and that she definitely did not want to have a PEG tube inserted for feeding. Mrs Hedley also had a son who was very upset about the imminent death of his mother and the decision not to use a PEG tube, and told his sister that she was killing their mother by refusing to feed her.

1   What is Amandeep's duty of care for Mrs Hedley?
2   What should Amandeep do with the information that Mrs Hedley's daughter had supplied?
3   What should Amandeep do to advocate for Mrs Hedley?
4   What ethical and legal issues might arise in this situation?

4.5 Open disclosure processes

open disclosure
The acknowledgement that harm has occurred to a client while being cared for in a health-care facility

The **open disclosure** process is undertaken when an adverse event occurs to a person in the health-care facility. The staff member involved, the supervisor and/or the doctor speaks with the person and their family. The person is able to verbalise what happened and the result of the action. The staff are able to apologise and explain how the event occurred and the steps that have been taken to address the situation.

For more details on open disclosure visit https://www.safetyandquality.gov.au/opendisclosure.

As an enrolled nurse it is important to be honest about incidents that occur while looking after a person. If something goes wrong, verbally reporting it to the supervisor and fully documenting the incident following the organisation's policies and procedures will assist in determining if any further intervention is required. It is important to be guided by the supervisor of the area as to appropriate actions to take if an incident occurs.

Activity 4.6

Open disclosure in practice

Access the incident reports for the unit you are working on.
1　Is there an incident where the process of open disclosure was used?
2　Describe who was involved in this process.
3　What was the outcome of the incident?

Other health-care workers in relation to open disclosure

When something goes wrong for a person in a health-care facility there are a number of people who must be made aware. An incident report is filled in and this may go through different managers and also through to administration.

If harm has occurred to a person accessing the service, usually a meeting is held to analyse the incident and to decide on who is best placed to speak to the person. This could be the nurse, doctor, allied health member or a member of the administrative staff. Sometimes it is better that the person who was involved in the incident not be present as they may be experiencing a range of emotions. In open disclosure it is important to say sorry and show empathy for the person but not discuss who was right or wrong; this is a legal aspect that is not part of the process.

CASE STUDY 4.5

When things go wrong

Amanda was completing her aged-care placement and one of the key objectives was to administer oral medications. Amanda had successfully passed all the theory and practical skills at school and had been supervised by the clinical teacher on two occasions and was deemed to be competent.

Amanda had formed a strong friendship with one of the graduate nurses on the unit and arranged to work with her on the second week, despite the clinical supervisor telling her that it was not an appropriate arrangement

as the nurse was still very junior. Amanda decided not to follow this instruction. Amanda had been buddied with another more experienced nurse but told her that she would help out in a different section after completing the personal care requirements for the residents in their area. Her buddy was not convinced that this was appropriate and wanted to consult with the clinical facilitator. The buddy put in a call to the facilitator but she did not leave a message and could not reach the facilitator as she was busy supervising another student and resolved to call back after morning tea.

>>

At the midday medication round Amanda asked her friend if she could administer the oral medications with her supervision. Amanda and her friend were of a similar age and shared many interests and chatted about them while administering the medications. One of the residents they were caring for, Mrs Ethol, was scheduled for a procedure mid-afternoon, as she had ongoing pain following a laminectomy performed earlier that year. Mrs Ethol was being transferred to the local acute hospital for the procedure and would require a full anaesthetic and overnight stay. This had been arranged last week. Amanda and her friend were asked for some pain relief by Mrs Ethol and noted that there was an order for IM pethidine 50mg on the once only section of the medication chart. They prepared the medication and both checked the order and signed the DD register.

Later in the shift at the DD count it was noted that an error had been made and an ampule of 100mg of Pethidine was missing while the 50mg amps counted over by one ampule. Both Amanda and her buddy were questioned about the medication that was given to Mrs Ethol. It also was communicated to the registered nurse in charge of the facility that Mrs Ethol was returning to the facility as the operation had been cancelled due to the consent form not being able to be signed.

1   What legal and ethical issues are present in this scenario?
2   What consequences could Amanda and her buddy be subjected to as a result?
3   What documentation would need to be completed?
4   Who would be involved in the open disclosure process with Mrs Ethol?
5   Why should open disclosure be undertaken?

SUMMARY

- To act professionally, the nurse must be aware of legislation and guidelines that underpin nursing practice in the Australian health-care environment.
- The professional actions of a nurse involve obtaining informed consent before undertaking any interventions with clients.
- Legal and ethical requirements need to be considered when undertaking nursing actions that impose restrictions on clients or lead to injury of a client.
- Client information is protected by the *Privacy Act 1988*, which is a component of professional nursing practice.
- Ethical issues can arise in nursing practice and strategies need to be in place to resolve the issues and implement ethical nursing practice.
- One of the roles and responsibilities a nurse has is to be an advocate for a client and their family, and support their rights, interests and needs.
- If harm occurs to a client while undergoing treatment or intervention, open disclosure practices are put in place.

SELF-TEST QUESTIONS

1   What actions do you need to implement to perform nursing interventions that ensure you act within your scope of practice?
2   Can you identify the nursing actions required when undertaking nursing actions that are underpinned by legislation?
3   How can you ensure that your nursing practice is based on ethical concepts?
4   How can you support the rights, interests and needs of the person and their family?
5   What is involved in the process of open disclosure?

BIBLIOGRAPHY

Australian Government Department of Health and Ageing (2012). *Decision-making tool: Supporting a restraint free environment in residential aged care*. Retrieved from https://agedcare.health.gov.au/sites/g/files/net1426/f/documents/09_2014/residential_aged_care_internals_fa3-web.pdf.

Clarke, L., Gray, S., White, L., Duncan, G. & Baumle, W. (2016). *Foundations of Nursing: Enrolled Division 2 Nurses* (ANZ edition). Cengage Learning: South Melbourne.

Gray, S., Ferris, L., White, L., Duncan, G. & Baumle, W. (2018). *Fundamentals of Nursing* (2nd edition). Cengage Learning: South Melbourne.

Tollefson, J., Watson, G., Jelly, E. & Tambree, K. (2016). *Essential Clinical Skills: Enrolled Division 2 Nurses* (3rd edition). Cengage Learning: South Melbourne.

Clinical assessment and planning nursing care

LEARNING OUTCOMES

After reading this chapter, you should have an understanding of:

5.1   Collecting and interpreting health data

5.2   Admission and discharge procedures

5.3   Planning the nursing care of a person

5.4   Ongoing development of individual nursing care plans

Looking the part

I was so excited the day the class was given the equipment for undertaking client assessment.
I felt that with the stethoscope I was really a nurse. I soon learnt that it was one thing to look like the nurses on television with the stethoscope draped around my neck and another to competently use the stethoscope to obtain an accurate blood pressure measurement. I felt that I was all fingers and thumbs and wished I had another set of hands to perform this task.

5.1 Collecting and interpreting health data

It is important to undertake assessment in a professional manner. Not only do you need to perform physical assessment tasks but you must also establish a **therapeutic relationship** with the client to facilitate open communication.

Introduction and explanations

In Australia it is customary to introduce yourself, establish eye contact and smile. Before touching the person it is necessary to explain the actions you are going to do and obtain the person's consent.

Australia is a multicultural society and cultural safety and respect is important to nursing care. For example, where a person speaks a language other than English, use written material in that language or engage interpreters to assist in communication.

Gathering information

Communication and interview skills are important in gathering information. The family and carer are important to include in this process, but ensure that confidentiality is maintained. When interviewing individuals it is important to note cultural issues or communication difficulties that may require additional strategies to elicit the required information.

Asking the person open questions is a good way to get the most information about their care needs. The organisation will have pre-printed documentation to use to prompt you in this area.

The therapeutic communication between you and the person can be impacted by a variety of factors, for example, a person experiencing pain may need special assistance to fully participate in this process (Gray et al., 2018, p. 731).

What to include in the primary health assessment

During the interview there will be a large volume of information that is shared by the client. It is important to accurately document the information during the interview. The interview is **holistic** in nature and includes cultural, religious and spiritual aspects as well as physical data.

You will conduct physical assessments such as analysis of urine and blood, and also gather **subjective** and **objective data** about the person.

---

therapeutic relationship
A relationship that encourages the patient to express their feelings, facilitates trust and reduces the anxiety that he or she may be experiencing

Oral communication

holistic
Encompassing all aspects of a person, including physical and mental health and wellbeing, spiritual, religious and environmental considerations

subjective data
Include the person's sensations, feelings, values, beliefs, attitudes and perception of personal health status and life situation

objective data
Data that can be seen and measured, and are obtained through both standard assessment techniques performed during the physical examination and laboratory and diagnostic tests

---

CASE STUDY 5.1

Subjective and objective data

Susan was a 20-year-old university student who had been admitted with lower abdominal pain for investigation. Maree, the nurse, noted during the admission that Susan appeared pale and her fingernails were also pale. Maree also noted that Susan held onto her stomach and had facial grimacing. Susan told Maree that she had just had her period a week ago and that this was normal.

Susan also stated that she felt 'very stressed with examinations at university'. Maree asked Susan how long she had endured the pain and on a scale of 1–10 to rate its severity. Susan told Maree that she had experienced this pain on and off for the last eight weeks and the pain was around eight out of 10. Susan also told Maree that the pain was occurring with more frequency over the last two weeks and at times she was unable to get out of bed.

>>

Maree then asked if anything had occurred and Susan told her that she had had an episode of gastroenteritis after eating a chicken burger at the food court at her local shopping centre. Susan told Maree that since that time she had noticed that her bowel motions were sticky and black in colour. Maree asked Susan to call the next time she needed to open her bowels so that she could obtain a sample from her. Maree then took Susan's vital signs and recorded them.

1   What subjective observations did Maree make in the admission process?
2   What objective observations did Maree make in the admission process?

Review the skill in Tollefson *Essential Clinical Skills* 2 Assessment

temperature
Measurement of internal body warmth

pulse
The number of times the heart beats per minute

respiration
Breathing air both in and out of the airways

TIP 5.1

Preparing for admissions
Ensure before undertaking initial assessment that you have gathered all equipment and paperwork to facilitate a smooth and professional interview.

Vital signs

Physical assessment is undertaken when the therapeutic relationship is established. **Temperature**, **pulse**, **respiration**, **blood pressure**, **oxygen saturation** and **blood glucose level** are routinely taken on admission. The nurse will prepare the client for other assessments such as **urinalysis**, **electrocardiogram (ECG)** and **blood tests** that may be ordered by the doctor. Depending on the health problems that the client is admitted or being treated for, specialist assessments may be necessary. These may include neurological assessment, neurovascular assessment and pain assessment process (Gray et al., 2018, p. 739).

Activity 5.1

Assessments on admission

Choose one of the clients that you are caring for and review the assessments that were taken on admission.
1   Identify if any assessment was outside the normal parameters.
2   How does this assessment reflect the medical diagnosis?
3   Were other assessments ordered by the doctor as a result?
4   Did the nursing diagnosis and plan of care address actual and potential problems the person may have?

blood pressure
A measure of the pressure exerted by the blood on the wall of the artery

oxygen saturation
The percentage of haemoglobin binding sites in the bloodstream occupied by oxygen or the amount of oxygen that has combined with the haemoglobin in the red blood cell and is circulating in the blood

Developmental stages

The **developmental** state of the client will affect the assessment and care provided. The normal range of physical assessment data levels that is collected varies according to the developmental stage. The person's developmental stage will also affect their ability to give the required information (as in the case of children). At placement you will need to show that you can adapt to the needs of the person.

A person's **physical development** occurs in tandem with their **cognitive development** and **psychosocial development**. The way you provide education and nursing care provided will depend on the client's level of development. An example of this is educating a child as opposed to a middle-aged adult. For children, play assists them to make sense of the word while an adult may prefer to read information process (Gray et al., 2018, p. 738).

Activity 5.2

Learning through play

1   How would you educate a child of eight years regarding insulin injections?

2   How would you educate a teenager on the dangers of alcohol and drugs?

3   What education on smoking would be appropriate for a 26-year-old?

Reflective practice 5.1

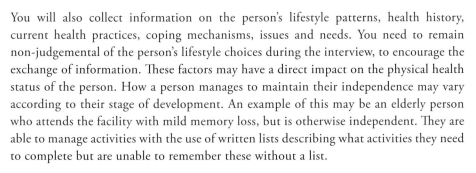

Admission process for clients

Principles such as confidentiality, privacy and ethical conduct are important to construct the therapeutic relationship. The nurse needs to balance these with legal constraints. Refer to the following examples. When are these concepts not required to be adhered to?

1   An elderly man with visual and hearing difficulties

2   A 16-year-old girl presenting for contraceptive measures

3   An eight-year-old boy with a fractured arm.

Other data to collect

Learning

You will also collect information on the person's lifestyle patterns, health history, current health practices, coping mechanisms, issues and needs. You need to remain non-judgemental of the person's lifestyle choices during the interview, to encourage the exchange of information. These factors may have a direct impact on the physical health status of the person. How a person manages to maintain their independence may vary according to their stage of development. An example of this may be an elderly person who attends the facility with mild memory loss, but is otherwise independent. They are able to manage activities with the use of written lists describing what activities they need to complete but are unable to remember these without a list.

blood glucose level
A measurement of the amount of glucose (the principal blood sugar) circulating in the blood

urinalysis
Analysis of the urine using an indicator strip

Reflective practice 5.2

Questioning techniques

A 76- year-old Japanese woman has been admitted to the aged care facility. The client does not speak fluent English.

1   Why is it important to use open questions?

2   What type of information will you obtain?

3   What actions do you need to employ to gain the information?

electrocardiogram (ECG)
Graphical recording of the heart's electrical activity

blood tests
A scientific examination of a blood sample for the diagnosis of illness or detection and measurement of other substances or cells

See next page, Definitions *Continued*

>>

Reflective practice 5.3

Other issues

Describe what activities the elderly person needs to complete to independently use a dossette box for medication administration.

1   What nursing interventions might be considered for this person?

CASE STUDY 5.2

The impact of lifestyle choices

Jane was reading through the information in the case file of the new patient, Mr Richards, an elderly man who had been admitted with exacerbation of chronic obstructive pulmonary disease. Mr Richards had been admitted numerous times over the last three years and there had been notations about his difficult manner when counselled about the need to stop smoking.

Jane noted that Mr Richards had been a heavy smoker in the past but had stopped smoking for the last three months.

1   Should Jane inform Mr Richards that his condition was most likely brought on by his lifestyle choice of smoking?

2   Is it appropriate to make judgements about his manner? What effect could this have on the interaction between the nurse and patient?

development
The growth of the individual from simple to complex functions and skill strengths to enable survival

See next spread, Definitions *Continued*

Families and carers

The needs, both emotional and physical, of the family and carer are important to note and document. The nurse needs to obtain permission before undertaking any conversation with the family or carer. Separate interviews may be needed, if there appears to be conflict between the person and the carer.

For families it can be an emotional time. The role the person held in the family may have altered leading to a change in family dynamics and lifestyle changes.

CASE STUDY 5.3

Needs of others

Mrs George, a 74-year-old Greek woman (78 kgs), was admitted with advanced cancer of the breast. Mrs George had undergone a *bilateral radical mastectomy* five years previously and completed a course of *chemotherapy*. Over the last four months Mrs George had felt extremely tired and lost more than 10% of her body weight. Her family had noted that Mrs George at times did not appear to know what was happening. On assessment it was found that the cancer had returned and spread to the lungs, bone and brain. Mrs George was now being treated with a *palliative* approach.

The health-care team had wanted to arrange *hospice* accommodation for Mrs George but her family was against this and requested to care for her at home. Mr George stated that his daughter would be able to provide

this care. Mrs George had always stayed at home and prepared the meals and took care of the family. The daughter had three children still at home and worked part time. The daughter expressed a fear of not being able to care appropriately for her mother, especially in the areas that required her to move her mother, as her father suffered from severe *osteoarthritis* and her two brothers worked in the family business full-time.

1   Define *bilateral radical mastectomy*, *chemotherapy*, *palliative*, *hospice* and *osteoarthritis* and describe the pathophysiology of each disease state that is italicised above.

2   What issues and needs does this family have in relation to Mrs George's illness?

3   What emotions might the father and daughter have in this scenario?

Critical thinking

Writing, problem solving

Review the skill in Tollefson *Essential Clinical Skills* 7.1 Documentation

Analysis of the data is undertaken to determine if the results fall within the normal levels, or if intervention is needed. The doctor needs to be notified immediately or a specialist referral, for example, to the physio or social worker, may be required.

Critical thinking is how nurses make decisions to solve problems. Nurses, through reflection and applying problem-solving techniques, demonstrate critical thinking. Refer to **Figure 5.1** to see the components of critical thinking that nurses apply through the decision-making process.

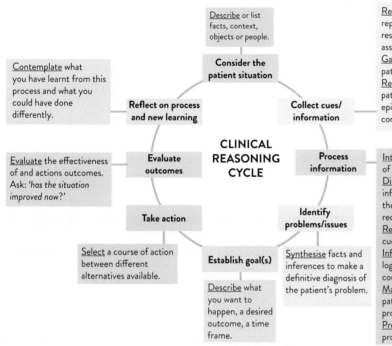

FIGURE 5.1 The clinical reasoning cycle

Source: Estes, M.E.Z., Calleja, P., Theobald, K. & Harvey, T. (2016). *Health Assessment and Physical Examination* (2nd edition). Cengage Learning: South Melbourne, Figure 1.1, p. 6.

CASE STUDY 5.4

New admission of respiratory patient

Jo, a student nurse, was allocated the responsibility of completing the assessment process for Amanda, a 19-year-old female who was admitted to the ward with an exacerbation of asthma following a cross-country run. Jo established a therapeutic relationship with Amanda and completed all the assessment data required. Amanda confessed to Jo that she had a cold in the days leading up to the run and knew her peak flow meter readings were not optimum but wanted to take part in the run with her boyfriend. Jo reported the data to the registered nurse also assigned to Amanda to review. 'Well done, you have also managed to obtain the details of her asthma management

plan', said the nurse complimenting Jo. 'I will let the team know that Amanda is having her medication by her bedside, in line with the asthma management plan. I will make the referral to the physiotherapist Amanda saw the last time she was admitted.'

1   How will the asthma plan impact on Amanda's care plan?

2   What nursing interventions would be appropriate to care for Amanda?

3   Why is it important to remain non-judgemental about lifestyle choices?

4   Can being non-judgemental affect the therapeutic relationship?

Table 5.1 provides an overview of the normal parameters for adult vital sign monitoring. The heart foundation sets the normal parameters for blood pressure each year and these are accessible from their website at https://heartfoundation.org.au/your-heart/know-your-risks/blood-pressure.

Numeracy

TABLE 5.1 Normal parameters of vital signs for adults

Temperature	36.2–37.2
Pulse	60–100
Respirations	12–20
BP systolic	100–139 mmHg
BP diastolic	60–89 mmHg
BGL	3.5–8 mmol
O$_2$ statistic	95–100%

Communication when a person's condition deteriorates

If the patient's observations are outside normal parameters these need to be immediately reported and actions taken to address them. A person's condition can change very quickly. The baseline observations are an objective measure of the person's progression towards wellness or deterioration.

CASE STUDY 5.5

Deterioration of a person

Mr Stokes was admitted to the medical ward with angina. Brad, his nurse, took his vital signs that were within normal limits and documented these along with the fact that Mr Stokes was not experiencing any chest pain. Mr Stokes' temperature was 37.2, pulse was 86 and regular, and blood pressure was 140/80. Brad went to have his tea break and on his return found Mr Stokes pale, very sweaty and incomprehensible. Brad took a set of vital signs and rang the Medical Emergency Team. Mr Stokes' pulse was too rapid to count and very irregular and his blood pressure was elevated to 175/104.

1 What do you think Mr Stokes may be experiencing?
2 What actions should Brad now implement?
3 What changes were noted with Mr Stokes' physical health status?

5.2 Admission and discharge procedures

You provide pre-admission care to ensure good use of resources and provide timely care for people. At discharge the person needs to be provided with the appropriate care and supports to assist them to maintain and improve their health status.

Data for admission and discharge

The assessment data is used to plan care for the person after discharge. The discharge planning is often commenced before the person is admitted, for example, if it is a planned admission such as in the case of surgical patients.

Issues that may impact on discharge

Many people after discharge and feeling better cease to follow the care plan or take medication and this can lead to readmission or a recurrence of their symptoms. In some instances, such

CASE STUDY 5.6

Data for admission and discharge

Mrs Green, a 55-year-old woman, was being admitted for a *dilatation and curette* and removal of a *uterine polyp*. Mrs Green was privately insured and was an *elective admission*. The *pre-admission* nurse contacted Mrs Green and began the collection of data for an elective admission. Mrs Green had undergone several tests, including a *uterine ultrasound*, *chest x-ray*, blood tests and an *ECG*. Mrs Green was also asked to provide details of next of kin and who would be picking her up post-

surgery as she was required to have a light *anaesthetic*. Questions about previous disease states, medication, previous surgery and who would be home to care for her on discharge were also asked.

1   Define the italicised terms in the scenario.
2   Why does the nurse need to know these things before Mrs Green is admitted?
3   Why are some of the tests already completed before admission?
4   Why is it important to have a person available to take Mrs Green home?

---

as with antibiotic therapy, it can lead to a resistant infection that will take longer to recover from and require stronger antibiotics to combat the infectious agent.

It is also important to realise that the majority of clients want to follow to the letter the discharge instructions and this could lead to different health issues occurring if education is not given. For example, a client may be told to rest to aid their recovery and takes that quite literally and stays in bed till review appointment. This could lead to serious health issues such as deep vein thrombosis or chest infections, especially if the client is elderly.

At times clients may need ongoing education for specialist care such as in the case of chronic diseases such as diabetes. The amount of lifestyle change may be significant with modification to diet, exercise and medication. Trying to educate on all these areas may be overwhelming. It may be a better plan to chunk the information and have follow up by a diabetes educator.

Discharge planning includes lifestyle modifications, level of compliance and the education that may be required for the individual. Discharge planning will be discussed in more detail in Chapter 14.

CASE STUDY 5.7

Paul's discharge

Paul was a 36-year-old man who was divorced, lived on his own in an apartment close to the city and held a position as head chef for a successful restaurant that he and his friend had set up. Paul had been admitted for stabilisation of his *type 2 diabetes*. Paul stated that he loved food and found it impossible not to try the new creations that he was designing in the restaurant. Paul's occupation also meant long hours and this impacted

on his ability to undertake social activities, especially physical activities such as sport that he enjoyed previously. Paul also stated that drinking wine was an essential part of his lifestyle in the restaurant business. On admission Paul's *BGL* was HI and his *BMI* was 38.

1   Define the italicised terms in the above case study.
2   What are the normal parameters for a BMI and BGL?
3   What lifestyle factors may impact on Paul's discharge from hospital?

Community supports

Care is given to enable the person to achieve goals quickly and return to their normal environment. An example of this is the newly diagnosed diabetic person. Once they have been stabilised, the diabetes educator will review the client when they have returned to their

psychosocial development
The ability to understand emotional responses for both self and others and the ability to interact with others

normal behavioural patterns to assess further health needs. Returning to the community prevents the person being subjected to harm in the health-care environment (falls, medication errors, infections, etc.) and allows resources for other individuals to be available.

The health-care team is responsible for organising community supports during the recuperation period.

Community support services and resources are provided to the level of care and support the person requires after discharge.

Reflective practice 5.4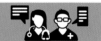

Meals on Wheels

Consider the following scenario: 'I was so nervous about ordering meals on wheels for a patient being discharged. I felt such responsibility as I knew the patient could not get to the shops or do cooking and I did not want her to be left without any food. I also did not want the Meals on Wheels (MOW) staff turning up and finding no one at home. I asked my buddy when

MOW should be notified and I was relieved that the referral had already been sent and I only needed to notify them the morning of the discharge'. Thinking about this scenario in relation to the people you are caring for:

1   Identify those you would require community supports for.
2   What type of community supports would be suitable for these clients?

Activity 5.3

Support services

Choose one of the clients that you are caring for.
1   What supports will they require on discharge?
2   How do they need to be contacted?
3   Is there specific documentation that needs to be completed?

Review the skill in Tollefson *Essential Clinical Skills* 7.4 Admission, discharge and patient transfer & 7.5 Health teaching

Requirements for discharge

The person can often feel overwhelmed with all the information and instructions given to them on the day of discharge. All information is given both verbally and in written form to support the person if they have any queries when they arrive home or at their discharge destination. Their GP also needs to be notified of their discharge and given relevant information that relates to changes to their condition and care.

5.3 Planning nursing care for clients

An individualised care plan needs to be formulated for each person on admission. Each person is unique and the care plan reflects the individual needs of the person.

Identifying risks and the health care that is required

Reading

The assessment data is used to identify areas in which the person will need support to achieve their activities of daily living. These areas are critically analysed and a problem-solving approach is used to address them. A care strategy is formulated, and a risk assessment is performed to assess the most appropriate action.

Activity 5.4

Clinical pathways

Obtain a **clinical pathway** for a condition that is used in caring for persons admitted to the health-care facility.

1   Do all people with this condition progress according to the pathway? Explain why or why not.
2   Where should deviations from the pathway be documented?

   Critical thinking can assist in the identification of care or address other issues required by the person. Nursing care plans require evaluation, critical analysis and reformulation of care strategies to meet the person's changing needs. If the individual is supported by family and/or carers their needs have to be considered alongside the individual's needs. Often including the carer in the care planning process will assist in achieving a holistic approach. Another person's perspective of the person's interests, physical, emotional and psychosocial needs allows the nurse to plan appropriate care. Refer to the Nursing and Midwifery Board of Australia's website for information related to the decision making for nursing staff. Go to http://www.nursingmidwiferyboard.gov.au/Codes-Guidelines-Statements/Frameworks.aspx.

Activity 5.5

Meeting the needs of people in care planning

Choose one of the people that you are caring for and review their care plans.

1   When do the care plans get evaluated?
2   Has there been a change in the care plan since the person was admitted to the facility?
3   What factors brought about the change to the care plan?

5.4 Ongoing development of nursing care plans

Ongoing development of individual nursing care plans includes analysis of the rationale behind specific actions, assessment that care meets a person's needs, principles of best practice, risk assessment, and communication between the whole health-care team.

Analysis of rationale behind decisions

Nurses analyse the best action to take to achieve a desired outcome for a person. The rationale is an important component of the planning process and is what nurses use to justify, educate and explain nursing actions. An example of this is encouraging a person to sit out of bed. The person may not feel 100 per cent and would like to lie down and curl up for comfort. The nurse will explain that sitting out of bed assists the respiratory and circulatory systems of the body and prevents further complications.

clinical pathway
a standardised, evidence-based multidisciplinary management plan that identifies the sequence of clinical interventions, timeframes, milestones and expected outcomes for an homogenous patient group. (Queensland Health Clinical Pathways Board definition 2002) accessed https://clinicalexcellence.qld.gov.au/resources/clinical-pathways 10.7.2018

Reflective practice 5.5

The reason for nursing actions

Think about the tasks you have undertaken for your clients. Identify one action that is completed for a specific reason but may not have the person's full support till education is given.

1   What was the action and what was the reason behind doing it?
2   When the person was made aware of the rationale were they more accepting of the intervention?

Confirming that nursing interventions are meeting client's needs

The evaluation component of the nursing process is the process of reviewing the care given and assessing if we have met the client's needs and assisted them to progress to achieve their goals.

- Have we achieved what we set out to achieve?
- Is the person improving in their health status?
- Has another problem occurred for the person as a result of the nursing intervention?

The nursing care plan tells the story of the person during their time in hospital. And over the time spent in hospital we could see an improvement or decline in the client's health, depending on their admission diagnosis, prognosis and response to therapy.

Activity 5.6

Meeting the person's needs

Identify one of the clients you are providing care for. Review their care plan.

1   Has that person improved over their stay of hospitalisation?
2   How has the care plan altered since admission?
3   What goals have they achieved?

The nurse uses the principles of best practice and risk assessment to ensure that nursing care is undertaken in the safest and most competent manner.

Best practice is the most current evidence-based practice that is available to nurses on which to base their clinical interventions. Each intervention is assessed singularly for the risk and the outcome. The nurse then decides if the nursing intervention is appropriate.

Reflective practice 5.6

Sitting the person out of bed

Best practice indicates that if there is no clinical reason for the person to rest in bed, it is beneficial to restoring strength and wellbeing to sit the person out of bed. Choose a person that requires assistance with the standup lifter to get out of bed onto a chair.

1   If the client is suffering from delirium is it still appropriate to use the standup lifter?
2   What is the criteria for using the standup lifter in the facility?
3   Is using the standup lifter still demonstrating best practice?
4   What might be a risk when using the standup lifter with this person?

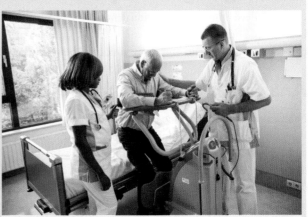

Science Photo Library/Arno Massee

Implementation of equipment resources as part of planned nursing care

Conflicts between the nursing care plan and the already prescribed plan of care

A collaborative approach to planning nursing care is a model of best practice. This means you are required to ensure that appropriate referrals to members of the allied health team are identified and actioned.

Using the same plan by the team avoids wasting of resources and prevention of harm through duplication or poor care that could result from two separate care plans being followed by different members of the team.

CASE STUDY 5.8

Jenny's wound care

Jenny was an 86-year-old woman admitted to the medical ward with a chronic leg ulcer.

A nursing care plan was organised for Jenny by Carla her admitting nurse. The wound care intervention required application of a zinc bandage, padding and combine for protection.

The following day Emma, the afternoon nurse caring for Jenny, could not find and review the care plan but thought that it was an inappropriate dressing and replaced it with a non-adherent gauze, combine and bandage. Emma then completed a new care plan and placed it in the folder. This alteration between different dressings continued for the next two days before it was noticed that there were two care plans in the file. On review Jenny's leg ulcer had not improved.

1   What problems occurred in the above case study?
2   What was the outcome for Jenny?
3   What actions should now be taken to assist the healing of the wound?

SUMMARY

- It is important that a person is assessed holistically to ensure best practice.
- Assessment is how nursing care can be formulated to address areas of concern for an individual.
- Assessment is an ongoing activity that can be commenced before admission and continues after discharge.
- Therapeutic communication is vital to the process of assessment.

SELF-TEST QUESTIONS

1   Why is the establishment of a therapeutic relationship important in the collection of client information?
2   How does expertise in the use of specialised equipment assist in collecting and interpreting health data?
3   Why is it important to commence discharge planning before or on admission to a health facility?
4   After assessing an individual, discuss why a collaborative approach is important.
5   Why is it important to consider lifespan development when assessing the individual?
6   What type of approach does nursing implement when undertaking care planning? How does this assist the client?

BIBLIOGRAPHY

ANMC National Competency Standard for Enrolled Nurse (2016), http://www.nursingmidwiferyboard.gov.au/Codes-Guidelines-Statements/Professional-standards.aspx.

Estes, M.E.Z., Calleja, P., Theobald, K. & Harvey, T. (2016). *Health Assessment and Physical Examination* (2nd edition). Cengage Learning: South Melbourne.

Gray, S., Ferris, L., White, L., Duncan, G. & Baumle, W. (2018). *Fundamentals of Nursing* (2nd edition). Cengage Learning: South Melbourne.

Tollefson, J., Watson, G., Jelly, E. & Tambree, K. (2016). *Essential Clinical Skills: Enrolled Division 2 Nurses* (3rd edition). Cengage Learning: South Melbourne, VIC.

Communication skills in nursing practice

LEARNING OUTCOMES

After reading this chapter, you should have an understanding of:

6.1   Effective communication skills in complex situations

6.2   Identifying and addressing actual and potential constraints to communication

6.3   Using information technology to support communication in nursing practice

6.4   Leading small group discussions

6.5   Giving and receiving feedback for performance improvement

6.6   Evaluating effectiveness of communication in complex situations

Communication in nursing

Ensuring you communicate clearly and effectively is incredibly vital in delivering safe care. Not explaining a point or using words that cannot be understood can create confusion, distress and mixed messages. Consider the following example:

Nurse – Hello, are you Mrs Jones?

Mrs Jones – Yes, where is my husband?

Nurse – He is in the operating room. He will be out soon, and the doctor will talk to you then when it is all finished (walks off).

Although the nurse in this example communicates where Mr Jones is, she does not give any insight into what Mr Jones' condition is or any information regarding time frames. Imagine receiving this as an update!

Now consider this example:

Nurse – Hello, are you Mrs Jones?

Mrs Jones – Yes, where is my husband?

Nurse – Mr Jones right now is having an operation. He had an injury in the accident that caused bleeding into his abdomen. So the surgeons are repairing that now. He has been in the operating room for about an hour. I will call up now and get an update for you, then I will take you to the waiting room.

Mrs Jones – Oh, thank you.

Communication can make or break any situation, not just in nursing.

6.1 Effective communication in complex situations

Everything we do in nursing involves **communication**. We communicate thoughts, feelings, desires, respect, happiness, uncertainty, delight, misery, and a whole host of other emotions through body language, verbal and non-verbal communication. Seventy per cent of all communication is body language. Twenty-three per cent of communication is in the tone of your voice and only 7% of communication is the words we actually convey. It is surprising how heavily we rely on non-verbal cues to guide us in effectively communicating (Balzer Riley, 2016).

communication
The exchange of information, thoughts and feelings using both verbal and non-verbal methods

Activity 6.1

How tone of voice can change the message

Tone of voice is incredibly important. Try saying hello in different tones and think about how that could impact on your communication with patients and colleagues.

Nursing staff within any health-care setting will typically spend a significantly large portion of their time communicating with others to relay often vital client information; thus, it is no surprise to find that the basis for many errors in the health-care environment is related in some way to poor communication. Effective communication is an essential component of client care whether it is at an interpersonal, intrapersonal, transpersonal, small group or public level.

Communication in nursing practice is a two-way process of giving and receiving information through any number of channels such as verbal (as shown in **Figure 6.1**), non-verbal or written information. Effective communication is required in nursing practice for the exchange of health-related information and ensuring your client's best interests are always at the forefront. Although we have all been communicating since we were born, and often we believe quite effectively, the process of transmitting and receiving information from an individual or group is quite a complex one that we rarely consider in detail.

Explore the theory in *Foundations of Nursing*, Chapter 7: Communication

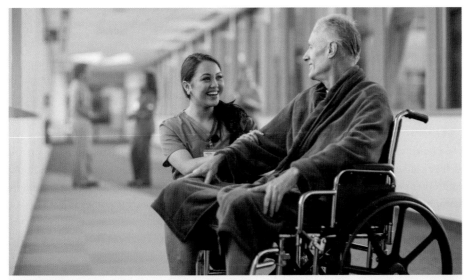

FIGURE 6.1 Communication in nursing

While on placement you will observe and be involved in many forms of communication. Communicating in complex situations can relate to a grieving family, an aggressive or angry client, an emergency situation, or even the birth of a child. All communication needs to focus on being clear, professional, respectful and concise. Communication also includes documentation, so being effective in communicating is a holistic approach to patient care, encompassing more than just direct conversations with the patient.

To summarise the roles and responsibilities, enrolled nurses:

- work as part of the health-care team to advocate for and facilitate the involvement of individuals and groups, their families and significant others in planning and evaluating care and progress towards health outcomes
- fulfil the duty of care by identifying and clarifying enrolled nurse responsibility for aspects of care in consultation with registered nurses and other members of the health-care team
- liaise with others to ensure that the rights of individuals are maintained, seeking assistance from other members of the health-care team to provide care and resources that are sensitive to the needs of the individual
- consult with registered nurses and other members of the health-care team to facilitate provision of accurate information to protect the patient's rights, and enable informed decision making for patients
- recognise their level of competence, and ensure care is provided within their own level of competence (ANMC, 2002; NMBA, 2016).

Good communication between health-care professionals and clients depends on each being able to understand the other. A wide range of factors can aid or create obstacles to that understanding, for example, age, gender, social and economic circumstances, health status, education, cultural background, disability and literacy. Failing to recognise and meet communication needs can lead to clients:

- not understanding their medical condition and the risks and benefits of treatment options
- becoming unduly anxious about their condition and treatment options
- being unable to discuss their condition with health professionals or participate in discussions, as much as they would like to about their health-care needs.

Activity 6.2

Communicating with a patient

Your patient asks you if an operation they are scheduled to have is dangerous. It is a routine, elective hernia repair. How would you explain the procedure to the patient? What type of terminology would you use?

interpersonal skills
The ability to interact and communicate effectively with other people

Health-care professionals utilise communication and a team-based approach in the delivery of health care. As a nurse, it is your role to report abnormalities, changes in conditions and other pertinent clinical issues regarding your patient. To do this, you must be able to communicate utilising appropriate medical terminology, respectful communication, and effective **interpersonal skills**. We will now look at listening and other skills concerned with the delivery of information and associated communication.

Listening skills

Listening is often considered a passive way of receiving information. In reality it is actually an *active* process that requires the nurse's complete attention. Good listeners show a strong desire to reach a common understanding with the person with whom they are communicating. Their **active listening** behaviour informs the speaker that the message was heard, it was understood and its context was evaluated appropriately.

Good listeners confirm another person's sense of self-worth by sending the message that 'what you have to say is important and I am listening to you'.

In summary, effective listening behaviours assist you to learn about the other person, and enhances your ability to relate with them, thus changing attitudes and behaviours because others know you are actively listening and understanding them.

To improve our communication skills we need to practise, especially our listening – Table 6.1 outlines some of the skills you can practise.

listening
Interpreting the sounds heard and attaching meaning to them

active listening
A technique used to reflect on what a patient has said and can help patients feel more deeply understood

TABLE 6.1 Listening skills

Communication skills		
Attending skills	**Following skills**	**Active or reflective listening skills**
• attentiveness • postures and gestures of involvement • appropriate body motion • positive body language • gazing and eye contact • minimising distractions in ourselves and the environment	• conversation starters • minimal responses and encourages vocal expressions • infrequent questions – open and closed questions • attentive silence • concentration • short-term memory • long-term memory	• paraphrasing • clarifying • summarising • reflecting feelings • reflecting meanings • statement (relating feelings to content)

Activity 6.3

Communicating professionally

Observe your buddy, registered nurse, doctor or allied health-care team member interact with the client for whom you are providing care and support.
1 What type of language skills do they use?
2 Observe their body language. What cues can you see with the person interacting with the client? Is their posture open or closed? What type of eye contact do they employ when interacting with the client?
3 What verbal communication cues do they use, for example, paraphrasing, reflecting?
4 All of these interactions are part of the communication process. See if you can record yourself with one of the other students. What communications cues do you use?

Listening behaviours are not the same as hearing. The process of hearing is a physiological process that happens when vibrations in the air impact the eardrum. The important thing to note is that hearing is a passive process that occurs without any attention or effort on part of the hearer.

Listening also involves paying attention to the speaker's body language, tone of voice and facial expressions. These all contribute to the overall message that is being sent.

Review the skill in Tollefson *Essential Clinical Skills* 7.5 Health teaching

CASE STUDY 6.1

Complex communication

Hayden is a 28-year-old male who has been hospitalised for the past few days with a traumatic fracture to his femur as a result of a motor vehicle accident. Also involved in the motor accident was Hayden's brother, Brendan, who is currently in the operating room having a fracture reduced. Hayden is speaking in a raised voice, fidgeting and looking about the room.

1   What factors do you think are contributing to Hayden's behaviour?
2   How could you, as a nurse, communicate with Hayden?

TIP 6.1

Constraints on effective communication

Remember that a shared ward can be a very public space so be conscious about the volume of your voice when you are having private and confidential conversations with a patient.

6.2 Identifying and addressing constraints to communication

Workplace factors such as noise, temperature extremes, distractions and lack of privacy or space may result in patient confusion, misinterpretation of what has been said, and frustration and discontent with the situation. In the health-care setting these workplace factors may very easily affect communication with patients, relatives or visitors, and other health-care professionals more readily than perhaps we believe. Workplace distractions are common in workplace settings and can interfere with messages sent between people, so nurses need to reduce these factors where possible to create the ideal environment for *effective* communication.

Let's take a look at actual constraints to effective communication in **Figure 6.2**.

Workplace noise
• People noise, equipment noise, white noise. There is a great deal of noise in a ward environment.

Workplace temperature
• It is difficult to regulate any environment to suit each individual. For example, air conditioning is sometimes too cold or too hot for some staff or patients.

Workplace distractions
• Due to the time pressures you will face, it is easy to be distracted. There might be a phone enquiry, a patient call button or another nurse requiring your assistance to check a medication.

Workplace privacy/space
• The environment itself can be an actual constraint to effective communication – for example, curtains are not soundproof, and you are asking patients if their bowels have opened, or how much pain they are in, or any number of other personal questions.

FIGURE 6.2 Constraints on effective communication

Other constraints to communication include:
• external factors affecting your thoughts (for example, your cat died this morning)
• your working relationship with colleagues (you may feel harassed or bullied by a co-worker, making it difficult to communicate effectively in the workplace)
• if you have a patient that has a non-English-speaking background and the organisation cannot find an interpreter
• language barriers between health-care professionals
• sick leave of staff at short notice may result in you taking on more patients than usual, increasing your time pressures
• sudden facility evacuation for a fire that you have not prepared for.

6.3 Using information technology to support communication in nursing practice

In today's health-care environment, it is essential for nurses and all health professionals to understand and utilise the vast availability of information through computers and information technology. There is a great deal of information available to help guide nursing and health-care practices. In particular, information technology has had a revolutionary impact on health because it has allowed widespread dissemination of health information throughout the world.

Rapid trends and developments in portable technology, the miniaturisation of handheld and portable computer devices, and high quality voice-activated inventions will continue to drive the use of computers and developing technologies in nursing practice. This dramatic increase in the nature and extent of communication and information technology use worldwide has also changed the way in which health care is managed and delivered. Communication and information technology skills are an important adjunct in the provision of quality patient care.

Reflective practice 6.1

Information technology

Principles such as *confidentiality*, *privacy* and *ethical conduct* are fundamental to nursing care delivery. With the instantaneous notion of social media, what are some concepts you need to keep in mind when using social media? Of the following examples, which are not appropriate?

1   Emma Crawford checked in @ All Pines Aged Care....time for another fun day being treated like crap....#studentlife

2   Emma Crawford checked in @ All Pines Aged Care.....yay! Day 3 of placement – learning heaps, wish me luck!

3   Emma Crawford checked in @ All Pines Aged Care.....why...Mr J will be walking around swearing all day, Mrs P will be stealing stuff from other residents and my RN will be a sour cow because she did not win her eBay bid....FML

For further information, refer to the social media policy from AHPRA at http://www.nursingmidwiferyboard.gov.au/Codes-Guidelines-Statements/Policies/Social-media-policy.aspx.

6.4 Leading small group discussions

Most group discussions that you will participate in or lead within the health-care environment are usually 'smooth sailing' as the people who turn up or are invited to small group discussion are there because they have an interest and can see the benefits of the meeting. However, given the non-authoritative and flexible nature of small group discussions, sometimes issues that are raised can heighten participant sensitivities, particularly if it is about an individual/facility/unit/ward performance matter. Therefore, those who lead small group discussions need to stay alert to group dynamics and be prepared to deal with them when they arise.

CASE STUDY 6.2

Clinical handover

Clinical handover is an example of a group discussion. You will need to deliver information, answer questions and understand information being conveyed to you. Often handover is undertaken at shift changeover times. This can lead to an 'I need to get out of here' attitude and is why the National Safety and Quality Health Service has identified clinical handover as an area of focus (Standard 6 – Clinical Handover).

Consider the following information:

'Fifty-six-year-old female, Caitlyn Ross, admitted five minutes ago from emergency. I don't know what is wrong with her but she has already buzzed for pain and I have not made it there yet so you will need to sort that. I did not get a full

handover from the ED staff as they had to leave for a medical emergency call. All I know is that she was in an accident and the airbags were deployed in the car. I don't know if she was driving. I think she might have theatre tomorrow or that might be the other patient coming. Sorry, it has been one of those nights, ahh, her ADDS is, actually I don't know'.

1   If you were to follow the ISBAR format (go to https://www.safetyandquality.gov.au/wp-content/uploads/2012/02/ISBAR-toolkit.pdf) – is there enough information in this 'handover' to determine patient safety and needs?

2   What would you ask the nurse who is leaving? What clarification would you seek?

3   Is this an acceptable handover? If not, why not?

---

clinical handover
The transfer of information, accountability and responsibility for patients from one health-care worker to another

Review the skill in Tollefson *Essential Clinical Skills* 7.3 Clinical handover – change of shift

6.5 Giving and receiving feedback for performance improvement

There are many types of feedback that can be used; here are some examples of the types of feedback you may encounter or use while on placement:

* observation of performance
* audit of documentation (for example, care plans, clinical notes in medical record)
* interview/personal reflections
* 360-degree feedback
* peer review
* testing (for example, drug calculations)
* incident/event/near miss reporting
* client feedback – verbally or via compliments (for example, thank you letters, cards)
* outcome indicators of care (for example, client outcome measured against care planned and delivered)
* annual performance review.

Activity 6.4

Providing feedback to a colleague

You are involved in handover and your buddy has given incorrect ADDS scores for your patients. How would you correct her?

Performance review

In nursing, and in nursing education, you will be evaluated using performance review and structured feedback. *Performance review* is a planned, structured process that is aimed at highlighting areas for improvement, learning and support. It is also a forum to provide feedback to your manager or facilitator on your insight into your role and your clinical development. *Structured feedback* is focused on the standards for practice and scope of practice and how your practice relates to these in your performance review.

Performance review is not a negative tool – it is a positive tool aimed at empowering staff to find ways to achieve professional satisfaction. It is also great to hear positive and encouraging feedback from your manager or facilitator who you may not work closely with.

As part of this process you will need to communicate verbally and in writing in an assertive manner to ensure that your attributes are identified. This may pose a problem for anyone who is not confident and who might feel intimidated by discussing their performance with a nurse in a senior position or a facilitator.

While a performance review can feel overwhelming, it is also a great opportunity for you to express your wishes with respect to ongoing training, skills that you require further education or in-service on, or other issues that relate to your role.

Self-evaluation

Self-evaluation and appraisal is an excellent tool in nursing – and it is used regularly in the daily roles of the enrolled nurse. It is a component of annual registration and ongoing continuing education – both now as a student and in the future as an enrolled nurse.

Using SWOT analysis for self-evaluation

SWOT analysis, as shown in **Figure 6.3**, is a useful tool to use for self-evaluation. It can be applied to any aspect of your life. You might like to jot down your answers to view them when you complete reading the prompts.

Activity 6.5

SWOT self-analysis

Complete the SWOT analysis template for your own self-analysis as a student nurse.

Strengths	Weaknesses	Opportunities	Threats
• Are there skills or educational components that make you stand out? Do you have a natural ability in some skills? • How do you view your strengths? What are they? • What resources do you have available to you? • What have previous employers stated that your strengths have been?	• What are some aspects you think you could improve on? Being on time, non-verbal communication and confidence are all good examples. • What do you think you should avoid? This could be things like fatigue (so no short shift turnarounds such as finishing at 11 pm and starting at 7 am), attitudes or body language when talking to colleagues. • What do you think people around you may view your weaknesses as?	• What opportunities are available that build on your strengths? • What opportunities are available that will minimise your weaknesses or help you improve on them?	• Do you have any obstacles? • Do any of your weaknesses threaten your progression?

FIGURE 6.3 Using SWOT for self-analysis

Sometimes it is quite confronting to list your *strengths*. Try writing some characteristics about yourself that you believe – 'strong', 'reliable', 'honest' are all strengths as well as characteristics.

Weakness can often be more confronting than strengths, because we are generally unaware of them. When writing this list, think about it as a process, not an attack.

It is always difficult to analyse our own weaknesses, but there is something that is also empowering about it. It is a great way for identifying things to improve upon. Another way to review weaknesses would be a comparison to colleagues – are you always taking longer to perform tasks? Do you have areas of practice that you do not understand or know how to complete?

Opportunities can be reviewed by looking at your strengths and thinking about what opportunities this opens up for you. For example, do you show a natural affinity to information technology in the workplace? How can you create more opportunities using this as a basis?

Opportunities, particularly in health care, can result from social change/s and changes in government. Funding is particularly relevant, so keeping that in mind also will assist in reviewing opportunities.

Another way to review opportunities is to analyse your weaknesses and use this list positively by focusing on opportunities to minimise weaknesses.

Threats are aspects such as obstacles, changing technology or processes, or the impact of any weaknesses you may have.

Reviewing potential threats can be a great way to put your weaknesses and threats into perspective (Manoharan, n.d.).

Reflecting on feedback

Have you ever had an unexpected negative response when interacting with another person? Most of us believe that we are good communicators, but how many of us actually reflect on our performance or seek feedback from those we communicate with? Feedback helps us to see how people are reacting to our communication style.

Most people, when they receive negative feedback about their performance, become defensive and reject the feedback. This, in turn, can appear to the person providing the feedback that the receiver is unwilling to accept constructive criticism. This is not ideal because sometimes you need to hear feedback that is not always positive in order to learn and grow in your position (Lloyd, 2017).

The initial reaction of being defensive is often instinctive but being aware of the need for feedback is essential and this can assist you in accepting feedback, as well as identifying if there is anything in the negative comments that you can take on board and use to improve your performance. In nursing, this is generally a component of reflective practice and our everyday communication. As a student, you will often feel as though you are not progressing – but you will be. It is difficult to see how far you have come some days when you are focusing on a single skill. Always look to the bigger picture and communicate your concerns, questions and comments appropriately. As a student, effective communication will always ensure your learning needs and your patient's needs are being met.

6.6 Evaluating effectiveness of communication in complex situations

The ability of a nurse to deliver complex information in a manner that is clearly understood by clients, carers, colleagues and others requires a unique skill set. It is essential that you understand your client and their needs to ensure any information you provide is interpreted accurately and has not been misunderstood.

While on placement you will observe many complex situations – and you will be involved in some too. Keeping a reflective journal is a good method of being able to see your progress and also deconstruct situations that were new and possibly frightening to you. Simply jotting down a few sentences or adding them to your journal can be very helpful.

CASE STUDY 6.3

Identification of a patient

The emergency buzzer has sounded. You attend the bedside and note that there is a female on the ground, unconscious. She is laying next to bed 31. You are the second person on the scene and you go to obtain the emergency trolley.

As the patient was found next to bed 31, it is presumed that she is Nikki Savage. During the course of resuscitation, other staff members contact Nikki's family. They immediately present to the hospital to find their loved one watching television in the day room and are incredibly distressed. The patient on the floor being

resuscitated is Joanne Ross. No one has checked her ID band during the course of resuscitation. Joanne is also allergic to amiodarone and has received some during the resuscitation. She has gone into anaphylactic shock and has been transferred to the intensive care unit for adrenaline and monitoring.

1   What are the concepts of patient identification?
2   In complex communication situations, such as emergencies, what are some factors that increase the likelihood of communication errors?
3   What is open disclosure? How is it appropriate in this case study?

SUMMARY

- Health care is ever changing – no two days are the same! Health-care delivery is undertaken through effective communication and continuous improvement through constant assessment, reassessment and evaluation of patient needs and goals.
- All events and occurrences must be documented, and a basis in communication ensures that all aspects of nursing care are documented.
- Communication is the foundation of all nursing care, and requires an ongoing and evolving approach to ensure efficacy.
- Ensuring documentation is contemporaneous is essential.
- Verbal handover is the handover of responsibility – ensure yours is safe!
- Communication is complex and in nursing is often conducted in challenging environments due to changing patient needs, conditions and events.

SELF-TEST QUESTIONS

1   What are the different types of communication?
2   How can you ensure a message is received?
3   What communication strategies are used to work collaboratively with other members of the team?
4   What constraints to communication are you aware of when interacting with colleagues and clients?
5   When should you report difficulties with communication to your supervisor?
6   What legal and organisational requirements apply to documentation in the workplace?

BIBLIOGRAPHY

Australian Nursing and Midwifery Council (ANMC) (2002), *National Competency Standard for the Enrolled Nurse,* Retrieved from http://www.nursingmidwiferyboard.gov.au/documents/default.aspx?record=WD10%2f1349&dbid=AP&chksum=aljeSkQ0D2Yzm4jBCcBhtg%3d%3d.

Australian Commission on Safety and Quality in Healthcare, http://www.safetyandquality.gov.au/.

Balzer Riley, J. (2016). *Communication in Nursing* (8th edition), Mosby: Sydney.

Lloyd, J. (2017). *The art of receiving feedback.* Retrieved from https://www.joanlloyd.com/People-Skills/The-art-of-receiving-feedback.aspx.

Manoharan, P. (n.d.). *Education and Personality Development.* Retrieved from https://books.google.com.au/books/about/Education_And_Personality_Development.html?id=0vfwcs5_d1MC&redir_esc=y.

Nursing and Midwifery Board of Australia (NMBA) (2016). *Enrolled nurse standards for practice.* Retrieved from http://www.nursingmidwiferyboard.gov.au/Codes-Guidelines-Statements/Professional-standards/enrolled-nurse-standards-for-practice.aspx.

Nursing and Midwifery Board of Australia (NMBA) (2017). *Social media policy.* Retrieved from http://www.nursingmidwiferyboard.gov.au/Codes-Guidelines-Statements/Policies/Social-media-policy.aspx.

Tollefson, J., Watson, G., Jelly, E. & Tambree, K. (2016). *Essential Clinical Skills: Enrolled Division 2 Nurses* (3rd edition). Cengage Learning: South Melbourne.

Physical health status

LEARNING OUTCOMES

After reading this chapter, you should have an understanding of:

7.1   Obtaining information about physical health status of clients

7.2   Checking the physical health status of clients

7.3   Identifying variations from the normal physical health status of individuals

The human body

I found anatomy and physiology difficult at first. There was so much to learn. Before starting my nursing studies I had just accepted my body and its good health as a matter of fact. Learning about how the body worked and how the systems interacted made me more aware of the complex being I was. It gave me knowledge of the impact on a person's health when individual systems are not functioning properly, and how it can change the functioning of other systems within the human body. Before this I had always felt sorry for people in ill health with multiple health problems but had thought it could never happen to me.

This chapter is cross referenced to Gray et al., *Foundations of Nursing* 2e, Chapter 30.

7.1 Obtaining accurate information about physical health

In the admission process you must use all of your own senses and knowledge to obtain a detailed picture of the health status of the person. You may notice the individual's gait and posture, an abnormal smell, or abnormal appearance of the integumentary system when conducting the admission. Information obtained is related to the appropriate body system and associated systems of the body.

Through questioning you may also note abnormal patterns of speech and thought as well as more detailed information that the individual has noted about the onset of symptoms.

When using the organisation's documentation for admission of an individual, additional information may be elicited through specific questioning of both the individual and their carer or family. The information obtained by the nurse can be of two types, *subjective data* and *objective data*, as first discussed in Chapter 5.

Once all the information has been collated from the different members of the health team, the team can then begin to formulate a care plan that is based on the specific problems and potential problems of the individual. The nurse can use the basic human life processes of **metabolism**, **nutrition**, **body temperature regulation**, **biological maturation**, inheritance and ageing as a basis to identify the problems the client may be having or may develop.

Interpreting information based on the structure and functioning of body systems

The information is then analysed according to the structure and functioning of the human body systems and their interactions. You must be able to differentiate the levels of organisation of the body. After identifying the variations from normal parameters, you are then able to make clinical judgements to provide safe and competent nursing care.

Structure of the body

A classification of the structure of the human body can be from smallest unit to the entire body. **Figure 7.1** is representative of this structure.

metabolism
The functional activities of cells that result in growth, repair and the release of energy by the cell

nutrition
All the processes (ingestion, digestion, absorption, metabolism and elimination) involved in consuming and using food for energy

body temperature regulation
The internal temperature of the body after the excess heat produced is lost by the body

biological maturation
The process of progressing towards the mature state that occurs in all body systems, organs and tissues

Review the skill in Tollefson *Essential Clinical Skills*, 7.4 Admission, discharge and patient transfer

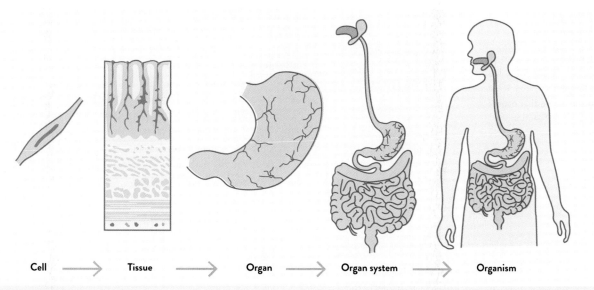

| Cell | ⟶ | Tissue | ⟶ | Organ | ⟶ | Organ system | ⟶ | Organism |

FIGURE 7.1 Structural organisation of the human body

Body systems and their functions

The human body is an integrated being with the different systems all interdependent on each other to maintain healthy body functioning. Each body system performs a specialised function to maintain the health of the body. **Table 7.1** provides an overview of the body systems and their function and **Table 7.2** shows how each system functions.

TABLE 7.1 Body systems and their function

Body system	Function
Cardiovascular system	Consists of the blood, heart and blood vessels. The heart is a pump, blood vessels transport blood and the blood is a connective tissue that takes nutrients and oxygen to every cell of the body and transports waste materials away from the cell to the excretory organs.
Respiratory system	Consists of the lungs and structures designed to take air into and expel air from the body.
Musculo-skeletal system	The skeletal component consists of bones, joints and cartilage. It provides a frame for the body, and protects and supports body organs. It also assists with movement, produces blood cells, stores minerals and produces heat.
Endocrine system	Consists of glands that secrete hormones and chemical substances that regulate body activities such as growth, reproduction, metabolism and water balance.
Digestive system	Consists of organs that ingest food, break it down into nutrients and absorb these nutrients into the body. It also eliminates waste material that cannot be absorbed by the body.
Urinary system	Consists of two kidneys, two ureters, a bladder and a urethra. It filters the blood, removes waste products, secretes hormones and helps maintain electrolyte balance.
Reproductive system	Consists of organs and structures that enable the human being to reproduce itself.
Integumentary system	Consists of the skin, hair and nails. It forms a protective covering for the body, helps regulate body temperature and assists in the process of touch and sensation.
Lymphatic system	Consists of the lymph nodes, lymphatic vessels, lymph and lymphoid organs. It assists in fluid balance and defence of the body against **pathogens** and foreign material.
Immune system	A defence system that protects the body from pathogens, other **allergens** and abnormal cells.
Nervous system	Consists of the brain, spinal cord and nerves. It collects information about the environment, both external and internal, and conveys the information to the brain where it is interpreted and the body's function adjusted.
Special senses	Vision, hearing, touch, smell and balance. They allow the person to process information about the world and assist in identifying hazards to the health and wellbeing of the person.

pathogen
A disease-causing microorganism (Rizzo, 2015)

allergen
A substance that causes an allergic reaction

TABLE 7.2 Functions of the body systems

Life functions/ body systems	Definition
Movement 　　　Muscle system	The ability of the whole organism – or a part of it – to move
Ingestion	The process by which an organism takes in food
Assimilation	The breakdown of complex food molecules into simpler food molecules
Digestion 　　　Digestive system	The transformation of digested food molecules into living tissue for growth and self-repair
Transport 　　　Circulatory system	The movement of necessary substances to, into and around cells, and of cellular products and wastes out of and away from cells
Respiration 　　　Respiratory system	The burning or oxidation of food molecules in a cell to release energy, water and carbon dioxide
Immunity 　　　Lymphatic system	The filtering out of harmful bacteria and production of white blood cells (lymphocytes)
Protection 　　　Integumentary system	The waterproof covering of the body
Growth 　　　Skeletal system	The enlargement of an organism due to synthesis and assimilation, resulting in an increase in the number and size of its cells
Secretion 　　　Endocrine system	The formation and release of hormones from a cell or structure
Excretion 　　　Urinary system	The removal of metabolic waste products from an organism
Regulation (sensitivity) 　　　Nervous system	The ability of an organism to respond to its environment to maintain a balanced state (homeostasis)
Reproduction 　　　Reproductive system	The ability of an organism to produce offspring with similar characteristics (this is *essential* for species survival as opposed to individual survival).

Source: Scott, A.E. & Fong, E. (2017). *Body Structures and Functions* (13th edition). Cengage: Boston, MA, p. 7.

Activity 7.1

Body systems and how they relate to each other

For each body system identify one other system that would be affected by the body system not functioning well.

Anatomical and medical terminology

Correct anatomical and medical terminology is used to document and relay information to other members of the health team. This is not only professional communication, but also gives clearer information to the person reading or listening to the information. Terminology relates to:

- relative positions – the position of one body part in relation to another as shown in **Table 7.3**

- planes and sections of the body as shown in **Figure 7.2**
- regional terms – the different regions or areas of the body (refer to **Tables 7.3** and **7.4**).

Terminology and communication

When using terminology it is important to consider the audience. Individuals outside the medical environment will often not understand medical terms. It can be helpful to explain and point to the part of the body you are referring to. Depending on the age of the individual some parts of the body may be referred to with special terms. Children often do not know the anatomical terms and have their own terms to describe parts of the body.

TABLE 7.3 Relative positions of the body

Positions	Explanation
Superior	A part of the body that is closer to the head than another part of the body
Inferior	A part of the body that is closer to the feet than another part of the body
Anterior/ventral	Towards the surface of the abdomen
Posterior/dorsal	Towards the back surface of the body
Medial	Towards the midline of the body
Lateral	Away from the midline of the body
Proximal	The body part is closer to the point of attachment than another body part
Distal	The body part is further away from the point of attachment than another body part
Superficial	The part is near the surface of the body
Deep	The part is away from the surface of the body
Central	The body part is located in the centre of the structure
Peripheral	The body part is located closer to ends of the limbs or structure

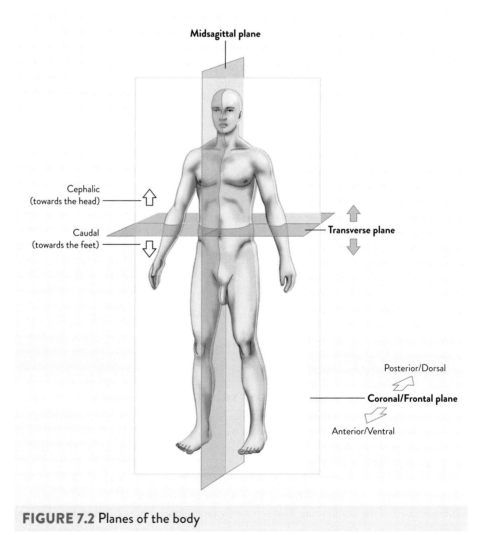

FIGURE 7.2 Planes of the body

Source: Scott, A.E. & Fong, E. (2017). *Body Structures and Functions* (13th edition). Cengage: Boston, MA, Figure 1-1, p. 3.

TABLE 7.4 Common regional terms used – matching the term to the descriptor

Terms	Location front of body
Abdominal	Anterior trunk located under the ribs
Antecubital	Area in front of the elbow
Auxiliary	Armpit
Brachial	Arm
Buccal	Cheek
Cephalic	Head
Cervical	Neck region
Cranial	Nearer to the head
Digital	Fingers, toes
Femoral	Thigh area
Flank	Fleshy area located on the sides of the body between the ribs and the top of the hip bone
Inguinal	Groin
Oral	Mouth
Orbital	Area around the eye
Patellar	Front of the knee
Pedal	Foot
Plantar	Sole of the foot
Pubic	Genital area
Sternal	Middle of the chest
Umbilical	Naval
Dorsal	Back of the body
Caudal	Lower region of the spinal column
Deltoid	Area of shoulder nearest the arm
Gluteal	Buttocks
Lumbar	Area of back between the ribs and the hip
Occipital	Back of head
Popliteal	Behind, or back of, the knee
Scapular	Shoulder blade area

Review the skill in Tollefson *Essential Clinical Skills* 7.4 Admission, discharge and patient transfer

Reflective practice 7.1

Handover

At handover I felt very uncomfortable. The staff were stating the diagnosis and using medical terminology to describe treatments and interventions. I could grasp some of the words but a lot went right over my head. I found it hard to understand what was wrong with the clients and what treatment I should take. After the handover I contacted my supervisor who went through the handover sheet with me. I looked up some of the terms that I was not familiar with and wrote down their meaning.

1   What strategies could you use to understand unfamiliar terminology?
2   As a nurse you will be expected to give a handover report. What can you do to ensure that you can pronounce the terminology correctly?

Body cavities

Descriptions and locations of organs or body systems can also be used by referring to the different **body cavities**. The body cavities are the *dorsal cavity* and the *ventral cavity*. The ventral cavity is further subdivided into the *thoracic cavity* and the *abdominopelvic cavity*. These two cavities are separated by the diaphragm.

As the abdominopelvic cavity is large, in order to identify the specific location the cavity can be divided into quadrants or regions as shown in **Figure 7.3**.

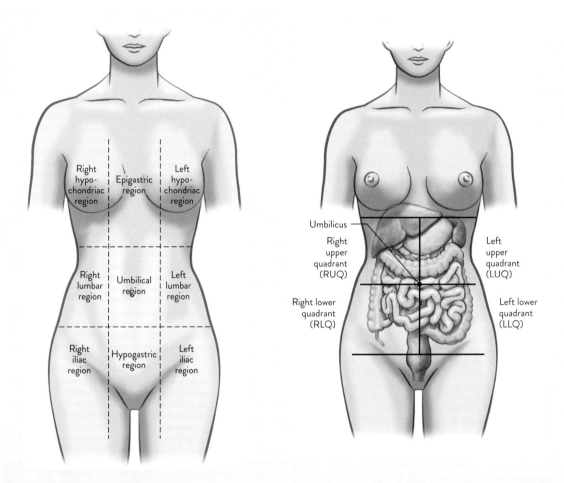

FIGURE 7.3 Regions and quadrants of the abdominopelvic area

Source: Scott, A.E. & Fong, E. (2017). *Body Structures and Functions* (13th edition). Cengage: Boston, MA, Figure 1-5 and Figure 1-6, p. 6.

Using information obtained to identify actual or potential health problems

The nursing care plan consists of five distinct stages known as the nursing process. The stages of the nursing process, as outlined in **Figure 7.4**, are constantly reviewed to correspond with the actual health status of the client. In the

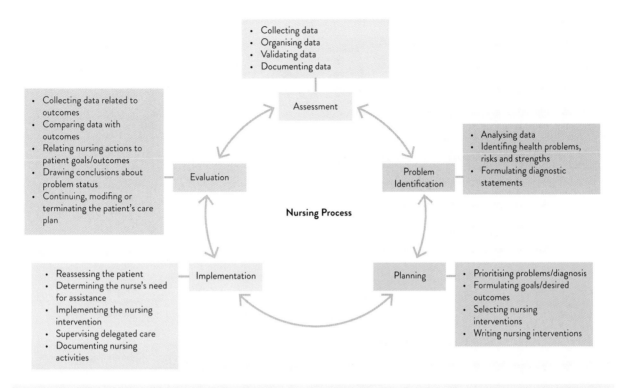

FIGURE 7.4 Components of the nursing process

diagnosing stage, the problems identified may be both actual problems the patient has and potential problems that may arise. These problems can be due to the disease process or from the treatment and care required to assist the client.

Factors that can impact on physical conditions

It is important that you adopt a holistic approach to the assessment of each individual to correctly identify the factors causing actual health problems. Each person reacts differently to factors that contribute to and cause disease, and the care plan needs to reflect the individual's needs along with best practice for treatment of the actual disease process. The causes of disease can be categorised as physical, mental and emotional, and you need to address each component to provide individualised nursing care for the client.

Pathogens

A number of bacteria live in harmony on and in the body and can assist in the healthy functioning of the body. When a pathogen – a microorganism that can cause physical disease – broaches the body's defences and resides and multiplies in other areas of the body, infection occurs. For example, urinary tract infections occur when the *E. coli* bacteria, which resides in the gut, is able to transfer to the urinary bladder where conditions are favourable for growth of the organism.

The human being has a number of defence mechanisms to overcome this invasion but *a susceptible host* (elderly, those with chronic illness, infants) with poorly functioning immune systems becomes ill. The **chain of infection**, as shown in **Figure 7.5**, is the phenomenon of an infection developing through an interactive process involving the host, the pathogen and the environment.

chain of infection
The circumstances of an infection occurring

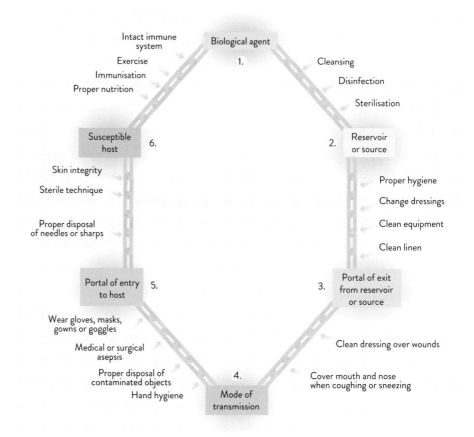

FIGURE 7.5 The chain of infection

Source: Clarke, L., Gray, S., White, L., Duncan, G. & Baumle, W. (2016). *Foundations of Nursing: Enrolled Division 2 Nurses.* ANZ Edition. Cengage Learning: South Melbourne, Figure 20.2, p. 457.

mitochondria
The energy producing structures in the cells of the body

Genetic conditions

Some conditions arise through the inheritance of genetic makeup from parents. **Table 7.5** outlines types of genetic conditions.

TABLE 7.5 Genetic conditions

Type of genetic condition	Disease state caused by genetic condition
Single gene disorders	Inheriting genes that lack a component of a particular gene such as haemophilias (X-linked recessive). Another example of a single gene disorder is vitamin D resistant rickets (X-linked dominant).
Multi gene disorders	A genetic disease where an individual has two recessive genes that give rise to the physical manifestations of a disease process such as cystic fibrosis is known as autosomal recessive.
Chromosomal abnormalities	A genetic disorder where an individual has additional or missing chromosomes. An example is an individual with Down's syndrome.
Mitochondrial inherited disorders	A genetic disorder where an individual has a condition that has resulted in damaged genetic material being used in the reproductive process, such as damaged **mitochondria** seen in cardiomyopathy.
Multifactorial disorders	Due to the interaction of genes and the environment. An example of this is spina bifida.

Trauma, toxins and other environmental hazards

Trauma is a physical or mental injury that can affects a person's health status. It can be a wound, bruise, cut, laceration, lesion or a broken bone that results in a physical injury that can lead to disease or an altered functioning of body systems. Examples of this are fractures where the person no longer can use a body limb (musculoskeletal system) appropriately, or the ingestion of a caustic substance, such as swallowing batteries, that damages the gastrointestinal tract.

7.2 Checking the physical health status of clients

Checking the client's physical health status is one of the most important tasks you will undertake. The human body is in a constant state of change as it tries to maintain a healthy balance. By checking the client's health status the nurse can identify any changes in their health and indicate a need for review of health interventions by the team. Examples of this are seen in surgical patients who require strong pain relief delivered intravenously immediately post-surgery but recover to the extent that a smaller dose of oral analgesia is only required to manage the degree of pain.

Importance of checking client's physical health status before delivery of interventions

Interventions that are developed and implemented need to be continually monitored and evaluated before the delivery of each intervention. If a change has occurred in the health status of the client, if the previous intervention has caused an adverse reaction or if the intervention has not had any impact, it is identified and nursing interventions are replanned and implemented.

Health issues may continue to progress where there are further degenerative changes to vital organs. This will require a review of the current interventions and a new plan put into place. Cancer is an example because it can lead to the loss of normal control mechanisms and the uncontrolled growth of cancer cells.

If the client's health status has deteriorated, it is important to document and report your findings to the supervisor. The client may have other needs, such as increased pain control, that have to be addressed by the team.

FS Numeracy, analysis, technology

Job role and organisation requirements for interventions

The nurse operates and performs interventions that are within their scope of practice and organisational guidelines. At times an organisation may not have the required resources to adequately care for clients in a safe manner. An example of this is when a person is coming back from theatre. It is important that the post-surgical bed and nurse are ready to receive the client.

Depending on their physical health status clients may need to be transferred to another health-care facility or to a different area of the health-care facility. The organisation's guidelines need to be followed and all the required documentation completed to enable smooth transition of the client from one environment to another.

When a specific intervention is ordered for a client you must analyse the requirements of the intervention, the equipment required and the needs of the client. It is important that you recognise the limitations to your practice. The decision-making process that you follow can be found at http://www.nursingmidwiferyboard.gov.au/Codes-Guidelines-Statements/Frameworks.aspx.

 Technology, IT

Clarification of client's physical health status

A number of checking procedures are undertaken before implementing an intervention to ensure safe nursing practice. The nurse considers all the communication that has been documented in the client's file and through verbal handover from other members of the health-care team. This information is then analysed in conjunction with the care plan for the client. If there are any discrepancies further clarification may be required. An example of this is a client who is on a full ward diet, meaning that they can eat and drink as they desire, but is also ordered to undergo a fasting blood test that morning. The nurse must ensure that the patient does not eat or drink till after the blood has been collected.

Clients often experience significant change in their physical health status and as a result their health status requires re-evaluation and nursing interventions adjusted accordingly. For example, a client who has been admitted with exacerbation of asthma may have required support initially with supplemental oxygen therapy. After administration of medications the client may show a marked improvement with their respiratory status and no longer require this intervention.

The nurse accurately monitors the physical health status of the client and communicates the client's health state both in documentation and through verbal reports to other members of the health-care team. The accurate collection and documentation of the client's vital signs in the graphical charts provide a pictorial representation of the client's physical health status.

7.3 Identifying variations from normal physical health status

Variations from normal health status may arise as a result of functional changes that are associated or arise from disease or injury. When undertaking care planning for an individual the nurse will identify both the actual problems that a client has and also the potential problems that may arise for the client and provide nursing care that addresses both. Monitoring and critically evaluating the client and their response to treatment and care is vital.

Identifying variations from normal health status using standard methods and protocols

One of the ways that nurses can identify variations from normal health status is through the constant monitoring of vital signs. An increase in temperature may indicate an infection or inflammatory process occurring within the body. The pulse rate and blood pressure represent the functioning of the circulatory system while the respiratory rate monitors the client's ability to adequately take in and expel air. Oxygen saturation levels monitor the ability of the client to transport blood to and from the cells of the body.

Activity 7.2

The relationship between clinical investigations and assessments

For one of the clients that you are caring for, list the assessments that you are responsible for completing. Then identify what other investigations the doctor has ordered to assess and monitor the patient's condition. This might include blood test results, x-rays and other investigations. Why are these assessments taken?

If the client has received test results, review the results and identify the abnormalities and try to identify the cause. An example may be the client who has a low level of iron stores and has a low Hb level as a result. List two abnormalities and why they have occurred.

All health-care facilities have specific documentation that assists the health-care team in assessing and monitoring a client's physical health status. The nurse is required to complete a number of risk assessment forms that will identify potential problems and body systems that are not functioning within normal levels. These can include but are not limited to the Glasgow coma scale, blood glucose level (BGL) charting, fluid balance charting, skin assessment forms and falls risk assessment/mobility assessments. **Table 7.6** identifies some of the common assessments that nurses undertake to identify variations to physical health status. If any of these assessments show a variation from normal, the nurse must report these to the supervisor or doctor who will then order a more specific assessment test.

Review the skill in Tollefson *Essential Clinical Skills 2.1* Head-to-toe assessment

Reading and writing

TABLE 7.6 Body system, type of assessment

Body system	Assessment	Information obtained	Disease that may be indicated	Skills for assessment
Nervous system	Glasgow coma scale	Assesses the person's conscious state	Brain injury	2.7 Neurological observation
	Reflexes for infants (adults if required)	Assesses neurological function	Brain or spinal cord injury	As described in assessment procedures of the facility for individuals
Cardiovascular system	Pulse	Assesses the rate, volume and pattern the heart is working at	Heart failure Atrial fibrillation Cardiac arrhythmias	2.3 Temperature, pulse and respiration (TPR) measurement
	Blood pressure	Assesses the amount of pressure exerted by the blood on the arterial wall	Hypertension	2.4 Blood pressure measurement
	Electrocardiogram	Assesses the electrical conduction of the heart	Heart failure Atrial fibrillation Cardiac arrhythmias Conduction problems	2.10 12-lead ECG recording
Respiratory system	Respirations	Assesses how often the client breathes in and out. One inspiration and one expiration = one respiration	Neurological function Respiratory disease- COPD, asthma	2.3 Temperature, pulse and respiration (TPR) measurement
	O_2 saturation level	Assesses how much oxygen a single RBC is carrying on each haemoglobin molecule	Respiratory disease- COPD, asthma Anaemia	2.5 Pulse oximetry
	Peak flow measures	Assesses the amount of air the client can move into and out of their airways in one expiration	Asthma	As described in assessment procedures of the facility for individuals
Urinary system	Urinalysis	Tests for abnormal constituents of urine	For all clients	3.8 Urinalysis and urine specimen collection

>>

Body system	Assessment	Information obtained	Disease that may be indicated	Skills for assessment
	Mid-stream specimen of urine	Urine will be collected from the midstream for micro and culture to identify bacteria (a doctor needs to authorise this test)	Suspected urinary tract infection	3.8 Urinalysis and urine specimen collection
Digestive system	Weight	Assesses the person is at a healthy weight	Obesity and nutritional state	As described in assessment procedures of the facility for individuals
	BMI	Assesses if body mass index is within normal levels	Obesity and nutritional state	As described in assessment procedures of the facility for individuals
	Waist circumference	Assesses if the waist measurement falls within normal levels	Obesity and nutritional state	As described in assessment procedures of the facility for individuals
	Stool chart	Assesses if normal bowel motion – usually against the Bristol Stool Chart	Absorption disorders of the gut Constipation/diarrhoea Crohn's disease/IBS GIT bleeding	3.9 Faeces assessment and specimen collection
Endocrine system	BGL measurement	Assesses if blood glucose levels are within normal levels	Diabetes	2.6 Blood glucose measurement
Musculoskeletal system	Gait	Assesses if the person is able to move in normal pattern	Strength and coordination – related to intact joints, muscles and bones	2.8 Neurovascular observation 3.14 Active and passive exercises
	Falls risk assessment	Assesses if the person is at risk of falling	Strength and coordination – related to intact joints, muscles and bones	As described in assessment procedures of the facility for individuals 3.14 Active and passive exercises
Integumentary system	Skin assessment: – Norton – Waterloo – Braden	Assesses whether the person has an intact skins-barrier to infection, maintenance of internal systems	Pressure areas Skin infections Chronic wounds Traumatic wounds	As described in assessment procedures of the facility for individuals
Immune system	Temperature	Assesses if within normal parameters	If the person is at risk of infection or other disease processes	2.3 Temperature, pulse and respiration (TPR) measurement
Lymphatic system	Check for peripheral oedema	Assesses if circulatory system is functioning well. Assesses electrolyte balance	Cardiac failure Hormonal diseases such as Addison's disease	As described in assessment procedures of the facility for individuals

Activity 7.3

Admission and assessment

For the clients you are caring for, review the admission assessments that were made.

1   Were all assessments within normal parameters?
2   If some assessments showed abnormal results, what disease or pathophysiology were they attributed to?
3   What system of the body or function of the body do the assessments relate to?

Potential factors responsible for variations in health status

When a person is assessed, if any of the assessments show a variation from normal parameters it is due to a homeostatic imbalance. This means that the person is suffering from a disease or a malfunction of a body system. This has been outlined in **Table 7.6**. Another term used to describe this is **pathophysiology**.

One of the observations that you must make is inspection of the oral cavity. Tooth decay has been linked with serious cardiac disease and nutritional deficits that can lead to serious disease states. You should note the colour of the oral mucosa, note if teeth are present and intact or have **caries** and what condition the tongue is in.

A normal tongue is moist, pink with small **papillae**, while a person who is unwell may have a swollen, red shiny tongue or one that is coated with a white material known as **thrush**.

pathophysiology
The altered functioning of an organ and the resultant symptomology that occurs in a disease state

caries
Decay of the tooth

papillae
Small projections on the tongue's surface that allow the person to identify the different tastes of food, for example, the sourness of lemon

thrush
Infection of *Candida albicans*

CASE STUDY 7.1

Identification of disease

John, a 46-year-old male, was admitted to the acute medical ward with anaemia for investigation. John told Amelia, the nurse admitting him, that he could not get enough to eat and was constantly eating chocolate bars to give him more energy. John also told Amelia that he felt he was becoming more tired because he could not get a good night's sleep as he constantly had to get up to go to the toilet overnight. Amelia did the routine vital signs assessment and recorded that John's:

–   pulse was 106 beats per minute
–   blood pressure was 90/50

–   respiration was 24
–   O₂ saturation was 95% on room air
–   BGL was 17.6
–   urinalysis showed glucose +++
–   bowel action showed the presence of blood.

1   What disease states do you think that John was showing on admission?
2   What factors are due to the anaemia?
3   What should Amelia do in this instance?

Risk factors associated with variations from normal health status

There have been intensive studies to determine risk factors that are associated with variations from normal health states. Risk factors are those that increase the likelihood of a person developing a disease. There are both behavioural risk factors and biomedical risk factors, as outlined in **Figure 7.6**.

- Smoking
- Alcohol consumption
- Inadequate fruit and vegetable consumption
- Physical inactivity

Behavioural risk factors

- Overweight or obesity
- High blood pressure
- Abnormal blood lipids
- Impaired fasting glucose levels

Biomedical risk factors

FIGURE 7.6 Behavioural and biomedical risk factors associated with variations from normal health states

Review the skill in Tollefson *Essential Clinical Skills*, 7.5 Health teaching

Reading, oral communication, documentation

Authoritative information and statistics to promote better health and wellbeing can be found through the Australian Institute of Health and Welfare at http://www.aihw.gov.au/risk-factors/.

These factors are important to consider when admitting and assessing a person as they offer opportunities for the nurse to provide health education and counselling. Another area that may be affected by these factors is medication administration. It is always important that the client is assessed on an ongoing basis as interventions may cause a change in the level of medication required. An example of this is where the client loses a significant amount of weight through diet and exercise and as a result their blood pressure is lowered. This will require the doctor to alter the prescription of medication that was ordered for the client.

When to refer issues

As a health professional it is important that you undertake tasks and duties within your scope of practice. You are a member of the health team and can refer clients to other members of the team if a client requires a specialist intervention or intervention from a more experienced practitioner. This occurs in all facets of the health-care environment, such as referral to a wound specialist or to a speech pathologist.

Review the skill in Tollefson *Essential Clinical Skills* 7.4 Admission, discharge and patient transfer

The time when a referral is made is important. You should make documented notes regarding any variations from normal functioning of your client as well as reporting the variations to the appropriate member of the health-care team. The organisation will have standard forms, policies and processes to assist in the referral of the client, so that all members of the health team are kept informed and the client receives the appropriate care. Early intervention from the health team may prevent more severe consequences for the client.

When a client is admitted to hospital the discharge planning happens either at the same time or even before admission if it is elective. It is important that the client is referred to the specialist member of the health-care team in a timely manner to ensure that the discharge of the person is not delayed due to inadequate supports being organised.

Documentation

CASE STUDY 7.2

Graham's discharge

Graham was admitted via the emergency department following a fall at home. Graham was 76-years-old and a widower. Graham lived in a first-floor apartment by himself. Before admission Graham was independent and enjoyed taking part in community social activities where he had a number of friends. It was found that Graham felt dizzy on occasion at home but told Adam, his nurse, that he just waited for a couple of minutes before going downstairs. Graham was diabetic and also had been prescribed antihypertensive medication for high blood pressure.

1   What members of the health-care team need to be involved with Graham?
2   What assessments should the health-care team make to ensure that Graham will be safe at home after discharge?
3   Describe the disease processes that Graham has presented with.
4   What post-discharge community supports need to be organised for Graham?

SUMMARY

- Assessment of the client involves observation, questioning and review of documentation to obtain information about their physical health state.
- Observations of clients are undertaken to assess body systems and identify assessments that lie outside normal physiological parameters and are documented to formulate a plan of care for the client.
- It is important to document and verbally report assessments that lie outside normal physiological parameters.

SELF-TEST QUESTIONS

1   When planning care for a client, how can you use the body system assessments to identify actual or potential nursing diagnoses?
2   What nursing actions are required when checking the physical health status of a person?
3   Why is it important to have knowledge of the normal parameters of the systems of the body when undertaking assessment of clients?
4   List the normal parameters for the assessments taken to assess the systems of the body.
5   What factors can impact on the assessment process?

BIBLIOGRAPHY

Australian Institute of Health and Welfare, *Behaviours and risk factors*, http://www.aihw.gov.au/risk-factors/. Accessed 4 March 2017.

Clarke, L., Gray, S., White, L., Duncan, G. & Baumle, W. (2016). *Foundations of Nursing: Enrolled Division 2 Nurses* (ANZ edition). Cengage Learning: South Melbourne.

Gray, S., Ferris, L., White, L., Duncan, G. & Baumle, W. (2018). *Fundamentals of Nursing* (2nd edition). Cengage Learning: South Melbourne.

Nursing and Midwifery Board of Australia (NMBA) (2016). *Frameworks*. Retrieved from http://www.nursingmidwiferyboard.gov.au/Codes-Guidelines-Statements/Frameworks.aspx.

Rizzo, D. (2015). *Fundamentals of Anatomy and Physiology* (4th edition). Delmar Cengage Learning: USA.

Scott, A.E. & Fong, E. (2017). *Body Structures and Functions* (13th edition). Cengage: Boston, MA.

Tollefson, J. (2012). *Essential Clinical Skills* (3rd edition). Cengage Learning: South Melbourne.

Nursing within the Australian health-care system

LEARNING OUTCOMES

After reading this chapter, you should have an understanding of:

8.1   Applying principles and knowledge of nursing practice to work in the health-care system

8.2   Identifying and discussing funding sources for health care in Australia

8.3   Identifying and responding to factors and issues affecting health in Australia

8.4   Working in the context of professional nursing practice

8.5   Contributing to a professional work team

The role of nursing in the Australian health-care system

In the beginning of the course my favourite subjects were those that contained the practical aspects of delivering nursing care. I really felt like a nurse when I mastered the skill of taking a blood pressure reading. As the course progressed we learnt more about how the profession of nursing came into being and evolved to become a profession that met the needs of people and the health-care system that we are part of. I was surprised at the different influences that had affected nursing in Australia, but I was also pleased that I was now almost one of a group of individuals who made up the nursing population in Australia. One of the most interesting things that we learnt was the expansion of the scope of practice for enrolled nurses in Australia and the many contexts that enrolled nursing could now participate in. I had never really given much thought to the influence of politics or finance on nursing but it really opened my eyes to see how nursing is affected by decisions on a national political level.

 This chapter is cross referenced to Gray et al., *Foundations of Nursing 2e*, Chapter 6.

8.1 Principles and knowledge required of nurses in a health-care system

The health-care system is constantly evolving due to political and economic impacts on health-care delivery. The Australian community is also constantly changing due to the increasing numbers of individuals immigrating to Australia. This diversity within communities requires the nurse to constantly evolve their nursing practice and knowledge to encompass non-Western approaches to health and cultural impacts on health.

You must be able to problem solve a diverse number of health needs and to be able to assess if the solution is within the scope of practice of enrolled nursing. To do this you need to be familiar with standards of care and be able to apply these standards to all nursing practice.

Maintaining knowledge of current health issues impacting upon clinical practice and health policy development is vital for nursing to survive and to provide best practice for individuals accessing health-care services.

Principles of primary health and wellness

The aim of primary health care and wellness is to *decrease the risk of disease or dysfunction to a person*. Two key approaches required to achieve this are *health promotion* and *preventative care*, which focus on social, economic and environmental factors of a society that can lead to illness or dysfunction. These two approaches proactively encourage healthy lifestyle habits that increase an individual's wellbeing.

Developing a therapeutic relationship with clients is an important part of both of these approaches to health management. Your assessment of the client will allow you to review their health, identify factors that could lead to ill health, educate, and also refer to other health-care workers or services as required.

Reflective practice 8.1

Primary health care and wellness

All nursing care is undertaken with the goal of preventing further harm to an individual or to improve the functioning of the individual. Choose one nursing intervention that you have undertaken during your placement and identify how you applied the principles of primary health care and wellness promotion. Did you achieve both principles? Why or why not? If you did not include these principles, what could you do next time in your nursing interventions to ensure that you do?

Agencies that facilitate positive health outcomes

The health-care system not only consists of primary health care but also contains secondary and tertiary care facilities.

It is important that the enrolled nurse is able to identify and access appropriate agencies that can address the individual's health-care needs. Early detection of illness and intervention by appropriate health-care workers can facilitate positive health outcomes for the individual. Some individuals may need referral to all three types of health care to address their health issues. An example of this is a person who presents to their local GP and a routine screening test identifies an endocrine imbalance leading to an elevated blood glucose level. The individual has initially accessed primary health care to address his needs but will now require access to secondary care facilities to undertake more specific screening and diagnostic testing and also tertiary care facilities to obtain specialist education from a diabetes educator.

You will need to explain how these health-care facilities can assist the individual and how the person can access them. In order to meet the client's needs you will need to have knowledge of the facilities in the local area and how to complete a referral to these facilities.

Activity 8.1

The different levels of health care

For one of the clients that you are providing care for, investigate what types of health care the individual accessed before being admitted to the current health-care facility.

Sociocultural and social influences that affect health

Australia is a multicultural society with a diverse community of people. There are a number of different cultures present in today's society representing both people who have lived in Australia for many years and others only recently arrived as refugees or migrants. The 2011 Census found that there were over 300 different ancestries within the Australian population. For more information see the Australian Bureau of Statistics at www.abs.gov.au/ausstats/abs@.nsf/Lookup/2071.0main+features902012-2013.

As well as differences in language, different cultures have different beliefs that directly impact on health. An example is a culture that believes it is harmful for a mother who has delivered a baby to take a shower post-delivery. This is in direct opposition to the current practice of health care in Australia. Culture can affect the person's perception of health, the cause of disease and the type of treatments a person will take. The Chinese concept of Yin and Yang is an example of a belief that health is a state of proper balance of hot and cold energy. **Table 8.1** provides some religious beliefs and customs of individuals that influence the person's health-care choices.

TABLE 8.1 Examples of how cultural customs can influence health care

Culture	Cultural customs
Jewish	Views medical treatment positively. Does not countenance suicide or help others to commit suicide. Does not endorse experimental or speculative treatment.
Hinduism	Elders of families have a strong influence on decision making related to health matters. Cultural customs related to birth – father places a dot on the infant's forehead and whispers mantras into the infant's ear. Hindus may request that health-care visitors to the home remove their shoes. Sanctity of life is central to Hindu teachings.
Muslim	Muslims when unwell are happy to receive many visitors. Cleanliness is part of Islamic faith. Where choice exists medicines containing alcohol/pork derivatives should NOT be used. Health professional the same sex as the patient whenever possible.
Jehovah's Witnesses	Accept medical and surgical treatment. Blood transfusions are forbidden but they can accept other blood products such as albumin, immune globulins and haemophiliac preparations. Carry on their person an Advanced Medical Directive/Release.
The place of spirituality and religion in health care	Most Australians have a religious affiliation or spiritual connection. Spirituality/religion is important when a person is ill and rituals can help at these times.

Reflective practice 8.2

Caring for a person from a different culture

Choose one of the clients that you are caring for.

1   What is their cultural identity?
2   Does this particular culture have an impact on health for the person?

Political and economic impacts on health

The Australian health-care system constantly evolves due to the political and economic impacts of society. Because of reforms in Australia, Casemix and Diagnostic Related Groups (DRG) and Activity-Based Funding (ABF) have been developed in an effort to provide a quality and cost-effective health-care service. The impact of these funding models is shown in **Figure 8.1**.

PROFESSIONAL TIP

Impact of DRGs and ABF

* Decreased length of client stay in hospitals
* More emphasis on preventive care
* Increased concern about client's response to care
* Increased number of critically ill clients in hospitals
* Clients sicker upon discharge from hospital
* Increase in outpatient care
* Client and family more responsible for care
* Greater need for home health care

FIGURE 8.1 Impact of DRGs and ABF

Source: Clarke, L., Gray, S., White, L., Duncan, G. & Baumle, W. (2016). *Foundations of Nursing: Enrolled Division 2 Nurses* (ANZ edition). Cengage Learning: South Melbourne, p. 111.

Economic and political changes can mean a change in the enrolled nurse's job role requirements. Working within aged care has seen enrolled nurses now caring for the complex needs of the older person, while a nurse working within an emergency department may be required to cannulate clients presenting to the facility.

At other times health-care services can change due to political pressure from the community. Two examples of this are:
* legalisation of abortion
* costly medications being added to the Pharmaceutical Benefits Scheme (PBS).

Currently new legislation regarding the ending of life is being developed for use in Australian society. See this link for the End of Life and Palliative Care Framework now operating in Victoria: https://www2.health.vic.gov.au/hospitals-and-health-services/patient-care/end-of-life-care/palliative-care/end-of-life-and-palliative-care-framework.

Medications and the PBS

For one of your clients, make a list of medications that have been ordered. Research the list of medications to check if all are on the PBS.

1   What does this mean for the client?
2   What cost applies for PBS medications for a person receiving the aged care pension?

alternative therapy
Therapies used instead of conventional medical therapy

complementary therapies
Therapies used in conjunction with conventional medical therapy

Non-Western approaches to health care and nursing practice

Western medicine traditionally uses medicine, surgery and other technological interventions. In today's society there are many **complementary therapies** that are used with traditional medicine or as an alternative to traditional Western medicine, known as **alternative therapy** (see **Figure 8.2**).

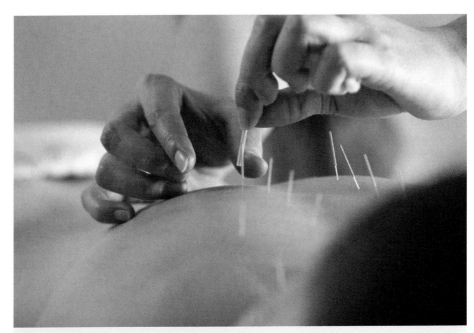

FIGURE 8.2 Complementary and alternative therapies are becoming more popular in today's society

Alamy Stock Photo/Konstantin Shishkin.

TIP 8.1

Complementary and alternative treatments

It is very important when prescribing medication that all complementary and alternative medications are listed for the doctor to review. Some alternative medications can have a strong impact on traditional medicine.

Table 8.2 provides examples of alternative therapies that influence a person's choice of alternative treatments, depending on their cultural beliefs.

TABLE 8.2 Examples of alternative therapies

Alternative therapy	Explanations of alternative therapies in health care
Homeopathy	Therapy is selected on how closely symptoms mirror symptoms of the patient's disease.
Oriental medicine	Harmony between positive and negative energies within the body. Treatment can consist of the following therapies: • acupuncture • herbal medication • oriental massage • energy therapy.
Naturopathy	Aims to treat the mind and body. Treatment may consist of education and cognitive-behavioural approaches such as: • meditation • hypnosis for certain uses • dance • music • art therapy • prayer. These are considered as complementary and alternative to Western medicine.
Biofeedback	Mind-body therapy where patients are taught to control certain involuntary body responses. Used in Western medicine to treat certain conditions such as high blood pressure, incontinence and headaches.
Massage	Manipulation of the tissues of the body to return muscles and tissues to normal states. Used to treat muscular conditions.
Hypnotherapy	Altering a person's state of consciousness. Used by Western medicine to relieve the symptoms of a number of diseases and conditions.

Strategies the nurse can use to maintain standards of care

Practising as a nurse in today's health-care system requires you to maintain current and up-to-date knowledge of different therapies and treatments, to provide education to clients and to contribute to the health-care team in providing input to the client's care plan.

An important resource for the enrolled nurse to ensure they practise within the boundaries of their role is the Enrolled Nurse Standards for Practice (www.nursingmidwiferyboard. gov.au/Codes-Guidelines-Statements/FAQ/Enrolled-nurse-standards-for-practice.aspx). By ensuring their practice reflects these standards, the nurse is able to competently provide best practice care to all individuals accessing the health-care facility.

Other ways the enrolled nurse can maintain currency is through:
• computer research
• reading of journals
• accessing experts
• attending conferences
• attending professional development activities.

Reflective practice 8.4

Changes to work practice

Consider wound care management strategies and describe how nursing practice in this area is undertaken. Try to review what strategies were undertaken 10 years ago. What changes have occurred for this work activity that you are aware of?

Current health issues for health-care delivery

The health of communities is constantly evolving due to changing factors that affect the community and/or the environment that people are living in. Different factors such as immigration involve people with different levels of immunity while local disasters such as leakage of chemicals into the environment can directly impact the health of the community.

When the community experiences a change that affects the health of its population, the government responds by changing health policies and the clinical practice of nursing.

Enrolled nurses had their scope of practice extended initially to give medication and later to include complex nursing care and intravenous medication administration. This came about through policy changes that sought to meet the perceived need of nurses that would be practising in the health-care system in coming years.

Changing technology has resulted in changing medical treatments and interventions requiring you to maintain current clinical practice in order to function using new equipment and approaches.

CASE STUDY 8.1

Caring for people from a non-Western culture

Lynn was an enrolled nurse working on the medical ward of the local hospital. The ward saw many elderly people admitted with a variety of respiratory or cardiac conditions. One of the clients that Lynn was allocated to care for was an elderly woman with end-stage renal failure. Mrs Wong was 86 and had migrated to Australia five years ago from China. Mrs Wong lived with her daughter and family.

Mrs Wong was a tiny woman, not even five foot tall, but had severe oedema in both of her legs. Any exertion left Mrs Wong extremely breathless, even though she had oxygen supplied via nasal prongs at all times. Mrs Wong did not speak English and it required a lot of miming and pointing to communicate in a basic manner with her if her daughter was not present to interpret for her. An interpreter service was sometimes used to communicate with Mrs Wong if the conversation was of a technical nature and her daughter was usually present in such instances.

Mrs Wong had chronic leg ulcers on both of her lower legs and these caused her pain, especially when they required new dressings. Lynn hated causing pain to Mrs Wong and decided to research new dressing materials that might assist in reducing the pain. Lynn spoke to the unit manager who organised a referral to the wound management nurse. The wound management nurse suggested a new dressing that had just recently come onto the market, one that she felt would reduce the number of times the dressing needed to be changed. Lynn asked the wound specialist a lot of questions about

the dressing material and also researched the literature given by the manufacturer. This knowledge assisted Lynn in explaining the changes to Mrs Wong's daughter, who then explained it to her mother. The dressing material was only previously used in very limited cases as it was extremely costly. The government had recently put this material onto the subsidised list so that it was more affordable but it was still restricted and required the doctor to obtain permission to order it.

Mrs Wong's daughter also asked if it was possible for Mrs Wong to take some traditional Chinese medication for pain relief. Lynn was not familiar with this medication but asked Mrs Wong's daughter to provide the name of the medication. Lynn told Mrs Wong's daughter that she would pass on the information to the doctor but that until the doctor approved the medication it would be safest to not give it to Mrs Wong because it may interact with the other medications that she was taking.

1 What wellness principles should Lynn incorporate into her work role when caring for Mrs Wong?
2 What other health professionals did Lynn access for Mrs Wong? Describe how this facilitated a positive health outcome for Mrs Wong.
3 What sociocultural and social influences impacted the health status of Mrs Wong?
4 What political and economic impacts were affecting Mrs Wong?
5 What non-Western approaches did Mrs Wong wish to take and were they appropriate in this situation?
6 What strategies did Lynn employ to maintain standards of care for Mrs Wong?
7 How did Lynn acquire knowledge of new clinical practice?

8.2 Funding sources for health care in Australia

Australia has both a public and private funding system that operates to accommodate the needs of the Australian population. Medicare was introduced to Australia to provide a health-care system that provides care and services to all people in the community. This service is funded in Australia through the tax system, via a levy imposed on everyone that earns a taxable income. Government funding in the public system is based on the Diagnostic Related Groups (DRGs) and Activity Based Funding (ABF) models. ABF is a hospital funding rewarding timely access while delivering both efficient and quality services in relation to the volume of clients and the type of illness or procedure as determined by using the DRG coding system (Clarke et al., *Foundations of Nursing*, p. 111).

Awareness of appropriate sources of funding

Private health-care insurance allows the person to access health services, for non-emergency health care, quicker than that of the public health-care system. A privately insured person can choose their doctor, health-care facility and the services they require.

Private health insurers partner with a variety of health-care providers, such as dentists and physiotherapists. If a person visits one of those partners, they often have a reduced out-of-pocket cost.

There are also many different types of funding that a person may be eligible for, such as veteran affairs, worker's compensation or TAC funding. It is important that the nurse is aware of the type of funding the person is entitled to in order to provide the most accurate costs for the individual and the appropriate services that the person can access as part of their insurance or cover.

To obtain accurate information on costs for a person the nurse may:
- access the business department
- access private health insurance companies
- review the cost of different services.

Some individuals still opt for private health providers regardless of insurance costs so it is important that they are provided with accurate information to enable them to make an informed choice of health care.

Activity 8.2

Health insurances

In your workplace are most individuals funded privately or publically?

   Describe all the types of funding that individuals accessing this service may have.

Discussing health-care services

Individuals in today's Australian society have many ways to access information. Previously the doctor or the nurse at the clinic were the main sources of information, but today the Internet and social media provide a wealth of information that the individual can access.

As a nurse it is important to always have accurate information about the cost of services that the person, family or carer might want to have before making a decision about treatments, facilities or doctors. At times this can be very complicated and often printed literature can provide helpful information. The cost of medical treatment can place a burden upon the person and carer, and it is important that they have current, accurate information in order to make an informed decision.

CASE STUDY 8.2

The cost of hospitalisation

John was a 28-year-old man who had been admitted to the hospital from the emergency department following a car accident the previous night. John had suffered a compound fracture of his right leg and internal bleeding from a ruptured spleen. After being assessed in the emergency department. John had been taken for emergency surgery and was transferred to the intensive care department (ICU).

After a couple of days in intensive care John was able to be transferred to the surgical unit but there were no beds available. John was moved to a private hospital as a public patient. John was worried that this would cost a lot of money that he could not afford. David, his nurse, arranged for John to be visited by the business department. This was not common practice as most of the clients had private health insurance.

John was reassured that he would not face any out-of-pocket expenses as his stay in ICU was in the public system and TAC was funding the bed in the hospital. John progressed well and suffered no complications. Arrangements had been made on John's admission to the public hospital for John to be transferred to the regional rehabilitation centre when he was well enough to go. John was surprised that everything was arranged so quickly but was happy to agree to the plan as it represented a step back to recovery.

1   What funding sources did John have access to for his hospitalisation?

2   What action did David take to give John accurate advice on costs?

3   Why is discharge planned early in the admission of patients?

8.3 Identifying and responding to factors and issues affecting health in Australia

It is important that the nurse working in a community is able to identify factors that may affect health for a range of people and groups. This can mean that health education and health promotion activities are prioritised to meet the needs of the community.

In order for you to develop effective health promotion strategies, risk factors need to be identified for the community and monitoring of effectiveness of the strategies must take place and the strategies adjusted if required.

Factors affecting health

A person's state of health and wellbeing may be affected by a wide variety of different factors as shown in **Table 8.3**.

TABLE 8.3 Factors that affect health

Factors	How they affect the health status
Age	Infants – do not possess the immunity status to combat illnesses Children – prone to falls, accidents, childhood illnesses Teenagers – risk-taking behaviours Adults – fertility issues, stress from workplaces and financial pressures Older adults – the ageing process affects the body's ability to maintain health due to ageing of the organs and body systems
Financial	Individuals may have different financial states that influence: – type of nutrition – accessing preventative or other health-care services such as aged care facilities – medicine or complementary services
Level of education	Awareness of good preventative health-care measures
Language	Access to health-care services and literature
Geographical location	Access to services
Mental health issues	Different awareness of health-care needs due to the mental health issues experienced
Ethnicity	Some cultural groups are more likely to experience specific types of health issues

Reflective practice 8.5

Factors that affect health status

Choose three of the clients you are caring for. Are there any common factors that these individuals have that affected their health status? Do the clients you have chosen have different needs for health care? What strategies would you implement to assist them?

Risk factors for health

When the nurse has achieved a therapeutic relationship that includes families and/or carers' information, risk factors and social circumstances that impact on their health may become known. There are a series of questions that the nurse asks a person on admission to the health-care facility that are designed to identify risk factors for a person's health state. It is important that all the information is documented on the appropriate forms and filed in the person's case notes. This will allow all members of the health-care team access and have input into the care planning of the individual. Usually the admission process can last for 24 hours to obtain all the required information, but the nurse should ensure that the information obtained is entered in a timely fashion.

Existing health services

Health-care services in Australia provide an outline of the services they offer people. In some cases this information is provided through the type of service on offer or the geographical location of the service. The health department for each state or territory will also provide up-to-date information on services that support current health matters and may issue alerts to health situations that arise (for example, 'Bird flu').

Health-care services have both a preventative focus and health promotion focus. The government runs information on health issues through a variety of media forums (see http://www.health.gov.au/internet/main/publishing.nsf/Content/state-health-services.htm).

TIP 8.3

Admission

All sources of information are important to include. Remember the patient's privacy and confidentiality rights. Do not be tempted to skip any areas on the admission form.

Therapeutic communication

Review the skill in Tollefson *Essential Clinical Skills* 7.4 Admission, discharge and patient transfer; 7.5 Health teaching

Reflective practice 8.6

Health promotion

Identify two health promotion campaigns that you are aware of. Does the information have a direct relationship to the health of the people you are caring for?

Effectiveness of community health promotion

There may be a specific focus on a type of health promotion activity in an area or at a specific time (see **Figure 8.3**). It may seem that this health promotion activity is not having an effect

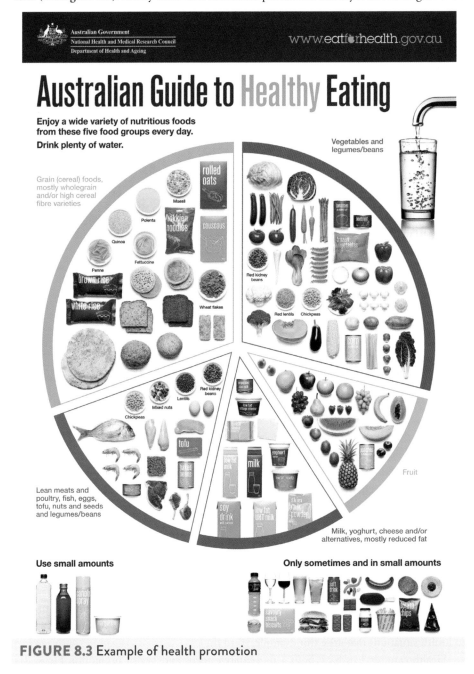

FIGURE 8.3 Example of health promotion

Source: National Health and Medical Research Council. Australian Guide to Healthy Eating, https://www.eatforhealth.gov.au/sites/default/files/content/The%20Guidelines/n55_agthe_large.pdf. © Commonwealth of Australia.

on the behaviour or cause of illness or dysfunction. One way the government can evaluate the effectiveness of the health promotion activity is to keep statistics on the prevalence of a particular health problem in the community.

At other times providing education to individuals on a specific health-care need and re-evaluating how well the person has taken on the desired learning is an area in which nursing may have a positive effect. During a health education session a person may share information that may identify why they are continuing problematic behaviour. You can then provide further education or refer the individual to the health-care professional who can provide more specific education.

Review the skill in Tollefson *Essential Clinical Skills* 7.5 Health teaching

Reflective practice 8.7

Health education regarding antibiotic use

For a while it was identified that individuals who were prescribed antibiotics for infections were failing to complete the course. When people felt better they discontinued the medication. Health promotion activities and education by doctors, nurses and pharmacists have had an effect and now most people are aware of the need to complete the course of medication. Are there any other areas of behaviour that you are aware of that directly impact on the health state of individuals? What strategies are being used to address these?

Emotional and social wellbeing

When considering the health needs of the individual, you should adopt a holistic approach that addresses the emotional and social wellbeing of the individual as well as the physical.

One way to accomplish this is to have patient-centred care planning. The individual is at the centre of all interventions that are planned and implemented. The other way you can address the person's emotional and social wellbeing is to be an advocate for them, ensuring that their rights are upheld.

CASE STUDY 8.3

Emma's story

Emma was a 34-year-old woman who was diagnosed with advanced breast cancer. Emma was aware that she had a lump in the breast but decided to ignore it. The doctor wanted Emma to have a radical mastectomy and chemotherapy. The doctor felt that it would lead to a positive outcome for Emma but she refused this treatment as she believed getting back to nature and eliminating toxins from her environment would be the best way forward.

The doctor could not accept this belief and sent Emma to a psychiatrist for a mental health evaluation. The psychiatrist found that Emma was of sound mind and was able to make decisions as she wished.

Emma discharged herself from hospital and lived in an environmentally friendly community with her partner. Her family were estranged because they had argued that Emma should go along with the doctor's plan. As Emma became more frail the family reunited to a degree that gave Emma and her mother some comfort.

Unfortunately the cancer progressed and Emma lost her eyesight and her ability to ambulate was affected. It was found that the tumour had metasised from her breast to her brain and Emma was experiencing severe pain due to the growth of the brain tumour. Emma went back to hospital for pain relief and wanted to access some traditional treatment to prolong her life. Unfortunately it was too late for treatment to change the outcome but Emma was able to access palliative care. Emma died two weeks later.

1   Is breast cancer a common concern for women in this age group?
2   What health promotional strategies are in place in Australian society to address this disease?
3   What cultural factors impacted on Emma's decision?

8.4 Working in the context of professional nursing practice

It is an exciting time to be a nurse in Australia. Advances in health care, new technologies and changing requirements of the community ensure that nursing is a profession that offers challenges and opportunities for development.

However, it is also important to have an appreciation and knowledge of the history and evolving nature of nursing.

Historical development and current perspectives of nursing

Nursing has evolved to become a scientific profession that is founded on evidence-based theory. **Table 8.4** shows some significant changes that have occurred over time. It can be seen that religion and politics have always influenced nursing.

TABLE 8.4 Nursing throughout time

Period	Types of information
4000 BC	Primitive societies believed illness arose as a punishment from the gods or was a curse
700 BC	Greece: the source of modern medical science
711	Spain: field hospital utilised nursing
1633	Daughters of Charity founded
1811	Sydney hospital founded with convicts as nursing staff
1859	Florence Nightingale's *Notes on Nursing* published in England
1863	Lucy Osburn arrives with four other nurses in Sydney
1902	Royal Victorian Trained Nurses Association founded New Zealand the first country to implement *Nurses Registration Act*
1924	Australian Nursing Federation established
1983	International Council of Nurses (ICN) defined, in a new constitution, two categories of nursing: the first level being Registered Nurse (RN) and the second level, Enrolled Nurse (EN)
1990s	Australian nursing training transferred to the tertiary education sector and delivered at a degree level

Source: Clarke et al. (2016). *Foundations of Nursing*, p. 50.

Nursing theorists

It is important for nursing staff to maintain up-to-date knowledge of nursing theorists and incorporate theoretical concepts related to nursing care into nursing practice. One of the major changes that nursing has seen has been the adoption of evidence-based practice that influences all nursing care provided to clients. Roles and work practices have also changed throughout the years with a move away from task-assigned nursing with rigid routines to nursing practice that places the individual at the centre of the nursing process.

Professional nursing bodies

Nursing has moved away from the image of the nurse being the doctor's helper to the nurse being a health-care professional in their own right. There are a number of regulations and professional nursing bodies that work to ensure that nursing maintains its high professional standard in the community. **Table 8.5** notes some of the professional nursing bodies that are part of the nursing environment in Australia.

TABLE 8.5 Professional nursing bodies

Professional body name	Types of information about the professional body
Australian Health Practitioner Regulation Agency	Governs and registers health professionals Supports the national boards in the role of protecting the public National register of practitioners Accepts and processes complaints about individual practitioners Registration standards and codes and guidelines for the boards Provides advice to ministerial councils
Nursing and Midwifery Board of Australia and Australian Nursing and Midwifery Accreditation Council	Sets policies and professional standards while also addressing complaints about individuals and making decisions about the registrations of individuals Develops the standards, codes and guidelines for the nursing profession Manages complaints, notifications, investigations and disciplinary hearings Assesses overseas nurses for registration
College of Nursing Australia	Provides quality nursing education that prepares the nursing workforce to meet the needs of diverse populations in an ever-changing health-care environment. Provides leadership and representation to political and policy development committees advocating for the nursing profession and the community
Australian Nursing and Midwifery Federation	The national union for RNs, ENs, midwives and AINs established in 1924
Nursing Council of New Zealand	Registration and governance of all New Zealand nurses and education accreditation
International Council of Nurses	Leads nurses internationally to ensure quality nursing care globally through sound health policies and education

Source: Clarke et al. (2016). *Foundations of Nursing*, p. 69.

The principles and parameters of nursing practice

Performing tasks that lie outside the principles and parameters of nursing practice can lead to a variety of problems for yourself, the client and the health-care facility. Utilising the Nurse and Midwifery Board's decision-making framework and ethical guidelines can help you determine if your actions are within the principles and parameters of nursing practice.

Activity 8.3

Code of ethics and decision-making framework

Select one of the policies and procedures that relate directly to your work in the health-care facility. Demonstrate how this policy and procedure uphold the code of ethics and decision-making framework for nurses.

Audits and accreditation processes

Activities that you might be involved with in the workplace are complying with an audit and the accreditation process. All health-care facilities aim to have accreditation which is a way the health-care facility can compare their performance against industry standards and implement continuous improvement activities.

The Australian Council of Healthcare Standards (ACHS) (2016) highlights five key elements to accreditation. These are:

- governance or stewardship function
- a standards-setting process
- a process of external evaluation of compliance against those standards
- a remediation or improvement process following the review
- promotion of continuous quality improvement (for more information visit https://www.achs.org.au/about-us/what-we-do/what-is-accreditation/).

Scope of practice framework

In an effort to assist nurses, the Nursing and Midwifery Board of Australia (NMBA) has released a Standards for Practice for Enrolled Nurses (2016) at http://www.nursingmidwiferyboard.gov.au/Codes-Guidelines-Statements/FAQ/Enrolled-nurse-standards-for-practice.aspx. This ensures that both nurses and the public are protected if nursing actions are maintained within the standards' boundaries. The standards also:

- communicate the standards that can be expected of the EN for the general public
- determine eligibility for registration for enrolled nursing students
- determine if nurses from countries other than Australia meet the requirements of registration
- assess ENs who wish to return to work
- assess competence of ENs (NMBA, 2016).

Reflective practice 8.8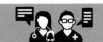

Enrolled nursing standards

Make a short list of some of the activities that you have undertaken as part of your role as an enrolled nurse. Access the enrolled nursing standards of practice.

Did all your actions achieve these standards? Is there any way that your practice could improve?

Role of the nurse

Each client who accesses the health-care facility is an individual and unique in their needs and expectations of what the facility can accomplish for them. It is the role of the nurse to adjust and care for each individual in unique ways.

Health-care environments vary and evolve according to the community's needs. These changes will have a direct impact on the type of activities and role of the nurse. For example, aged care used to be placed within an acute hospital setting and had a number of practices that related directly to the acute setting. A change in the community's expectations that aged care be situated within the community and reflect a home-like environment resulted in facilities being relocated away from the acute facility environment. This had two impacts – first, a number of nursing staff needed to be relocated within the acute hospital and retraining and skill acquisition in acute nursing care for these nurses became a priority; and second, the complex needs of individuals in aged care had risen requiring a greater number of complex interventions to be undertaken in a community setting.

8.5 Contributing to a professional work team

Nursing operates within a team environment that includes a number of other health-care professionals. It is important that nurses can establish collaborative relationships with other members of the health-care team.

Collaborative relationships

By establishing collaborative relationships with all members of the health-care team, the standards of nursing practice and outcomes for individuals are enhanced. The nursing standards reflect the need for collaborative practice.

Establishing collaborative practice includes respecting others, their culture and beliefs. One way that this can be achieved is by addressing team members by their preferred title or name.

Each person in the team has a specific job role. It is important not to duplicate effort as this will result in wastage of resources and may affect the early identification and treatment of the individual's health-care needs.

Activity 8.4

Teamwork

In the health-care facility, identify all the members of the health-care team. What specific role does each individual hold? How does this impact on your role as a nurse?

How reflective practice impacts nursing practice

Reflective nursing practice requires the nurse to analyse and evaluate nursing practice and the individual's response (this is discussed in more detail in Chapter 15). When documenting nursing practice it is important to include this type of reflective practice. This can give more insight into an individual's needs and will assist in adjusting the care planning that the team will undertake. An example of this may be: 'Mrs Jones ordered the correct items off the menu but did not eat all of the meal and stated she did not like some items. A referral has been sent to the dietician to assist Mrs Jones in food selection choices.'

Effective teamwork

When working as part of the team it is important to have group dynamics that support all members of the health-care team. Each team member has a role that is pivotal for the team to effectively meet the individual's needs.

Nursing staff are team members who interact with all members of the health-care team on a regular basis. Nurses can contribute to team effectiveness by modelling supportive group dynamics and professional standards of behaviour to all team members. An example of this is the adoption of cultural safety for everyone in the workplace. Modelling cultural safety involves all staff in the decision-making processes and communicating appropriately with all health-care team members.

CASE STUDY 8.4

Contributing to the team

Joni had just completed her Diploma of Nursing and had been lucky enough to secure a graduate year at a major teaching hospital. On her first day Joni was greeted by the nurse unit manager and introduced to the other members of the team. Joni was surprised at the professional behaviour extended towards her as a new member to the team. Each person identified their role and explained how they contributed to the team. Joni noted that each member of the team, from ward assistant to the consultant, listened to each other without interruption or trying to hurry the interaction.

Joni had initially felt quite nervous approaching other team members, especially more senior members who had a wealth of experience. The nurse unit manager told Joni that everyone who had input or interacted with the client was important. The manager told Joni that she needed to ensure that she communicated regularly and professionally with all members of the team if they were to achieve their objectives.

The following week, Joni was present at the team meeting where all clients were discussed and their progress evaluated. The clients and their family were also present. Each member of the team introduced themselves and their purpose in the meeting for each of the clients discussed. Joni noted that all team members were awarded equal time to communicate in the meeting and that each member addressed the other by their preferred names. Joni noted that the doctor led the meeting and she asked the unit manager why the doctor assumed this role. The unit manager told Joni that it was the responsibility of the doctor on this team to provide leadership and assume responsibility for the team. The unit manager said that this was customary and a result of the responsibility of the job role the doctor held.

During the meeting, specific notes were reviewed to assess clients' progress. Joni was at first nervous when one of her notes was read out. However, the group responded positively to Joni's identification of the need to provide more health education requiring nutrition as a result of the patient ordering certain food groups from the menu that were not the best choices.

1   How did the team promote a collaborative relationship with other members?
2   Describe the importance of the reflective nursing documentation Joni had completed.
3   What strategies were employed to achieve effective teamwork and group dynamics by Joni's work team?

SUMMARY

- Practising nursing in today's health-care system requires you to have the knowledge and skills to employ the principles of primary health care and wellness. The health-care environment is constantly changing due to economic and political impacts.
- The nurse needs to work with the knowledge of funding sources that affect health-care environments to give clients choice over healthcare options.
- You need to be aware of individuals' preferences and culture to meet their needs and protect their rights.
- Nursing practice is always evolving to keep pace with technological and knowledge discoveries.
- The nurse plays an important role in maintaining relationships and group dynamics within the health-care team.

SELF-TEST QUESTIONS

1   What are the principles that underpin nursing practice in the Australian health-care environment?
2   How do cultural and societal factors affect the health and wellbeing of people and the Australian health-care environment?
3   List some of the existing health services in the Australian health-care environment.
4   What skills and knowledge are required to undertake nursing activities in the Australian health-care environment?
5   How does the nurse contribute to the professional work team in the Australian health-care environment?

BIBLIOGRAPHY

Australian Bureau of Statistics (2017). *2071.0 – Reflecting a Nation: Stories from the 2011 Census, 2012–2013.* Retrieved from www.abs.gov.au/ausstats/abs@.nsf/Lookup/2071.0main+features902012-2013.

Australian Council on Healthcare Standards (ACHS) (2016), *What is accreditation?* Retrieved from http://www.achs.org.au/about-us/what-we-do/what-is-accreditation/.

Clarke, L., Gray, S., White, L., Duncan, G. & Baumle, W. (2016). *Foundations of Nursing: Enrolled Division 2 Nurses* (ANZ edition). Cengage Learning: South Melbourne.

Gray, S., Ferris, L., White, L., Duncan, G. & Baumle, W. (2018). *Fundamentals of Nursing* (2nd edition). Cengage Learning: South Melbourne.

Guidelines for health care providers interacting with Jehovah's Witnesses and their families (2005). Retrieved from https://www.kyha.com/docs/PreparednessDocs/cg-jw-rev.pdf.

Islamic council of Victoria (2010).*Caring for Muslim patients.* Retrieved from www.icv.org.au/icvdocs/caringformuslimpatients.pdf.

Myjewishlearning (2018). *Jewish Health & Healing Practices.* Retrieved from www.myjewishlearning.com/article/jewish-health-healing-practices/.

Nursing and Midwifery Board of Australia (NMBA) (2016). *Enrolled nurse standards for practice.* Retrieved from www.nursingmidwiferyboard.gov.au/Codes-Guidelines-Statements/FAQ/Enrolled-nurse-standards-for-practice.aspx.

Nursing and Midwifery Board of Australia (NMBA) (2017a). *Decision making framework.* Retrieved from http://www.nursingmidwiferyboard.gov.au/Codes-Guidelines-Statements/Frameworks.aspx.

Nursing and Midwifery Board of Australia (NMBA) (2017b). *Codes of ethics.* Retrieved from www.nursingmidwiferyboard.gov.au/documents/default.aspx?record=WD10%2F1352&dbid=AP&chksum=GTNolhwLC8InBn7hiEFeag%3D%3D.

Queensland Health (2011). *Healthcare providers' handbook on Hindu practices.* Retrieved from www.health.qld.gov.au/__data/assets/pdf_file/0024/156255/hbook-hindu.pdf.

The Royal Children's Hospital Melbourne (2007). *Spirituality and religion in healthcare practice.* Retrieved from www.rch.org.au/uploadedfiles/main/content/cultural_services/spirituality_staff_resource.pdf.

Tollefson, J., Watson, G., Jelly, E. & Tambree, K. (2016). *Essential Clinical Skills: Enrolled Division 2 Nurses* (3rd edition). Cengage Learning: South Melbourne.

Victorian Government Department of Health and Human Services (2017). *What we do.* Retrieved from https://www.dhhs.vic.gov.au/what-we-do.

Victorian Government Department of Health and Human Services (2018). *Victoria's end of life and palliative care framework.* Retrieved from https://www2.health.vic.gov.au/hospitals-and-health-services/patient-care/end-of-life-care/palliative-care/end-of-life-and-palliative-care-framework. Accessed 13 March 2018.

Working with diverse people

LEARNING OUTCOMES

After reading this chapter, you should have an understanding of:

9.1 Reflecting on own cultural identity and perspectives

9.2 The benefits of diversity and inclusiveness

9.3 Communicating with people from diverse backgrounds and situations

9.4 Promoting understanding across diverse groups

Communication with clients in the health-care facility

I was nervous about my first day at placement in the health-care facility. I had practised all the skills in the nursing lab and felt confident in my ability to undertake these tasks, but I came from another country and English was not my first language. I had found it hard to always grasp what was said, especially in an Australian dialect where people spoke quickly and tied words together. I knew that I could talk and listen but was nervous about making conversation in this environment.

On entering the ward I was pleased to see staff members from diverse backgrounds and during handover was aware of other staff who also were from cultural backgrounds where English was not their first language. I found that my clients were very accepting of my culture. Two of them had suffered a stroke and their language had been affected. I was very pleased to be able to understand what they were communicating as I was used to listening very carefully.

9.1 Reflecting on your own perspectives

Reflecting on our own perspectives helps us understand ourself and also identify differences in others. Being aware of differences within the workplace assists us in gaining the other's perspective and helps to develop **empathy**. This will assist in identifying actions we can take to accommodate differences between people in the workplace.

Social and cultural perspectives and biases

Australia is a multicultural society where 4 in 10 Australians are migrants or the children of migrants, so as a nurse working in this society it is vital to have an understanding of what **culture** is and how it influences your own and your client's perspectives.

empathy
The ability to understand and share the feelings of another person, i.e. 'to stand in their shoes'

culture
Dynamic and integrated structures of knowledge, beliefs, behaviours, ideas, attitudes, values, habits, customs, languages, symbols, rituals, ceremonies and practices that are unique to a particular group of people (DeLaune et al., 2016)

Reflective practice 9.1

Understanding your own cultural identity

Culture as defined above covers a wide range of activities of daily living. **Figure 9.1** outlines some of the factors that can identify a cultural identity. Explain how your social and cultural identity is identifiable through these activities of daily living.

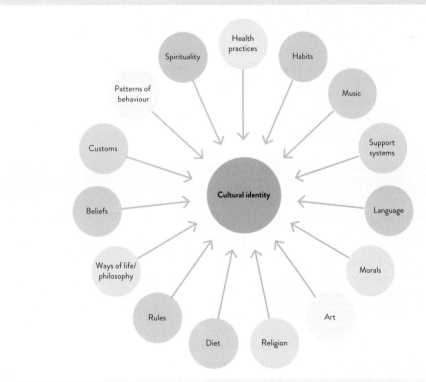

FIGURE 9.1 What makes a cultural identity?

cultural sensitivity
Being aware of differences
between people due to
their cultural identity

Being aware of our own social values and beliefs allows us to identify individuals who hold different values and beliefs. Having a basic knowledge of the health customs of the individuals you are caring for will allow you to put this knowledge into practice within the nursing care of the individual. If this does not occur, the nursing care may diminish or disempower the individual and would not create a safe nursing practice that is person-centred.

Socially and culturally inclusive nursing integrates the following:

1 **cultural sensitivity**
2 **culturally appropriate care**
3 **cultural safety** (Gray et al., 2018).

culturally appropriate care
Providing care that
is appropriate to the
patient's cultural context

Conflict can arise when your nursing care does not incorporate the cultural values and beliefs of the individual. This can be due to differences of verbal and non-verbal communication, accepted forms of courtesy, how you and the individual interact and how you perceive each other.

Activity 9.1

Differences in cultural identity

Choose a client from a different cultural background to yourself.

1 Identify areas of difference in values and beliefs that arise due to cultural differences.

2 What nursing actions can you take to address these differences and demonstrate cultural sensitivity to the person you are providing care for?

cultural safety
An environment that is
spiritually, socially and
emotionally safe as well
as physically safe for all
people within it

Improving self and social awareness

It is important to reflect on your own work practices and interactions with others. When conflict arises between yourself and others, both team members and clients, it is important to take the time to review the situation, understand the factors that caused it to arise and plan actions to address the situation.

The first step to achieving harmony with the other members of the group is to identify and clarify the problem. As discussed previously, reflection is central to this process. Reflection can also come through discussion with other individuals and can be a challenging process.

Reflective practice 9.2

How culture influences feelings and emotions

Think of a situation in which you felt uncomfortable. It may have been an interaction with another team member or a person that you are providing care for.

1 What was the issue that caused this feeling of being uncomfortable?
2 What feelings or emotions did you have in regard to this issue?
3 What perception did you have of the person as a result of this interaction?

How do we identify and act to improve our social awareness and the way we interact with people from different cultural backgrounds? First, it is important to know what are culturally damaging practices. These can include:

- acting without integrity towards individuals from a certain culture
- being critical of people from certain cultures
- lack of trust for people from other cultures
- refusing to listen to other points of view
- not listening or paying attention to people from other cultures

- being argumentative to people from other cultures
- not respecting other people's beliefs or cultural practices
- having no regard for the safety of people from other cultural backgrounds.

There are different ways that a nurse can become aware of behaviours that can lead to culturally damaging practices. This can be in the form of feedback from supervisors or clients. It can be either written or verbal feedback. Often the most effective method to identify social awareness is through the act of reflection.

Once identified there are ways that can be utilised to overcome conflict. These include

- Gather all the facts before making judgements.
- Be open to new ideas.
- Be a good listener.
- Be a good role model for others.
- Deal with the issue not the person.
- Do not bear grudges.

CASE STUDY 9.1

Knowing oneself

Rajpreet, a 23-year-old male student, was undertaking his Diploma of Nursing. Rajpreet had had no previous experience of caring for older people and had mixed feelings about his first clinical placement that was to be undertaken in an aged care facility. Rajpreet had applied to university for entrance to a physical education course. He had been unsuccessful but would be eligible to enter after completing his Diploma of Nursing. Rajpreet had come to Australia from India where he enjoyed an active lifestyle and came from a relatively well-off family. Rajpreet had told the class that physical education was his first preference as he loved sport and all physical activity.

At the placement Rajpreet was very caring and gentle but the clinical supervisor did not feel that he was very happy and, although meeting the objectives of placement, he did not appear to be very engaged. At debrief the clinical supervisor asked the students to describe the clients that they had provided care for. Rajpreet's description was very factual but brief. The supervisor asked Rajpreet how he enjoyed interacting with the clients but Rajpreet replied that he felt he could not engage with the residents as he did not feel they had much in common. Rajpreet in his reflective journal also described how he felt it was demeaning for people in this environment as he felt all they were doing was washing and changing incontinence pads for the elderly residents. Rajpreet did not feel that the residents had any joy or quality of life. Another aspect that the clinical facilitator identified was Rajpreet's dislike of the food and activities that the facility provided for the residents.

1 What cultural perspectives and biases is Rajpreet experiencing in undertaking this placement?
2 How are the cultural differences between Rajpreet and the facility affecting Rajpreet's interaction with residents and his enjoyment of the placement?
3 What could Rajpreet do to identify his own cultural perspectives?
4 What activities could Rajpreet undertake to gain more understanding of the different cultural environment he is experiencing?

9.2 The benefits of diversity and inclusiveness

Society is made up of individuals that are unique in the values and beliefs that they hold. Nurses also are a diverse group with their own values and beliefs. As a nurse all the people you encounter will be unique. This can make nursing a dynamic process, with job satisfaction and enjoyment through interacting with a diverse population. The different types of diversity between people can include:

- sexual preference
- racial and cultural diversity

- religious diversity
- political following
- physical and intellectual ability
- languages other than English.

As a nurse you will encounter clients with a multitude of different values, beliefs and lifestyles. This diversity can enrich the health-care environment and has a positive impact for all people who access the service.

Activity 9.2

Identifying cultural backgrounds

Take a quick survey of fellow students on placement with you.

1 What country did they come from?
2 Where did their parents come from?

Choose a student from a different culture to your own and research their cultural customs. Do they identify with a particular religion and how does this affect their life?

Professional relationships

As a member of the health-care team you will need to apply cultural safety and inclusion to all other members of the team as well as the clients for whom you are caring (see **Figure 9.2**).

Communicate professionally and respectfully with other members of the health-care team and clients. Be aware that stressful situations that arise in the workplace can lead to miscommunication among team members.

When working as part of the health-care team you may identify and form relationships with people who have the same cultural values as you, which can lead to the exclusion of other members of the team and give rise to negative attitudes.

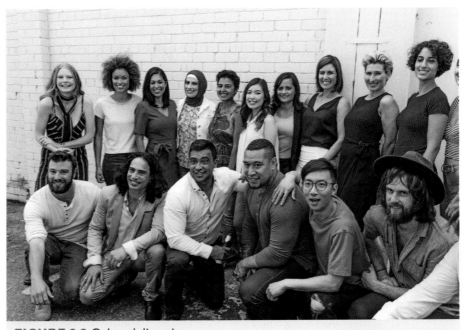

FIGURE 9.2 Cultural diversity

Source: Getty Images/Drazen_

Work practices for a safe environment

An integral component for best practice in nursing is to promote work practices that are culturally appropriate and inclusive. The nurse and other members of the health-care team can promote this by:

- developing cross-cultural work teams
- having different cultures represented on work committees
- reviewing all literature and written material to ensure it is free of cultural bias
- encouraging all cultures represented to participate in the decision-making processes.

Activity 9.3

Avoiding cultural bias and ensuring inclusivity

Choose one of the policies and procedures or a piece of written literature that you use in the clinical health-care environment.

1   How does this document ensure inclusivity and freedom from cultural bias?

CASE STUDY 9.2

Working together as a team

Sumit, a Muslim immigrant, had completed her Diploma of Nursing and had obtained work as an enrolled nurse with an agency that supplied replacement nurses to different aged care facilities and hospitals in a country area.

Sumit was required by her religion to wear a traditional dress and head covering. On arrival at the ward Sumit was ignored by other staff members who were predominantly from an Australian background, despite approaching the team leader and introducing herself professionally. The other staff did not invite Sumit to morning tea or lunch and she was left sitting by herself in the tearoom. Sumit also found that the clients she was caring for were also reticent, and one client yelled at her to get out of his room. Sumit went to the supervisor and explained what had happened. However, the supervisor told Sumit it was her fault and asked what did she expect coming to work dressed the way she did.

Sumit was caring for her clients when she noticed that one of the clients appeared to be having discomfort in the chest region. Sumit took the client's pulse and blood pressure and found that they were outside normal parameters and documented these in the client's notes. Sumit felt nervous approaching the supervisor after what had occurred previously, but knew that it was required. The supervisor heeded Sumit's concern and acted upon it according to the facility's processes. The doctor arrived to review the client and told the supervisor it was fortunate that the condition had been picked up and as a result he could investigate the problem quickly and provide treatment.

At handover the supervisor informed the incoming staff what had occurred for this client but made no mention of Sumit. When Sumit was leaving she informed the supervisor and asked her to sign her form. Sumit was hoping for some positive feedback on her performance but the supervisor made no mention of it and barely acknowledged Sumit. At the end of the shift Sumit reported to the agency that she did not want to return to this facility again.

1   How could the supervisor have made Sumit feel valued and part of the team?
2   What practices occurred that prevented appreciation of diversity and inclusion by the health-care team?
3   Was the workplace a safe environment for Sumit?

9.3 Communicating with people from diverse backgrounds and situations

When communicating with other people it is important to establish a professional or therapeutic relationship. In order to establish a therapeutic relationship, it is important to show respect to the other person (see **Figure 9.3**). The ways in which you can do this will

Review the skill in
Tollefson *Essential Clinical Skills* 7.5 Health teaching

obviously vary depending on the situation, but there are some general rules that apply to all communication interactions:

- Always commence the interaction by addressing the person formally. If the person then tells you to address them by a specific name use their preferred name.
- Listen attentively to the other person and demonstrate that you have understood what they want to communicate. You can use the techniques of active listening to do this.

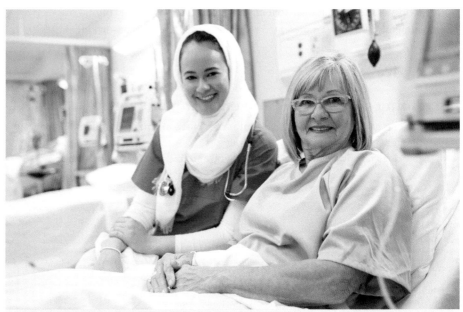

FIGURE 9.3 The therapeutic relationship is based on showing respect to the other person

Alamy Stock Photo/Hero Images Inc.

Reflective practice 9.3

Cultural diversity and communication

Reflect on an interaction that involved communication with a person from a different cultural identity. This could be racial, generational or another type of cultural identity.

1 Was the communication successful?
2 What strategies did you use to ensure effective communication?

TIP 9.1

Interpretation of body language

Do not assume a negative message is implied when communicating with clients from different cultural identities. Always check the cultural norms of the person to get the correct message.

Using verbal and non-verbal communication constructively

When interacting with a person from a different cultural background it is important to use the style of language that the person is familiar with. This may include not using slang words or jargon, speaking slowly and respectfully, and constantly checking that the message has been understood.

Non-verbal communication is also important to interpret correctly. The person may take offence to non-verbal behaviour that is unintentional. An example of this is eye contact. In Australian culture eye contact is important and shows that the other is attentive and listening. In some Asian cultures it may be considered rude and intrusive.

It is also important to note that our own cultural identity causes us to interpret behaviours in certain ways. In the previous example, not making eye contact may be viewed as secretive or showing a lack of interest.

Reflective practice 9.4

Cultural diversity and body language

Reflect on an interaction that involved communication with a person from a different cultural identity. This could be racial, generational or another type of cultural identity.

1 Was the communication successful?
2 What body language did you observe the other person using when communicating?
3 Did the body language you observed match the verbal message the person was sending?

Effective strategies to manage language barriers

At times a nurse may be required to care for individuals who speak in a different language. There are a variety of actions the nurse can take to assist with the communication process:
- ask the client's family to interpret
- use a communication board
- ask for help from other staff members who speak the same language as the client
- use non-verbal communication
- research the culture the person comes from.

TIP 9.2

Communicating

It is important when communicating with a person who does not speak English to maintain a friendly and professional approach. Allow additional time to undertake activities and if appropriate make eye contact and smile. This will depend on the individual's culture. At times the individual may rely on a relative to be part of the communication or may prefer that communication is directed towards this person.

Activity 9.4

Cultural diversity and language barriers

Locate the policies and procedures of the health-care facility that focus on communication with a person who cannot communicate in English.
1 What processes does the health-care facility have in place to manage this situation?
2 Is there a list of staff who can interpret information?
3 When is it appropriate to use untrained interpreter services or family members?
4 How can you gain consent from the person to share personal information in this instance?

Seeking assistance according to communication needs

At times complex communication may be needed. This can arise through explanation of technical testing that may be required or procedures in which the individual must give informed consent to undertake. At this time it is important to seek professional assistance from an interpreter service. Professional interpreters (see **Figure 9.4**) are trained to interpret complex issues and jargon to both parties, to ensure that the individual understands the communication and the communicator is assured that the communication is understood.

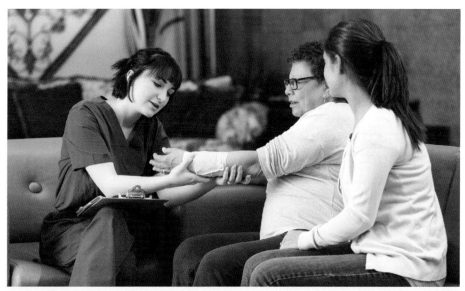

FIGURE 9.4 Interpreters help ensure that communication is effective

Getty Images/Steve Debenport.

Reflective practice 9.5

Communication of complex issues to speakers of other languages

Imagine that you are a patient in a different country. You are feeling unwell and no one speaks your language except for a cleaner who speaks halting English. The doctor and nurse come in and examine you and talk in another language and look serious. The cleaner tells you that you must have an operation.

1 What are some of the feelings you might have?
2 Can you give informed consent in this situation?
3 Has the nurse fulfilled their duty of care towards you?

CASE STUDY 9.3

Communicating with people from other cultures

Jason was a graduate enrolled nurse who had obtained his first position in an acute hospital in a major city. Jason was excited about his position and had researched the types of conditions and the population of the people who accessed the health-care facility. Jason noted that the hospital had a large number of newly arrived immigrants from China. Jason did not have any experience dealing with this population and did not know a lot about their culture. Jason decided to do some research on Chinese culture so that he could be prepared. Jason found that there was a lot of cultural differences between the Australian and Chinese ways of life.

In the ward to which Jason had been allocated a new client arrived. The client was an elderly man, who was being admitted for wound management for a large ulcer on his left lower leg that had not healed despite community visits from a nurse. There were notes about alternative treatments that the client had undertaken to try to heal the ulcer but it had not responded, and unless a good vascular supply could be established the prognosis was looking poor with a likely outcome of amputation.

Jason introduced himself but found that the gentleman did not make eye contact or verbally respond to him. Jason was told that the man had no English and that his daughter would be in shortly to interpret for him. His daughter was currently down at the office completing the administrative admission forms for her father. When his daughter arrived she told Jason that her father preferred to be addressed quite formally.

Jason knew from his research that this client did not like to be touched physically and decided to wait for his daughter to arrive to assist in settling the man into the ward. The doctor came and told Jason that he had

>>

ordered a series of tests to assess the vascular supply to the leg. The daughter came in and Jason introduced himself and assisted her to help undress and place the client into the bed. Jason found that the client responded well to body language signs and was more independent than Jason had first imagined. Due to the complexities and the need to gain informed consent, Jason discussed with the supervisor the need to obtain a professional

interpreter to relay the information about treatment and likely outcomes.

1   How has Jason demonstrated respect for cultural diversity in his communication with this client?

2   What strategies did Jason employ to achieve effective communication?

3   Was it appropriate for Jason to book a professional interpreter for this client?

9.4 Promoting understanding across diverse groups

A large component of nursing revolves around communicating with others. It is important that the messages being relayed between health-care team members, as well as between the nurse and the client, are understood correctly. In order to implement nursing care to best practice, the client and the health-care team all need to work together.

Issues that may cause communication misunderstandings

To avoid conflict when delivering or planning nursing care with individuals from another culture it is important to have an understanding of the person's culture, their view of health, how they express their emotions and what type of treatment is considered appropriate.

Other areas that can give rise to conflict are age, gender, level of education and socioeconomic status. Language is an obvious area where misunderstanding can occur, but without knowledge of the person's culture communication will not be effective.

Reflective practice 9.6

Misunderstandings

Consider caring for a person who is from a different generation but shares the same language and cultural identity as yourself. Your role is to educate the client, who is an 83-year-old man, on how to improve their health through restricting their fluid intake. The gentleman is deaf and requires glasses to see. You note

that the person was at sixth grade level when they left school to work as a truck driver for the local dairy.

1   Will they understand the words or concepts that you are trying to communicate?

2   What changes will you need to make to your communication with this person?

The impact of social and cultural diversity

Ethnocentrism is judging another culture solely by the values and standards of one's own culture. It is the belief that our culture is superior and that we are always right. It creates a divide by creating an 'us and them' mentality, and you need to be aware that people may live with different rules and priorities. At times when conflicts arise it may be necessary for you to take a step back and listen carefully to

TIP 9.3

Dealing with conflict

Do not get drawn into an argument with individuals. It is important to listen to what they are telling you. At times they may be giving you mixed messages, so you need to listen and watch their body language.

the individual to understand their point of view. Caring for people means creating a person-centred approach to nursing care. This will involve conducting interventions in a manner that is culturally acceptable for the person and you may need to accept practices that you believe are not the best.

Activity 9.5

Cultural beliefs and practices

Choose one of the clients you are caring for who identifies with a different culture and research cultural norms for this person.

1   Are there any cultural practices that are different to those of which you are aware?
2   Describe what impact these cultural differences make to the nursing care plan.
3   Are there any that you do not believe are 'right'? Give reasons for this belief.

Resolving differences

When differences do arise in the workplace, it is important to address the issues in a manner that supports the cultural safety of the person. Often differences or conflict can occur when communication is not effective or when interventions clash with a person's cultural beliefs.

It is important to be empathetic and remember it is an issue of difference not a battle where one person will be the winner.

TIP 9.4

Seeking
assistance

It is important to
remember that there
are no 'silly' questions
and the supervisors are
there to assist you.

Who should you refer difficulties to in the workplace? The most appropriate person to address any difficulties is the supervisor. The clinical educator is available to offer suggestions and support and you need to pass relevant information to them in order for the supervisor to support you.

When should you seek assistance? It is important to always seek assistance early. If there are any difficulties or misunderstandings then seeking assistance early may resolve the situation before conflict arises.

Activity 9.6

Dealing with difficulties

Describe the processes that are in place in the workplace for you to access when difficulties arise.

1   How do you contact the supervisor?
2   What documentation should be completed if there is a cultural difficulty in providing nursing interactions?

CASE STUDY 9.4

Difficulties with caring for a person with a different cultural identity

Susan found that she had been assigned to an aged care facility whose catchment area consisted of migrants from Asian cultures. The health-care facility provided both respite and long-term care to residents.

On arrival at the health-care facility, orientation consisted of a physical inspection of the facility and time to read the policies and procedures. At morning tea time Susan was assigned to Jessie, an experienced enrolled nurse who specialised in palliative care. Jessie explained that many of the families who had relatives in the facility held quite different health beliefs and practices.

>>

Jessie told Susan that they would need to communicate with both the residents and their families.

Susan was excited to be taking part in this activity and when one of the families came to visit their relative was eager to participate in the communication process. Susan smiled and introduced herself but felt confused when the client and her daughter refused to look at her. Susan had prepared well and had researched a variety of material for cultural care for clients from an Asian culture. Susan had gathered information on the aged care facility and how it could assist in maintaining a client's independence.

When the daughter came the next day to visit her mother Susan was disappointed to see that the pamphlets were still in the same envelope she had placed them in. Listening to the daughter Susan felt that the daughter had not taken on board any of the information contained in the pamphlets. Susan felt that the client and her daughter were withdrawn and reluctant to interact with her. Susan decided to talk through the situation with Jessie.

Jessie asked to see the pamphlets and found that, while they were recommended by the government and were in English they only addressed a Western dietary intake.

1   What issues in the above situation could cause communication misunderstanding or other difficulties?
2   What impact did social and cultural diversity have on the interaction of Susan and the client?
3   How can Susan resolve the difference she encountered, taking into account diversity considerations?
4   Should Susan have addressed the situation herself before liaising with Jessie?

SUMMARY

- It is important to reflect on your own perspectives to identify any social and cultural perspectives and biases to work inclusively and with understanding of others.
- Making the workplace safe for all who access it demonstrates the desire to create an environment that values and respects diversity and inclusiveness.
- Communication is essential in order to develop a therapeutic relationship with clients. It is important to develop strategies that can be implemented to assist with communication with people where language is a barrier.
- To identify issues that can lead to misunderstandings it is necessary to consider the cultural and social diversity of the individual.

SELF-TEST QUESTIONS

1   How does the practice of reflection assist the nurse to work inclusively and develop better understanding of others?
2   What work practices make the work environment safe for all?
3   How can the nurse use verbal and non-verbal communication to establish mutual trust and confidence in the workplace?
4   What social and cultural diversities lead to misunderstandings in the workplace?
5   What are two strategies that a nurse could use to communicate with people who have a language barrier?

BIBLIOGRAPHY

Australian Bureau of Statistics, http://www.abs.gov.au/. Accessed 9 January 2017.

Clarke, L., Gray, S., White, L., Duncan, G. & Baumle, W. (2016). *Foundations of Nursing: Enrolled Division 2 Nurses* (ANZ edition). Cengage Learning: South Melbourne.

DeLaune, S.C., Ladner, P.K., McTier, L., Tollefson, J. & Lawrence, J. (2016). *Australian and New Zealand Fundamentals of Nursing* (revised edition). Cengage Learning: South Melbourne.

Gray, S., Ferris, L., White, L., Duncan, G. & Baumle, W. (2018). *Fundamentals of Nursing* (2nd edition). Cengage Learning: South Melbourne.

Health and Human Services (2017). *How to work with interpreters and translators. A guide to effectively using language services*, https://dhhs.vic.gov.au/file/2351/download?token=hp9cTBWx. Accessed 5 April 2017.

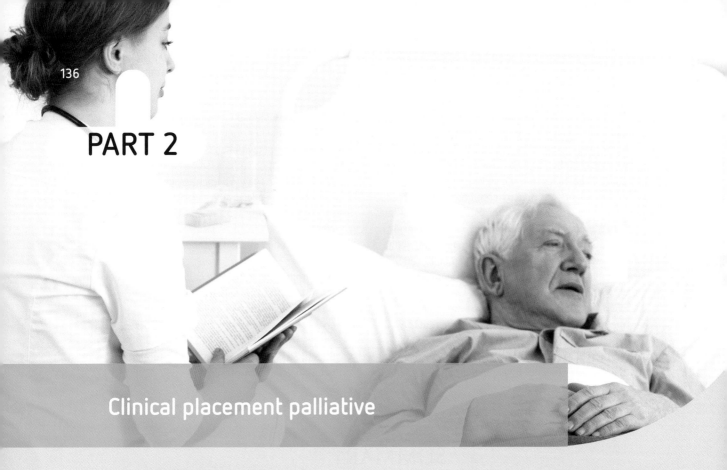

PART 2

Clinical placement palliative

Chapter 10: A palliative approach to nursing practice

The palliative care experience

To be honest, I was not at all looking forward to my palliative care placement. I was allocated to a hospice and my initial thoughts were it was just going to be standing around, with no real 'care' to be given. I cannot emphasise how wrong I was. On my first day, I think I had a case of 'bored face' as I assumed I knew all about palliative care – as in, how hard can it be? I was incredibly lucky, and my buddy nurse was obviously well used to students not understanding what palliative care 'is'. She took me aside, and she asked me what I thought end-of-life cares were, and what I thought was going to be nursing roles in a hospice. My responses were so far from the reality. I do not think I have ever learnt so much about a specialty before on this placement. I learnt not only about death and dying, but also about communicating effectively, providing support and comfort, and caring for an entire family who are all losing a loved one. I had patients so clearly tell me that it was okay that they were dying. Some days I left feeling so incredibly tired – tired emotionally as I had to wrap my head around the concept of death and being so brave when facing it like my patients were. By day three I was feeling so incredibly privileged to be a part of someone's death. I learnt the importance of listening, and of what it means to nurse a patient to their end of life. I worked with amazing nurses, who had all worked in palliative care for a very long time. One nurse was still 'new' having only worked in palliative care for 18 months. It was very interesting discussing the learning curve with them. It is absolutely a specialty I want to work in. I never had even considered it, figuring it was only for the elderly and was not really much work or interesting. My youngest patient was 28. And every day I went into placement wondering how each of my patients were and what the day would bring. It is a very rewarding aspect of nursing.

Your palliative care placement will generally be towards the end of your diploma. It will enable you to consolidate your learning from many subjects, such as complex, chronic, and of course, palliative care.

What is palliative care? Palliative care encompasses a large patient population and involves care of patients who have a life-limiting illness. Some patients who are palliative will receive their end-of-life care in an acute care facility, such as a hospital, while others may be in hospices or at home or in community settings.

What kind of patients are in palliative care facilities?

Palliative care is required by people of all ages. It is often delivered in the ward environment, for example, a patient may have an operation performed, such as a bowel resection, and suffer several complications post-operatively. The focus of care then turns from acute care to palliative care as the patient has conditions that are no longer curable. The focus of palliative care is not the model of curative medicine – it is focused on end of life.

In a hospital environment the patients you will come across will have a variety of illnesses or diseases that have contributed to their end of life. Cancer is a common cause of palliative care requirement. You will need to perform a thorough assessment of the patient and their family to determine their wishes, needs and expectations. Palliative care almost always has a specialty team in an acute care facility who will assist you in this process, and it is common for end-of-life pathways to exist to ensure that the patient care is holistic.

Common experiences of student nurses in palliative care

Palliative care is different for every patient. No two patients will have the same death, and this is why palliative care focuses on holistic health care. Your assessment will be of basic needs – nutrition, comfort, pressure area care and hygiene. The process of death has a different time frame for every patient, but you will soon see that there are signs of imminent death that are observable as the physiological processes shut down in the body.

Palliative care can be confronting as end-of-life care focuses on death – it is not a curative approach. Some patients are very much accepting of their imminent death, while others are not. Death affects everyone differently – including nurses. You will see death in this placement, and you will likely see the effects of that death in the form of grief in the relatives and loved ones. You will soon notice that you are caring not just for the patient, but also the family.

Palliative care will also have legal and ethical principles to consider – such as organ donation, advanced health directives and not-for-resuscitation orders.

Objectives

The objectives for this placement need to be contextualised to the palliative care setting, for example:
* how to identify the needs of the person, family or carers during a palliative approach to health care
* ethical and legal issues relating to a palliative care approach including decisions regarding advance care directives, conflicts that may occur in relation to personal values, and decisions made by or for the person, including organ donation and a request for an autopsy
* hydration and nutrition requirements during palliative care and at end of life
* pain management
* impact of loss and grief on the person, family or carers, and staff members.

Work allocation

In palliative care, often the same patients are allocated to a single nurse for several shifts in a row. Team nursing is not commonly used in palliative care to ensure continuity of care. Allocation takes into consideration the needs of the patient; for example, if they have many interventions and have not received adequate pain relief, then the nursing acuity is higher. Palliative care also takes time – time for listening and letting the family and the patient talk about their wishes, their life or their memories.

The student may administer medications if the unit HLTENN007 has been completed and the student is supervised. For more complex management there will be a registered nurse who will undertake specialised activities. All enrolled nurses and support staff work under the supervision of a registered Division 1 nurse.

Enjoy your placement and ensure you make good use of the valuable time you have with this specialty in nursing practice.

A palliative approach to nursing practice

LEARNING OUTCOMES

After reading this chapter, you should have an understanding of:

10.1 Recognising the special needs of a person requiring a palliative approach to care

10.2 Supporting the person, family or carers using the palliative approach

10.3 Identifying and responding to signs of deterioration and the stages of dying

10.4 Caring for the person's body after death and providing support for the family and others

10.5 Providing for your own self-care in palliative care role

A dignified death

I was very apprehensive when I was told that my next clinical placement would be on the palliative care ward. I had never seen a person die and the only funerals I had attended had been for my grandfather who was elderly and had been ill for a long time.

On the first day I tiptoed quietly after my buddy and was very nervous even touching one of the clients in case I caused them to die. One of the clients I was involved with was Eileen.

Eileen was an elderly person in the palliative care ward. During her final weeks she required oxygen for breathing difficulties and medication for pain relief and anxiety. The nurses were all aware of Eileen's advance care plan and accepted her refusal of any lifesaving treatment to allow her to die a dignified death. They provided comfort care to Eileen and her family and she died surrounded by her loved ones.

The nursing staff had all got to know Eileen during her stay and at the debrief session they exchanged many tearful hugs and talked about their feelings. Although Eileen's death was upsetting, in Eileen's case she appeared comfortable and did not die alone. This helped everyone cope with the experience. I felt privileged to care for Eileen and her family.

10.1 The needs of a person requiring a palliative approach to care

As a nurse you may be required to care for people who need palliative care. This specialised field of nursing aims to enhance the client's quality of life and positively influence the course of illness by treating pain and physical, psychological, social and spiritual problems in a holistic manner. Palliative care incorporates a positive and open attitude towards dying and death by the palliative care team.

Palliative care relieves the physical and mental distress of the dying person. Palliative care can be defined as:

> An approach that improves the quality of life of patients and their families facing the problem associated with life-threatening illness, through the prevention and relief of suffering by means of early identification and impeccable assessment and treatment of pain and other problems, physical, psychosocial and spiritual.
>
> World Health Organization (2002).

Principles of palliative care and the palliative approach

palliative approach
Meeting the needs of the whole person at the end of life – mental, emotional, spiritual relationship and environmental, as well as physical

A **palliative approach** is not simply confined to the final stages of an illness. It acknowledges that the quality of life of a person with a **life-limiting illness** can be maintained by early identification, assessment and treatment of pain, and by meeting the person's physical, cultural, social, psychological and spiritual needs. A palliative approach is taken when a person is moving towards the end of their life and there is no likelihood of extending life by curative means.

life-limiting illness
An illness that is expected to cause death

It is important to apply the principles of a palliative approach when supporting people with life-limiting conditions so that their holistic needs are met including their pain and comfort levels. This will enable them to experience the best quality of life until their death. Consideration must also be given to families and carers to ensure that they have the information and support needed to support the person in palliative care and their wishes.

The *National Palliative Care Strategy 2010 – Supporting Australians to Live Well at the End of Life* (the Strategy) represents the combined commitment of the federal, state and territory governments, palliative care service providers and community-based organisations to the development and implementation of palliative care policies, strategies and services that are consistent across Australia (Australian Government Department of Health, 2010). **Table 10.1** outlines the goals of this strategy.

TABLE 10.1 Goals of the National Palliative Care Strategy 2010

Goal	Description
Awareness and understanding	• To significantly improve the appreciation of dying and death as a normal part of the life continuum • To enhance community and professional awareness of the scope of, and benefits of, timely and appropriate access to palliative care services
Appropriateness and effectiveness	• Appropriate and effective palliative care is available to all Australians based on need
Leadership and governance	• To support the collaborative, proactive, effective governance of national palliative care strategies, resources and approaches
Capacity and capability	• To build and enhance the capacity of all relevant sectors in health and human services to provide quality palliative care

Source: Australian Government Department of Health (2010). *National Palliative Care Strategy 2010 -Supporting Australians to Live Well at the End of Life.* Retrieved from http://www.health.gov.au/internet/main/ publishing.nsf/Content/EF57056BDB047E2FCA257BF000206168/$File/NationalPalliativeCareStrategy.pdf.

Pathophysiological changes

In most people with a life-limiting illness, death is a consequence of systemic changes rather than the failure of a single organ. **Table 10.2** lists the common symptoms and pathophysiologies that are present in the palliative patient.

TABLE 10.2 Symptoms and pathophysiology

Symptom	Pathophysiology
Pain	Space-occupying lesions causing inflammation Bone pain causing nerve root compression or muscle spasm Abdominal distention from ascites or solid masses Constipation
Dyspnoea	Lung congestion, pleural effusion and pericardial effusion or tamponade
Anorexia, nausea, vomiting	Chemical abnormalities due to drugs or infection, impaired gastric emptying, obstruction, enteritis
Anxiety and depression	Response to the stress and worry associated with a terminal illness

Source: Krause, R. (2015). *Palliative Care in the Acute Care Setting, Emergency Medicine.* Retrieved from http://emedicine.medscape.com/article/1407757-overview#a2.

Pain management

Pain is the most common symptom of a person who is in the terminal phase of life. Pain that is not well controlled causes significant distress and disability, therefore the effective management of pain is a vital part of palliative care practice. Pain is managed best by a process of assessment, intervention using a range of drug and non-drug therapies, and evaluation of their effectiveness.

Types of pain

Understanding how pain is defined is important in order to learn how to better control it. Acute pain is defined as pain lasting less than three to six months, or pain that is directly related to tissue damage such as post-surgery. Acute pain disappears when the underlying cause of pain has been treated or has healed. Chronic pain results from chronic pathological processes, often has a gradual onset and becomes progressively worse. The person may appear depressed, withdrawn and lethargic. Treatment for chronic pain requires determining the underlying cause and providing pharmacological or non-pharmacological management.

Because pain is a subjective symptom, the most accurate evidence of pain is based on the person's description which may include aching, burning, heaviness, sharp 'pins and needles', tingling or tightness. The person may also experience nausea, vomiting, anorexia or dyspnoea due to pain.

Problem-solving skills

Pain assessment tools

Effective pain management requires careful assessment and regular review. Since pain is a subjective symptom, pain assessment tools are based on the person's own perception of their pain and its severity. A pain assessment tool gives a baseline from which to evaluate treatment interventions. It also gives the person a more active role in describing and dealing with their pain.

TIP 10.1

Signs of pain

Look for non-verbal clues to indicate discomfort or pain in the patient who can no longer speak. This includes restlessness, furrowed brow, and grimacing, crying or moaning and stiffened posture. Physiological signs that may indicate pain can include elevated blood pressure or rapid pulse.

Pain assessment tools include:

- Numerical Rating Scales (NRS), where numbers are used to represent the strength of the pain with 0 representing no pain and 10 representing severe pain (see **Figure 10.1**).

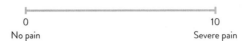

0
No pain

10
Severe pain

FIGURE 10.1 Numerical rating scale

- Abbey Pain Scale, which is an Australian-developed tool for people with dementia. Scores are totalled for vocalisations, facial expressions, and physical and psychological changes, with a score of 7–10 being assessed as severe pain.
- FACES Scale, where a number of faces are shown on a scale from a smiley face to a crying face (see **Figure 10.2**). This is useful for people who cannot verbalise their pain and in particular younger persons.

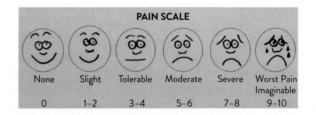

FIGURE 10.2 Wong-Baker FACES pain rating scale

Source: Wong-Baker FACES Foundation (2018). Wong-Baker FACES® Pain Rating Scale. Retrieved 21 November 2018 with permission from http://www.WongBakerFACES.org.

- Pain Assessment in Advanced Dementia (PAINAD) Scale, which is a pain behaviour tool used to assess pain in older adults who have dementia or other cognitive impairment and are unable to reliably communicate their pain.
- Brief Pain Inventory (BPI), which is a nine-item self-administered questionnaire used to evaluate the severity of a person's pain and the impact of this pain on the person's daily functioning.

Pharmacological management

The most common medications in palliative care are opioids – morphine and lesser-strength drugs including codeine and paracetamol for mild pain. One of the major considerations when opioids are used is that in the elderly liver and kidney function is reduced, which causes opioids to accumulate in the body with a higher chance of side effects. The use of multiple drugs in the elderly can also interact with opioids causing adverse reactions. Therefore, the use of opioids in the elderly requires caution and review.

Morphine can be given in a number of forms, including tablets and liquid, injection or via patches on the skin. When the person is approaching death and is unable to swallow morphine and other drugs, they may be given via a syringe driver, which is a battery-operated pump that provides a prescribed amount of medication continuously via a needle that has been placed under the skin.

Non-pharmacological management

Non-pharmacological approaches are increasingly playing a role in pain management. These approaches, such as complementary therapies, are being used in conjunction with analgesics to help support the holistic care of the person. Management may include:

- counselling
- positioning
- massage/relaxation techniques
- aromatherapy
- naturopathy
- therapeutic touch/Reiki/reflexology
- herbal/traditional Chinese medicines
- music therapy
- meditation/hypnotherapy
- acupressure/acupuncture.

CASE STUDY 10.1

Pain management

Brian was diagnosed with pancreatic cancer and was admitted to the palliative care unit with jaundice, uncontrolled pain, nausea and vomiting. A continuous subcutaneous infusion of morphine and anti-emetic was administered which provided relief.

The nursing staff regularly assessed Brian for signs of distress and agitation, which were controlled with additional doses of medication. As his disease progressed, Brian became increasingly withdrawn and no longer communicated verbally. He died a few days later.

1 What are the side effects of morphine and how can they be reduced?
2 What alternative opioids can be used for palliative patients?
3 How is anxiety reduced for palliative patients?

Social, emotional and spiritual needs

The palliative patient experiences physical and psychological stresses during the dying process. As the person moves through the stages of grieving they may experience anxiety, anger and depression. The way in which they exhibit or share their feelings will vary according to their spiritual, cultural and religious beliefs (https://www2.health.vic.gov.au/hospitals-and-health-services/patient-care/older-people/palliative/palliative-emotional).

Social and emotional supports for the palliative patient include:

- counselling and grief support
- assistance for families to discuss issues
- resources such as home-care help and equipment
- referrals to respite care services
- financial support services.

Spiritual and cultural support is also essential to a palliative approach and may help give access to rites and rituals that offer symbolic meaning to the palliative person. This will vary depending on the ethnicity, gender, social class and personal experiences of each individual. Spiritual support can be given by nurses through encouraging the person to reflect on parts of their life which are meaningful and allowing expression through prayer, meditation, rituals or any other activities that provide spiritual or religious connectedness. Spiritual and religious needs are an important part of the care plan, and should be reviewed regularly so that preferences and goals are met. All people are individual and unique. The dying person has lived a life that includes social, cultural and religious/spiritual beliefs. It is important that

Review the skill in Tollefson *Essential Clinical Skills* 3.11 Patient comfort – pain management (non-pharmacological interventions – heat and cold)

nursing care addresses these needs of the person during the dying process. This can also be important for the family/carer at this time and provide comfort and support to the person and their family/carer.

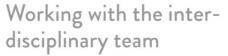

Activity 10.1

Applying a palliative approach

Choose a client that you have been caring for in the palliative environment.

1   How are their physical needs being met?

2   How are their social, emotional and spiritual needs being met?

3   Are there any additional needs that need to be addressed?

Listening

Collaboration

Working with the inter-disciplinary team

In delivering palliative care, the principle that nurses spend time with, and be available for, patients and their families as well as discussing and planning care within a multidisciplinary team framework should be included. The family and carers form part of this multidisciplinary team, with each having a role in providing holistic support for the palliative patient.

The health members of the multidisciplinary team are shown in **Figure 10.3**.

Psychosocial impact of palliative care on family and carers

Supporting family and carers of the dying person is an important aspect of end-of-life care – for both patients and their families. There are considerable psychological and emotional burdens for family members and carers when decisions need to be made or when the physical signs of dying are present.

Show respect for their needs by being inclusive, open, honest and available for them when they need you. Meetings may be organised to facilitate communication and decision making, and to support families and carers to identify realistic care goals, while also assisting them to deal with their own distress. Meetings also ensure that important information is relayed regarding the ongoing care of their loved ones. This information may include:

*   referral to a palliative care unit
*   discussion about disease progression
*   discussion about the patient's wishes for treatment
*   changes in the patient's condition with reassessment of goals.

It is important for the nurse to get to know family members and carers and include them in all communications and care decisions. By making them an integral part of the team and forming a relationship, you are more able to provide emotional and spiritual support, information about care and management, support during decision making on end-of-life issues, as well as support after the person's death.

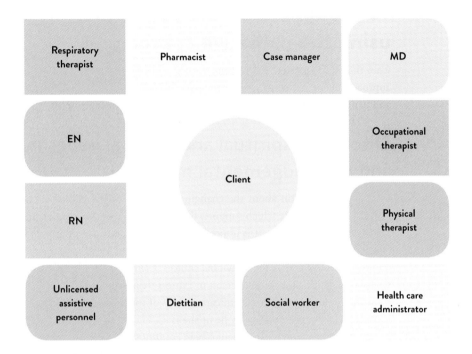

Responsibilities of the team include:
- Pain management and management of other symptoms such as depression and anxiety.
- Management of issues relating to nutrition and hydration because the person may stop eating and drinking towards the end-of-life.
- Support regarding advance care planning, i.e. planning and documenting the person's wishes for his/her end-of-life care.
- Education of the person and significant others in relation to the disease process and ensuring that they are fully informed about the likely path that the disease will take.
- Support for increasing disability, e.g. providing additional personal hygiene and toileting support; use of mobility aids when no longer able to walk.
- Spiritual support for the patient, carers and family as they proceed towards the end of the person's life.
- Support to ensure the patient, carers and family have access to bereavement care, referrals to community resources and support services.
- Providing information about medications and/or alternative medication.
- Assisting in dealing with death and offering help in talking about emotions and thoughts and helping find ways to manage concerns.

FIGURE 10.3 The multidisciplinary team

Source: Adapted from Clarke, L., Gray, S., White, L., Duncan, G. & Baumle, W. (2016). *Foundations of Nursing: Enrolled Division 2 Nurses* (ANZ edition). Cengage Learning: South Melbourne, Figure 6.2, p. 133.

CASE STUDY 10.2

Psychological and community intervention

Sheryl has been looking after her husband Daniel, who has a progressive motor neuron condition, for the last 18 months. He has been admitted for reassessment and the nurses note that Sheryl seems distressed and anxious. She admits that she is becoming overwhelmed and exhausted and she has had to resign from her job to help her husband with his care. She has become more isolated and lost contact with her friends and admits to feeling quite depressed at times.

She is referred to a psychologist and community palliative care service. The psychologist works on developing strategies to manage her anxiety and depression, while the palliative care service offers respite and gives her more information about how Daniel is going to die and how they can assist in preparing her and supporting her through the practical aspects of the death of her husband.

1. What relaxation techniques and cognitive behavioural strategies could be used to support Sheryl?
2. What additional community supports could Sheryl utilise to assist her in caring for her husband?

10.2 Supporting the person, family or carers using the palliative approach

Care that is focused on the patient, family and carers as a unit is essential for a palliative approach. By being inclusive with the patient and significant others, being open and honest and being available for them, you are showing respect for their needs.

Discussing spiritual and cultural issues in an open and non-judgemental manner

Open communication about the changing condition of the palliative person is the key to providing ongoing care which supports the person and their family and/or significant others. When providing support, it is important to listen without judgement and allow the person to feel and express themselves in any way that they need to. Remember that each person has unique needs and may make individual choices. Using a non-judgemental approach includes:

- listening and allowing the person to express their feelings
- using the non-verbal communication skills of touch and silence appropriately
- accepting the person the way he or she is
- maintaining a safe environment where emotions can be freely expressed
- observing the person's body language and maintaining an open posture to allow for open communication
- paying attention to the person's tone of voice.

Having as much information about the patient regarding their spiritual and cultural choices is vital to ensure any plans and decisions are inclusive and that staff are advocating appropriately for them. Strategies can include:

- asking the family/person to explain their rituals and beliefs
- asking the question 'Are you at peace?' or 'Where do you find strength in difficult times?' or 'Are there ways we might help with your spiritual needs or concerns'?
- referral to a member of the team trained specifically in spiritual or cultural care at the end of life, or someone from the person's own spiritual community or tradition.

Activity 10.2

Cultural considerations

When caring for a person from a specific culture it is important to discuss the culturally relevant requirements and preferences of the person who is dying. Many health facilities will have policies and procedures for supporting the palliative patient from different cultures. Choose a culture and research the following areas:

1. What other health workers can assist with a palliative approach in hospital and community settings?
2. Why is it important to acknowledge kinship and alternative treatments for some individuals?

Communication techniques and support services

As discussed in previous chapters, communication is both verbal and non-verbal, and both are dependent on the situation, environment, culture, physical and mental state of the people involved. In the palliative care environment you need to be able to decipher the message of the dying person using the cues given by the person and respond appropriately.

Communication involves emotional support and care. You should use the following skills:

- active listening
- open-ended questioning
- reflection of feelings
- empathy building
- being present
- silence.

Using empathy in communication involves listening to patients, understanding them and their concerns, and communicating this understanding to them so that they might recognise themselves more fully.

For more information on communication, see Chapter 6.

Speaking, listening

Monitoring the patient's condition and respecting their wishes

A palliative approach involves supporting the patient's choices and decision making and a focus on helping the patient, their carers and family to identify and achieve the outcomes they want wherever possible. By creating a supportive environment, you are able to provide accurate and timely information on the stages of dying and ensure that information-provision respects their wishes.

Advance care planning and directives

Nurses practice within legal boundaries. An understanding of the law supports critical thinking and provides a framework in which to work. Laws relating to health are constantly changing to keep pace with developing technology that in turn can pose ethical dilemmas. Advance care planning respects the right of an individual to decide how decisions are made about their care.

Advance care planning

An advance care plan is a plan that has been developed while a person is still able to make decisions about the type of treatment or interventions they wish to have if they are in a situation where they can no longer make decisions (NSW Ministry of Health, 2013).

Advance care directives

An advance care directive is a written or verbal plan that stipulates the person's decisions for their treatment in the event that they can no longer make decisions (instructional advance care directive) and also nominates a person (enduring guardian) to make decisions on their behalf when they can no longer do so (NSW Ministry of Health, 2013).

A person when making an advance care plan can make a decision about what treatments they do not want to have. This can be specific, such as refusal for life support but wanting other treatments such as antibiotic therapy, or wanting no further treatment at all (Advance Care Planning Australia, 2017).

In all cases the advance care plan will be followed if it reflects a person's expressed preferences and is advocated by their appointed guardian as the person's wishes and is in the person's best interests (Advance Care Planning Australia, 2017).

TIP 10.3

Advance directives

Health professionals consider Advance Care Planning for end of life as an expected part of clinical care and should understand the clinical and other requirements for doing so. Make sure that you understand the patients' wishes as documented in the advance care plan and ask your supervisor if unsure (NSW Ministry of Health, 2013).

End-of-life decisions

It is lawful for a competent adult to make their own end-of-life decisions and to refuse medical treatment, even if such a decision results in their death (see https://www.advancecareplanning.org.au/for-health-and-care-workers/legal-implications). It is also lawful for a substitute decision maker to ask that life-sustaining treatment be withheld or withdrawn from someone who no longer can decide on treatment for themselves.

For example, the 'legal framework in NSW supports end-of-life decisions and permits:

- refusal of any and all life-sustaining treatments by a person with decision-making capacity at the end of life
- advance refusal for a time of future incapacity, and
- decisions made by a doctor, in consultation with and preferably with agreement of an appropriate substitute decision maker, where a person has no decision-making capacity to withhold or withdraw life-sustaining measures so as to focus primarily on palliative care' (NSW Ministry of Health, 2013).

10.3 Signs of deterioration and the stages of dying

Physical death is a progressive process, during which there are some signs that usually indicate that death is imminent. Not all changes occur nor do they appear in any particular order as the body shuts down during the dying process.

Physiology of dying

Problem solving

Recognising that a person is deteriorating, and that death is imminent, is an important part of caring for that person. **Table 10.3** outlines symptoms of the dying process and suggested interventions.

TIP 10.4

Can they hear us?

We should assume that some nature of hearing/awareness/connection is maintained by the patient, and this should influence the nature of bedside conversations and behaviour.

TABLE 10.3 Nursing management of symptoms of the dying process

Symptom	Suggested intervention
Decreased appetite and thirst	Keeping the patient's mouth clean and moist is essential. Lanolin to lips can be applied. Lips can also be moistened with ice chips. Thirst is best treated by small amounts of fluid and ice chips offered frequently. If the person has a coated tongue, mucosa or teeth, remove debris with a soft toothbrush or mouth swab.
Changes to sleep and alertness	Communicate to the person when they seem most alert, and allow them to sleep when they want to.
Poor temperature regulation	Ensure good ventilation to circulate the air and providing cool damp towels can help if the person seems hot. If they feel cold, use light bedding to keep them warm.
Incontinence	Document daily the client's bowel habits. Provide medication to prevent constipation if fibre or fluid cannot be maintained. Provide protective continence pads, or external or internal urinary drainage devices to prevent discomfort and skin breakdown from urinary incontinence. Maintain skin integrity and clean and dry sheets.

>>

Symptom	Suggested intervention
Nausea and vomiting	When vomiting ceases, rinse the mouth, clean the teeth and offer small sips of water or ice cubes. Manage constipation if this is a causative factor. Keep food or other unpleasant smells to a minimum. Manage posture and avoid lying down straight after eating. Use appropriate anti-emetics.
Restlessness	Speak in a quiet way, massage the person's hand or forehead, or play familiar music. Give medications to reduce restlessness if necessary.

Source: Palliative Care Australia (2016). *The dying process*. Retrieved from http://palliativecare.org.au/resources/the-dying-process/.

Management of respiratory and swallowing difficulties

For some conditions dyspnoea (or breathlessness) is a symptom existing before the end-of-life period is reached. Interventions are available to relieve these symptoms:

- Low-dose morphine (subcutaneous injection) has been shown to reduce dyspnoea without significant respiratory depression.
- Anxiolytics (benzodiazepines) may reduce dyspnoea, especially when anxiety/fear is a contributing factor.
- Oxygen may relieve the dyspnoea associated with hypoxia.

Respiratory distress (dyspnoea) is managed in response to the underlying cause. However, in a conscious and cognitively intact person psychological factors related to the experience of dyspnoea will be a consideration. For the unconscious resident the primary management of dyspnoea in the end-of-life period is with morphine.

Noisy respirations, sometimes called 'death rattle', will occur in a large number of cases. This is due to retention of secretions in the pharynx and the upper respiratory tract. Management includes:

- giving medication to slow down the production of saliva and mucus
- sitting the patient upright supported by pillows to help with breathing, and if this is not possible, position on the side to prevent aspiration of secretions
- verbal reassurance
- avoiding the patient lying flat before and after meals
- maintaining good mouth care.

The person may have swallowing difficulties and a decrease in appetite and thirst, wanting little or no food or fluid. Do not try to force food or drink into the person, instead:

- Provide soft foods and thickened fluids (e.g. nectar) as tolerated.
- Stop feeding the patient if they are choking or pocketing food.
- If the person is able to swallow, fluids may be given in small amounts.

Malignant wound management

The management of symptoms in palliative wound care is critical. Wound care for malignant wounds must address haemorrhage, odour, pain, exudate and superficial infection. **Table 10.4** provides management strategies for malignant wounds.

TABLE 10.4 Wound symptoms and interventions

Symptom	Suggested intervention
Haemorrhage	Topical haemostatic agents, gentle cleansing
Odour	Metronidazole (systemic and topical) Silver dressings Honey Activated charcoal Debridement
Pain	Comfortable dressing Systemic analgesics Topical anaesthetics Topical analgesics
Exudate	Hydrocolloid dressing (low exudate) Alginate and foam dressings (moderate to large exudate) Dressings in layers
Superficial infections	Topical antimicrobial agents Silver dressings Honey Debridement

Source: Graves, M. & Sun, V. (2013). 'Providing quality wound care at the end of life', *Journal of Hospice and Palliative Nursing*, 15(2): 66–74.

Review the skill in Tollefson *Essential Clinical Skills* 8.15 Palliative care and end-of-life care

Signs of deterioration or imminent death

Impending death is often heralded by loss of consciousness and lack of responsiveness (days to weeks), with changes in breathing and circulation indicating a time frame of hours to days. Signs include:

- increased anxiety, restlessness and confusion, then the person becomes less responsive
- renal function declines and what urine is produced will be dark in colour
- **Cheyne-Stokes breathing** pattern is present until breathing ceases
- **stertorous breathing** if the person is unable to cough up secretions
- speech becomes increasingly difficult, confused or unintelligible and finally impossible
- pulse becomes rapid and weak
- extremities become cold and circulation slows with the development of cyanosis
- skin may become pale, cool, clammy and mottled as death approaches
- the person may involuntarily void or defecate
- the eyes stare and appear glazed
- consciousness is lost.

Cheyne-Stokes breathing
A breathing pattern where the breaths become progressively irregular and shallower, followed by periods of strong, deep breathing

stertorous breathing
Noisy breathing

Dignity in death

Shared decision making between the health-care team, the person and their families or carer is possible when everyone has an awareness of the person's approaching death. Clear information should be given to them about the dying process and what to expect because this can ensure that the person's preferences can be addressed. By listening to and respecting the choices made by the palliative patient and their family, a dignified death can be achieved. Some suggestions for achieving a dignified death include:

- maintaining open communication with the person, family and carers and being prepared to change care as required
- adhering to spiritual and cultural preferences
- making sure that the advance care directive is articulated and followed
- ensuring that the person remains in control where possible.

Ethical issues and concerns

In health care, and especially in end-of-life care, situations arise when health-care workers and families may become uncomfortable with treatment decisions or approaches. This discomfort may arise from a tension between our own values and those of others involved in the care of the palliative person.

Withholding treatment

Withholding or withdrawing treatment is part of providing palliative care. This is undertaken when the person decides that they no longer want to prolong their life. The patient is supported throughout the dying process. Euthanasia and assisted suicide involves an active intervention to advance the death of a person. Advance care directives may include discussions regarding 'not to perform CPR' and should be clearly documented to avoid confusion if the need to act on the decision arises.

Providing nutrition and hydration

Ethical issues may arise when the person can no longer take nutrition or hydration because of their terminal state. Some people request in an advance care directive not to receive artificial nutrition or hydration at the end of their life. Individuals who are dying do not feel hunger or thirst and the resultant dry mouths can be made comfortable with ice chips and lip moisturiser. This should be explained to the family members to reassure them if they are concerned about nutrition and hydration in the dying individual.

Analgesia

Proper administration of appropriate symptom-relieving medications is not euthanasia. Analgesia that is reviewed and adjusted in a systematic way in response to the patient's assessed need will provide comfort while the underlying progressive process of dying takes it course.

CASE STUDY 10.3

Palliative sedation

Trent has been admitted to the palliative care unit with end-stage bowel cancer. Over the last week his pain has worsened despite aggressive pain management. His suffering has caused distress to his wife and family, and the palliative team has proposed palliative sedation as a compassionate way to relieve his suffering. This has been agreed to by Trent and his family and documented in his care plan.

   Titration of pain-relieving medication commenced until Trent was deeply sedated and a continuous dose maintained him in a deep and continuous sedation. He

died five days later in a peaceful state with his family at his side.

   Palliative sedation is regarded as the use of sedation to reduce consciousness, relieving one or more unmanageable symptoms of pain and distress. It is important to emphasise that palliative sedation does not have the intent to directly hasten the end of life, but to provide comfort for the palliative patient.

1   Research the choices of sedative for palliative sedation.
2   What are the legal requirements for a patient or patient's family requesting palliative sedation?

Signs of clinical death

Death is defined as the cessation of all vital functions of the body, including the heartbeat, brain activity (including the brain stem) and breathing. The signs of clinical death are as follows:
*   the pupils do not respond to light and are permanently dilated
*   the jaw may drop

- eyes may remain open
- no pulse or respiration
- the body becomes cold
- blood pools with purple discolouration in the lowest areas of the body
- after two to four hours – **rigor mortis**
- fluids may leak from natural body openings, particularly if decomposition is allowed to occur.

rigor mortis
Stiffening of the joints and muscles of a body a few hours after death

10.4 Caring for the person's body after death and providing support for the family and others

When a person dies the body needs to be cared for and prepared for transfer to the mortuary or funeral directors. The facility will have a policy and procedure for you to follow that incorporates guidelines from the Australian Government Department of Health. A doctor needs to certify the death and complete a death certificate. There are some instances where death may have occurred unexpectedly or in specific circumstances, such as after surgery, where the body must be sent to the coroner. In such instances specific instructions regarding the care of the body must be followed.

Legislation (and policy and procedures)

In all cases a body is cleaned and dressed in clean clothing. Unless there is a specific reason, relatives may view the deceased person before transferring the body. At this time the nurse needs to provide the family with support. The relatives may request specific interventions according to culture and religion. It is important to allow these requests where possible unless there is a legal or health reason to prevent it. At all times the deceased person is accorded the same dignity as if they were still alive, for example, doors closed and body handled gently (NSW Ministry of Health, 2009).

Autopsy

In some situations a medical examination is undertaken after death (post mortem or autopsy). A coronial examination is done if the medical practitioner is unable to ascertain the cause of death or if the person died in unusual circumstances, and can be performed regardless of the family's wishes. A non-coronial autopsy is done to offer information to the medical profession on the deceased person's condition and can only be performed with the family's consent.

The immediate family may also choose to consent to an autopsy, but limit the extent of the examination. They can also decide whether or not organs or samples taken from the body may be kept for further study. Once the post mortem is complete, the body can be collected by the family's chosen funeral director before it is buried or cremated.

Organ donation

Many people register their wish to donate their organs after their death. This is registered through the Australian Government Organ and Tissue Authority's Donate Life program (see https://register.donatelife.gov.au/decide). At times families may consent to donate organs if there is no formal consent given by the person before their death. At all times if the family refuse to donate the person's organs their wishes are respected.

TIP 10.5

Viewing the body
If the family of the deceased person are not present, and if they wish to visit, the deceased person can be viewed in the hospital mortuary or holding bay or alternate facility. Check the hospital policy regarding where deceased people can be viewed.

CASE STUDY 10.4

Ethical and legal issues

Mina is 55 years old and has advanced ovarian cancer. She has written an advance care plan stating that she wants her pain managed with opioids and no active treatment when her condition deteriorates. She has no cognitive impairment and would like to donate her organs once she has died. Her husband does not want Mina's body to be touched once she has died and opposes organ donation.

1   What are the laws regarding consent to organ donation in your state?
2   Can the next of kin refuse organ donation for their partners?
3   What strategies can be implemented to resolve this ethical issue?

Care of the body after death

Learning

Care should be taken when attending to the person who has died. They are entitled in death to be treated with the same dignity and respect as any living person. It is a very emotional time for families and significant others and they all require special care during this time. After a person dies it is important to give their family the time that they need with the body. Some family members might like to stay with their loved one, while others might like to be involved with washing the body. Every death and every family is individual, therefore it is important to talk to the family and make them feel they are in a safe space to be with their loved one. It is important to respect cultural considerations or requests whenever possible.

Standard precautions

As with all individuals for whom you provide care, standard precautions are taken when caring for a deceased person. If the person was known to have an infectious disease, additional precautions are also implemented (http://www.icdkwt.com/pdf/policiesandguidelines/ICforSupportiveServices/MortuaryServices.pdf).

In general, unless culture or a coroner does not permit it, a body is prepared by washing the person, removing tubes and jewellery, and then placing them in a non-porous bag. Use gloves as a standard precaution.

Activity 10.3

Organ donation

Although the majority of religious and cultural groups do not oppose donation or transplant, some (for example, Islam, Orthodox Judaism and Buddhism) may not accept the concept of brain death before organ donation. Cultural issues may develop if the declaration of death by neurological criteria is opposed to cultural and/or religious beliefs. There is no right approach to resolve this dilemma.

1   Research the beliefs of cultural groups regarding brain death and organ donation.

Cultural and spiritual practices

Different cultures have different customs that are expected to be followed. Therefore, it is important to be aware of the religion and culture of the palliative patient.

For more information on different beliefs and appropriate care for persons after death, see http://www.alfredicu.org.au/assets/Documents/ICU-Guidelines/DeathAndDying/CALD MulticulturalCareDeathDying.pdf.

Support needs and resources for bereavement care

There are a number of social and community services available for clients and significant others who have experienced a loss. These include:

- support from family and friends
- bereavement counselling
- hospital and community health
- palliative care agencies
- volunteer groups
- church and religious groups
- specialist services including:
    - coping with the death of a child or baby
    - assistance available in dealing with SIDS
    - grief support groups for families involved in industrial or workplace accidents, victims of homicide and road accidents
    - support for children who have lost a parent or close relative, family separation, death
    - kids' help line
    - doctors
    - counsellors and social workers
    - grief line
    - National Association for Loss and Grief
    - IDSA industrial death support advocacy
    - road trauma support team
    - solace for bereaved partners.

Emotional support relating to grief, loss and bereavement

The management of clients and others experiencing loss and grief is best achieved by adopting a multidisciplinary approach. Members of the multidisciplinary team will need to have an understanding of family relationships and support networks which will enable effective emotional support to all members when clients and families are faced with grief and loss.

There are a range of strategies that can be implemented to manage and support clients and significant others who are experiencing loss and grief. These include therapeutic communication skills, counselling skills and knowledge of available community resources. Communication skills include:

- open and closed questions
- use of silence
- clarification
- reflection
- paraphrasing
- summarising
- active listening
- empathy.

Refer to Chapter 6 for more information regarding these skills.

Collaboration, listening, speaking

10.5 Self-care in the palliative care role

Dealing with death and dying can be challenging for members of the health-care team. It can add considerably to workplace stress and therefore must be managed effectively. It is important that systems are in place to facilitate access to peer support, mentoring and referral. Nurses should be supported to develop skills in self-care, reflective learning and if ethical issues arise, they should be raised with the appropriate person for discussion and management according to the organisation's policies and procedures.

Self management

Self-care and supporting wellbeing

Developing self-awareness is an important step in self-care. It assists you to identify your strengths and weaknesses as well as to understand why you react the way you do in certain situations. Being self-aware can assist you to manage your emotions and prevent stress, and by actioning self-care strategies, resilience can be achieved. You are then able to monitor your own levels of stress and identify and deal with issues that arise. Building self-care into daily routines can help to avoid a build-up of stress and burning out. Self-care strategies can include:

- identifying ways to leave the job behind to balance home and work life
- undertaking regular exercise or relaxation activities
- enjoying time with friends and/or family
- maintaining a balanced diet
- debriefing after difficult events
- seeking a mentor who can provide support
- accessing supportive services including counselling
- being proactive in raising and addressing concerns
- focusing on teamwork and a positive workplace culture
- acknowledging your grief and recognising that it is a normal reaction to the experience of loss.

> **TIP 10.6**
>
> Avoiding burnout
> Even if you have a great relationship with the palliative patient and their family and have looked after them for several days in a row, allow yourself to have a break sometimes and ask for a different patient load.

Support and professional debriefing

Nurses need to recognise their own feelings, values and attitudes when it comes to death and dying. Debriefing sessions can be used as an effective approach to supporting health-care professionals in managing their grief in caring for patients with life-threatening conditions.

When a death occurs it is normal for staff to be affected by the event. Debriefing is a supportive activity where staff can share their feelings and emotions with peers. Often the experience of sharing with peers can assist in acceptance and allay stress and anxiety. If a person finds that they are experiencing symptoms of stress that are ongoing and cause disruption to their day-to-day activities, professional assistance may be required (Hanna & Romana, 2007).

Reflective practice 10.1

Reflection about loss

1 What support does the workplace offer to staff if they experience the death of a patient?

2 How could you support your work colleagues when they are distressed due to the loss of a patient?

SUMMARY

- Caring for a person in palliative care involves knowledge of the pathophysiological changes that occur and the psychosocial needs of the person and their family/carers.
- Good communication skills are essential when providing care for a palliative patient and their families or carers.
- Palliative care involves identifying and responding to the signs of deterioration and the stages of dying a person experiences.
- Providing care for the person's body after death and support for the family or carer are essential aspects of palliative care.
- It is important to ensure you practise self-care when working in the palliative care area of nursing to ensure your own wellbeing.

SELF-TEST QUESTIONS

1   What special needs does a person receiving palliative care require?
2   How can the nurse support the dying person and their families/carers?
3   What are the stages of dying and the symptoms that the person may experience?
4   How can the nurse provide support to the family/carer after death?
5   How can the nurse ensure their own wellbeing when caring for palliative patients?

BIBLIOGRAPHY

Advance Care Planning Australia, © Austin Health (2017). *The legal implications*. Retrieved from https://www.advancecareplanning.org. au/for-health-and-care-workers/legal-implications.

ANMC (2016). *National Competency Standard for Enrolled Nurse*. Retrieved from http://www.nursingmidwiferyboard.gov.au/Codes-Guidelines-Statements/Professional-standards.aspx.

Australian Commission on Safety and Quality in Health Care (2015). *National Consensus Statement, Essential Elements for Safe and High-Quality End-of-Life Care*. ACSQHC: Sydney.

Australian Government Department of Health (2010). *National Palliative Care Strategy 2010 – Supporting Australians to Live Well at the End of Life*. Retrieved from http://www.health.gov.au/internet/main/publishing.nsf/Content/EF57056BDB047E2FCA257BF000206168/$File/NationalPalliativeCareStrategy.pdf.

Australian Government Organ and Tissue Authority (n.d.). *Donate Life*. Retrieved from https://register.donatelife.gov.au/decide. Accessed 22 March 2018.

Australian Institute of Health and Welfare (2013). *Palliative Care Services in Australia*. AIHW: Canberra.

Clarke, L., Gray, S., White, L., Duncan, G. & Baumle, W. (2016). *Foundations of Nursing: Enrolled Division 2 Nurses* (ANZ edition). Cengage Learning: South Melbourne.

DeLaune, S.C., Ladner, P.K., McTier, L., Tollefson, J. & Lawrence, J. (2016). *Australian and New Zealand Fundamentals of Nursing* (revised edition), Cengage Learning: South Melbourne.

Graves, M. & Sun, V. (2013). 'Providing quality wound care at the end of life', *Journal of Hospice and Palliative Nursing*, 15(2): 66–74.

Hanna, D. & Romana, M. (2007). *Debriefing after a crisis*. Retrieved from http://www.bhs.org.au/sites/default/files/finder/pdf/cnhe/journal%20club/2008/LeadingOpinions200802.pdf.

health.vic (2018). *Managing personal, emotional, cultural and spiritual needs in palliative care*. Retrieved from https://www2.health.vic.gov.au/hospitals-and-health-services/patient-care/older-people/palliative/palliative-emotional.

Krause, R (2015). *Palliative care in the acute care setting, emergency medicine*. Retrieved from http://emedicine.medscape.com/article/1407757-overview#a2.

NSW Ministry of Health (2009). *Respecting patient privacy and dignity in NSW Health*. Retrieved from http://www.health.nsw.gov.au/Performance/Publications/ct-8ways-booklet.pdf.

NSW Ministry of Health (2013). *Advance planning for quality care at end of life – action plan 2013–2018*. Retrieved from http://www.health.nsw.gov.au/patients/acp/Pages/acp-plan-2013-2018.aspx.

Palliative Care Australia (2016). *The dying process*. Retrieved from http://palliativecare.org.au/resources/the-dying-process/.

Palliative Care Australia (2016). *Understanding palliative care*. Retrieved from http://palliativecare.org.au/understanding-palliative-care-parent-menu/understanding-palliative-care/.

Tollefson, J., Watson, G., Jelly, E. & Tambree, K. (2016). *Essential Clinical Skills: Enrolled Division 2 Nurses* (3rd edition). Cengage Learning: South Melbourne.

World Health Organization (WHO) (2002). *WHO definition of palliative care*. Retrieved from http://www.who.int/cancer/palliative/definition/en/.

PART 3

Clinical placement rehabilitation/subacute

Chapter 11: Client health information

Chapter 12: Nursing care for a person with complex needs

Chapter 13: Principles of wound management

Chapter 14: Nursing care plans

Chapter 15: Improving professional practice

Chapter 16: Care for a person with chronic health problems

Chapter 17: Researching and applying evidence to practice

Chapter 18: Care for a person with diabetes

The rehabilitation experience

This was my second placement, and I was really looking forward to getting into some patient care! I was allocated to a rehabilitation ward, where the patient stay is generally two to four weeks and then, if further rehabilitation is required, the patients are then transferred to the rehabilitation centre, which is a separate entity. I definitely assumed that all patients would be post stroke or something similar, but what I soon learnt was that rehabilitation was for all types of things. Some people required rehabilitation after being hospitalised for pneumonia that turned into septicaemia, for example. Other patients were in rehabilitation post a motor vehicle accident, or a simple fall at work or at home that led to surgery and then the need to mobilise was complicated by factors. What was most astonishing was the difference between patients, and watching the anatomy and physiology in action. You could see the processes of musculoskeletal improvement or regrowth, or just general improvement in health status. Rehabilitation involved way more than just assisting people recover; it involved a complex history of events that led that patient to be in rehabilitation, and the journey to get them home. I found it incredibly rewarding and I felt it really assisted with consolidation of knowledge.

The subacute placement will generally be in the first component of your diploma. It will enable you to consolidate your learning from many subjects, such as anatomy and physiology, infection control, developing nursing care plans, and patient assessment.

What is subacute/rehabilitation nursing? Subacute/rehabilitation nursing is focused on restorative nursing to return the patient to their previous level of functioning, or as close to that as possible. Rehabilitation is required for patients who have had a variety of illnesses, complications or disease processes, or trauma. Rehabilitation is different for every patient and involves ongoing management and communication with the multidisciplinary care team.

What kind of patients are in the subacute/rehabilitation setting?

Subacute/rehabilitation care is for a broad range of nursing interventions. Patients will require rehabilitation for a variety of reasons. Common conditions include cerebrovascular accident (stroke) with resulting hemiplegia, recovery after a prolonged debilitating illness or injury, or patients who have an acquired brain injury as a result of an accident.

In this placement you will be working in either a hospital setting in a designated ward, or in a rehabilitation centre, which will be a stand-alone centre/facility. You will still need your acute nursing knowledge as you will need to assess your patients and review their progress. Patients will have input from a variety of allied health specialists and the role of the rehabilitation nurse is integral as the key communicator regarding the patient's progression or needs.

Common experiences of student nurses in the community setting

Rehabilitation/subacute nursing can be very demanding. Each patient responds differently to a challenge, and rehabilitation is challenging for all involved. You will be involved in caring for patients who may reach an 'all-time low' in their life, but the positive side is that you will be involved in enabling rehabilitation and improvement of their function. Your role will be in assisting patients with their activities of daily living (ADLs) and in health promotion and teaching. Patients may require analgesia and assessment of pain and mobility. Patients may have splints, wounds, mobility aids or other equipment necessary for their care.

Objectives

The objectives that are to be set for this placement need to be contextualised to the subacute/rehabilitation setting:

- conduct holistic clinical health assessments
- integumentary assessment
- pain assessment
- care planning
- wellness approach to health, including physiology and psychosocial aspects.

Allocation

In the rehabilitation setting allocation is undertaken with the complexities of the patient's needs in mind. There is no set ratio, as there are some patients who will require a great deal of nursing care. Team nursing may be utilised, but this will depend on each facility. As a student you may administer medications if the unit HLTENN007 has been completed and you are supervised. For more complex management there will be a registered nurse who will undertake specialised activities – such as administration of high-risk medications in the home environment. All enrolled nurses and support staff work under the supervision of a registered Division 1 nurse.

Enjoy your placement and ensure you make good use of the valuable time you have in this area.

Client health information

LEARNING OUTCOMES

After reading this chapter, you should have an understanding of:

11.1 How to assess a client's health status

11.2 Planning action to address the identified health status

Health information

I was going to a placement and I was both excited and nervous at the same time. I dreaded something going wrong, and I was sure someone would have a cardiac arrest and I was not sure that I would be able to manage this. I spent a lot of time reviewing my notes and practising my skills.

On the first day I was allocated to a cardiac ward. The butterflies in my stomach were doing somersaults. The clinical teacher told us to shadow our buddy and ensure that we researched the patients that we would be providing care for the next day.

I was allocated a gentleman of 72 years who had been admitted with chest pain for investigation. I noticed that he became slightly breathless while having a shower and on return to his bed appeared weak and pale. I took a set of vital signs and found that his pulse rate was over 124 beats per minute and it was very fluttery and hard to count.

I rang the emergency bell and reported it to my buddy. My buddy took an ECG, notified the doctor and applied some intranasal oxygen to the client. The registered nurse gave him an anginine and repeated this is in a couple of minutes as the client was complaining of an ache in his right shoulder.

The registered nurse praised me at handover, in front of all the staff, for the good job I had done in monitoring and following the policy and procedure for a client with chest pain. I felt six foot tall as I left the ward area that day.

11.1 Assessing clients' health status

Assessment of clients will soon become second nature to you. Tools for assessing your patient include:

- visual observation
- physical assessment
- questioning.

When you combine all these types of data, which are subjective and objective, you will be able to assess your client's current health status. Concepts underlying health status are views on health and wellness. The World Health Organization (WHO) defines *wellbeing* as a 'state of complete physical mental and social well-being and not merely the absence of disease and infirmity' (WHO, 2018, para. 1). Each and every person has their own definition of health in relation to their own expectations, experiences and values. We are constantly adapting to changes in both internal and external environments. Health and the maintenance of it is often related to daily activities and lifestyle choices. Another way to describe this concept is through the term *motivation*. Individuals are often motivated by factors such as self-fulfilment, joy, absence of disease, environmental hazards, exercise and diet. For example, if a patient is motivated to reduce their risk factors for heart disease, through alterations in diet and an increase in physical activity, we can observe the positive impact this is likely to have on the patient's health and wellbeing. Wellness refers to a balance between physical, social, psychological and spiritual factors in a person's life (Clarke et al., 2016).

Explore the theory in *Foundations of Nursing* Chapter 14: Wellness concepts

Planning services to meet a client's needs

Thorough assessment is the first step in identifying a client's needs. When we have identified what services the client needs we can then formulate interventions to address these. In all instances the nurse with the health-care team will assess the client's health and analyse the clinical findings to plan care.

The interventions will vary in response to actual or potential problems. One of the actions that the nurse may need to take is timely referral of clients to specialised health-care team members. As the client progresses towards their goal, the nurse needs to plan services for discharge to home. Depending on the client's condition, this may involve re-establishment of community services or accessing new supports for the client on discharge.

Some types of conditions you will encounter will require the client to have further interventions from members of the health-care team. These services may be assistance with personal care, or ongoing education if the client is diabetic or has another chronic condition.

Activity 11.1

Discharge care and the health-care team

Choose one of the clients you are providing care for and identify their discharge needs.

What members of the health-care team need to be involved with the client's care, both while in the health-care facility and on discharge?

Recognising normal readings for vital signs, tests and observations

The nursing process is how we derive our findings and obtain data. We do this by asking questions, measuring vital signs or performing other diagnostic testing. One of the most important sets of clinical skills you will undertake will be patient observations – temperature, pulse, respirations (TPR) and blood pressure (BP). These are often referred to as 'obs' or 'vitals'.

The nurse needs to be able to recognise what is normal and what is abnormal when assessing a client. Most client groups will have normal readings within set parameters. The nurse should always report and document abnormal results according to the policies and procedures of the health facility. In some cases the client may have normal readings for most of the time but at certain times they can be abnormal and this can form a pattern. Examples of this are an infection that causes the temperature to rise only in the evenings, or abnormal pulse and BP readings when the client experiences pain.

In our everyday lives we prioritise tasks without realising it. Whether you have a formal 'to do' list or plan out on a calendar, we all prioritise our needs on a daily basis. In nursing, we prioritise our workload and the urgency of interventions according to data and information we collect from our patients. Another method of obtaining data is that of a physical assessment.

Identifying pathophysiology through observation, physical assessment and analysis

The human body aims to maintain a balance, a state of homeostasis. Monitoring vital signs can identify if the client is suffering from a condition that is affecting their health. Most adults will maintain their vital signs within a set range. If there is a deterioration in health, the body will attempt to maintain homeostasis by altering the functioning of body systems. An example of this is when an infection occurs in the person. The vital signs will alter, the temperature will rise, the pulse rate will rise and there will be an increase in breathing.

All observations or assessments are completed to assess the health status of the client. A gait assessment will assess the functioning of the musculoskeletal system while an electrocardiograph (ECG) will assess the normal functioning of the heart muscle.

To fully assess the health status of the client you will use your special senses to detect abnormalities. Some examples of how the nurse does this are:

- visual – watching the patient mobilise, assessing skin colour
- hearing – listening for abnormal chest sounds
- touch – palpating the abdomen.

At other times you will use your specialised knowledge to analyse the client's health status. An example of this is when providing wound care and the assessment of the wound bed.

Review the skill in Tollefson *Essential Clinical Skills*, 2.3 Temperature, pulse and respiration (TPR) measurement & 2.4 Blood pressure measurement

Review the skill in Tollefson *Essential Clinical Skills*, 2.1 Head-to-toe assessment

TIP 11.1

Completing charting
Always carry a pen with you in order to note down the observations immediately. This will avoid errors in communication.

Review the skill in Tollefson *Essential Clinical Skills* 3.8 Urine specimen collection and urinalysis

---

Activity 11.2

Urinalysis and what it indicates

Select a client you are providing care for and undertake a urinalysis. What results did you obtain? What does this test indicate about the health of the client? Besides the indicator strip analysis, what else did you observe regarding the client's health status?

The impact of specific interventions

When an abnormal result from observations is obtained, the nurse and the health-care team will undertake specific actions that aim to address the underlying cause. For each action undertaken a response will occur. The nurse will monitor the client's response to assess the effectiveness of the interactions.

Each member of the health-care team will be involved in this process, depending on the cause. See **Table 11.1** for information on the different actions that other members of the health-care team may initiate and the likely impact of these interventions.

TABLE 11.1 Health-care team and their roles and responsibilities

Health-care team member	Problem	Action	Impact
Doctor	Elevated temperature	Will order specific medication or tests	Medications will have different effects, for example, Panadol will lower temperatures, antibiotics will treat underlying infection Specific tests will attempt to identify the cause of the problem
Physiotherapist	Decreased mobility	Will prescribe specific exercises depending on type of muscle weakness	Increase muscle tone and improve client's mobility
Counsellor	Anxiety/stress	Will listen and engage the client to share concerns. Will prescribe relaxation techniques	Alleviates stress and increases wellbeing
Dietician	Poor intake of food, resulting in loss of weight	Will prescribe a diet to address deficiencies	Maintain healthy weight and nutritional intake
Occupational therapist	Inability to undertake activities of daily living	Will assess ability to complete activities and recommend appropriate aids	Increase independence

Disease

When assessing a patient, we need to consider the concepts of disease processes in analysing our data and results. For example, a blood pressure of 170/80, which would normally be considered high, might be considered normal for an 82-year-old male with permissive hypertension related to the ageing processes. Other factors to consider, apart from ageing, are diseases.

Disease is a disruption in the normal structure or function of any aspect of a person – mind, body and emotions. Diseases are classified according to cause, acquisition, or body system affected. Disease signals an imbalance in the body between internal and external environments. Diseases can be caused by a single factor or a combination of factors.

Table 11.2 contains some examples you may encounter during your placement.

TABLE 11.2 Example of factors of disease

Factors of disease	Examples
Pathogens	Any microorganism capable of causing disease, for example, bacteria or a virus
Genetic conditions	Disease/s inherited or passed down from one generation to the next
Birth defects	Abnormality present at birth or earlier inherited due to environmental factors – foetal alcohol syndrome, drug use during pregnancy are some examples
Nutritional deficiencies	Deficiency of a single nutrient or vitamin, or many that results in disease. A good example is that of iron deficiency anaemia; that is, the person becomes anaemic due to the iron deficiency, and once this is corrected, the anaemia is also corrected
Trauma	Physical injury of cells or tissues, for example, temperature extremes, motor vehicle accidents, fractured bones, or any other mechanism of injury
Toxins	Substances that are harmful or poisonous to the body – chemicals, radiation etc.
Environmental factors	Pollution, insecticides, trace metals (for example, lead), alcohol and drugs
Degenerative changes	Gradual deterioration over time resulting in decrease or loss of function. The loss of normal control mechanisms, for example, the uncontrollable growth of cancer cells, and normal ageing also causes degenerative changes

In both health and disease, the ability to adapt physically and psychologically to stress is affected by age, health status and psychosocial resources. Successful adaptation is more likely when there is a gradual rather than a sudden change or deterioration in health status as the body has a greater chance to maintain internal and external balance. All the above factors play a part in health and wellness and affect us all as individuals differently (Clarke et al., 2016).

Health status

As a health-care professional, you will need to have an understanding of human anatomy and physiology and the function and purpose of each and every system in the complex and amazing structure that is the human body to ensure adequate care is provided. Refer to Chapter 7 for a review on anatomy and physiology.

Homeostasis

Homeostasis is the maintenance of the body's internal environment. Homeostasis refers to narrow limits or indices within which the body maintains normal functioning. Some examples of homeostasis in action are blood sugar levels, body temperature, heart rate and the amount of fluid in the cell environment. When our bodies maintain homeostasis we are healthy. When homeostasis is not able to be maintained, the body experiences disease and will respond by negative feedback mechanisms (Rizzo, 2015). These are automatic, that is, not under voluntary control, but are able to be observed or measured clinically. An example of a homeostatic response can be seen in **Figure 11.1**.

TIP 11.2

No two are the same!

When you are on clinical placement, you will notice that your patients may have similar medical conditions – such as hypertension, hyperlipidaemia or atrial fibrillation. What is significant is the difference in symptoms or lack of symptoms your patients will have. Some patients will have a blood pressure that is quite high – such as 180/100mHg – and not have any other signs or symptoms, while others may have a blood pressure of 160/90mmHg and have headaches and feel flushed. The variables between all humans is astonishing, so it is worthwhile remembering that the 'numbers' all need to be reviewed along with what the patient is reporting as signs and symptoms.

homeostasis
Balance or equilibrium among the physiological, psychological and spiritual aspects as an integrated whole (Clarke et al., 2016)

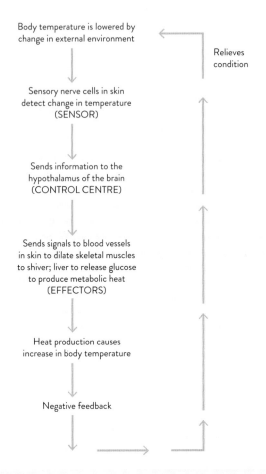

FIGURE 11.1 An example of how negative feedback controls body temperature

Source: Rizzo, D. (2015). *Fundamentals of Anatomy and Physiology* (4th edition). Delmar Cengage Learning: USA, Figure 1-10, p. 13.

Explore the theory in *Foundations of Nursing* Chapter 21: Fluid, electrolyte and acid-base balance

Electrolytes are inorganic substances such as acids and bases that are imperative for our survival. Electrolytes include potassium, magnesium and phosphates. They are all vital for cardiac conductivity and are measured in serum blood levels. Electrolyte imbalance/s can cause a myriad of symptoms in patients and should always be addressed. This can be assessed by pulse rate and in more detail by an ECG.

Acids and bases are chemical opposites. Acid base balance refers to the acidity or the alkalinity of the blood. Acid-base balance is assessed by looking at pH, bicarbonate and carbon dioxide levels in the blood. Acid-base balance is generally referred to in the act of respiration. This is yet another reason why assessing your patient's respiration pattern for a full minute is the better way to determine respiratory rate, pattern and effort (Tollefson et al., 2016).

One of the variables also important to cellular function is the normal blood pH range, which is 7.35–7.45. In order for normal metabolism to take place, the body must maintain this narrow range at all times. When the pH is below 7.35, the blood is said to be acidic. Changes in body system functions that occur in an acidic state include a decrease in the force of cardiac contractions. When the pH is above 7.45, the blood is said to be alkalotic. An alkalotic state interferes with tissue oxygenation and normal neurological and muscular functioning. Significant changes in the blood pH above 7.8 or below 6.8 will interfere with cellular functioning and if not corrected will lead to death.

Reflective practice 11.1

So much information

I can remember one of my first placements in an acute care facility. I had all these terms buzzing around my head like 'hypertension, hypotension, anaemia and hypocalcaemia' and I was so nervous that I would not remember what they actually meant. In my pocket I had a small dictionary and a note pad. The NUM told me immediately to remove both, as they were a *hazard*. I had a single piece of paper that I wrote terms on all during my shift – often spelt incorrectly as I was phonetically spelling them out. Each evening, I would look up each term and write down the definition.

On my second week, I was quizzed at handover about a disease – it was portal hypertension. The primary nurse did not know what it was. I was able to discuss very simply that it was hypertension due to hepatic insufficiency. I knew this only because for the very day prior to this I had written down the terms I did not know. I started an A-Z booklet, like an old address book pre-smartphones, and wrote them in. It stayed in my bag. It still stays in my bag four years post-graduation, and I still add to it. It is honestly one of the best things I have ever done, as there are so many diseases, processes and conditions, and remembering them all in the first year of practice is never easy.

Jane, 41, Enrolled Nurse

1   Why do you think it could be beneficial to write down terms you are faced with on placement?
2   Would you consider using an approach like this to manage and organise terms, diseases and experiences?

It is important to set priorities in nursing. It assists with your care plan and ensuring that the most important aspects of nursing care are delivered in a timely manner. For example, your patient needs to have a shower and has a low blood pressure with symptoms relating to this. Instead of showering the patient at that time you re-evaluate, assess and implement your plan.

There are several diagnostic tests that are routinely gathered on the ward environment that are incredibly important in establishing and planning care. Some examples are:

* *Blood Glucose Level (BGL)* – Blood glucose monitoring is an accurate method of assessing the effectiveness of diet, exercise levels and medication therapy on patients, and to gain information on the patient's current blood glucose level. Normal fasting glucose readings should be between 4–8mmoLs. Disease processes, medications, trauma and many other reasons can alter these readings.
* *Urinalysis (u/a)* – Testing the urine for abnormalities is referred to as urinalysis and is commonly performed when a patient is admitted to hospital or seen in the emergency department. Urine is examined by observation, by chemical testing in the ward and by further analysis in the laboratory. The frequency in which it is performed depends on the client's condition and prescribed management. Some patients will require daily urinalysis testing – an example would be a diabetic who has presented with ketoacidosis, or a pregnant woman in later stages of pregnancy when excess protein in urine needs to be monitored. The parameters in urinalysis are outlined in **Table 11.3**.

Review the skill in Tollefson *Essential Clinical Skills* 2.6 Blood glucose measurement

TABLE 11.3 The parameters in urinalysis

Parameters	Measures and indications
pH	Urinary pH may range from as low as 4.5 to as high as 8.0
Specific gravity	Measures urine density. Specific gravity between 1.002 and 1.0035 on a random sample should be considered as normal if kidney function is normal
Protein	Dipstick screening for protein is done on whole urine. Normally only small plasma proteins filtered at the glomulerus are reabsorbed by the renal tubule. Normal total protein extraction does not usually exceed 150 mg/24 hours or 10 mg/100 mL in any single specimen. More than 150 mg/day is defined as proteinuria
Ketones	Result from either diabetic ketoacidosis or from some other form of calorie deprivation (starvation, malnutrition, pregnancy)
Nitrite	A positive nitrite test indicates that bacteria may be present in significant numbers in urine. Gram negative rods such as *E. coli* are more likely to give a positive test
Leukocytes	A positive leukocyte test results from the presence of white blood cells as whole cells and can be detected even if the urine sample contains damaged white blood cells. A negative leukocyte test means that an infection is unlikely

Reference ranges for all serum blood/laboratory tests have slight variations between some providers due to machinery/equipment used. Any blood tests will come either through a computer-based program or printed and the values will be in parentheses next to the value. Any critical value (extremely high or low) will be called through from the laboratory to the test requestor to ensure intervention is made as quickly as possible. Tests specific to the haematological system are described in **Table 11.4**.

TABLE 11.4 Tests specific to the haemotologic system

Test	Explanation/normal values	Nursing responsibilities
	These ranges are averages and may vary from lab to lab and text to text. The lab report will have the range on it for that lab and client.	

Red blood cells (RBCs)	Number of RBCs × 10^{12} per litre of blood. May be low in clients with rheumatoid arthritis. Clients living in high altitudes may have an elevated RBC level.
	
	Normal:
	  Male: 4.6–6.2 × 10^{12}/L
	  Female: 4.2–5.5 × 10^{12}/L
		The client is not required to fast for the test.

White blood cells (WBCs)	Number of WBCs × 10^{9} per litre of blood. Elevation is associated with infectious processes. Normal: 5–9 × 10^{9}/L	The client is not required to fast for the test. Exercise, stress, last month of pregnancy, labour, previous splenectomy and eating may increase level and alter differential values. Note medications taken that may affect test; aspirin, heparin and steroids may increase WBC level, whereas antibiotics and diuretics may decrease WBC level.

>>

Test	Explanation/normal values	Nursing responsibilities
Differential count	Percentage of types of WBCs in 1 mm of blood.	The client is not required to fast for the test.
Neutrophilis segs (mature neutrophils) Bands (immature neutrophils)	Increase in bacterial infections and trauma. Normal segs: 50–65% Normal bands: 0–5%	
Eosinophils	Increased in allergic reactions or parasitic infestation. Normal: 1–3%	Corticosteroid therapy causes a decreased level.
Basophils	Increased in allergic reactions and during healing periods. Normal: 0.4–1.0%	Steroids cause a decreased level.
Lymphocytes	Increased in viral infections and other diseases, such as pertussis and tuberculosis (TB). Decreased in acquired immunodeficiency syndrome (AIDs). Normal: 25–35%	Steroids cause a decreased level.
Monocytes	Increased in chronic diseases, such as malaria, TB, Rocky Mountain spotted fever. May be low in clients with rheumatoid arthritis. Normal: 4–6%	
Haemoglobin (Hb)	Measures the oxygen-carrying compound in RBCs. Normal male: 135–180 g/L Normal female: 115–160 g/L Critical value: <5 g/L	The client is not required to fast for the test. Sample may be drawn from a finger of a child or the heel of an infant.
Haemoglobin electrophoresis	Detects abnormal forms of haemoglobin. Performed after positive sickle cell test. If the haemoglobin electrophoresis is negative, the client has the sickle cell trait. If the haemoglobin electrophoresis is positive, the client has sickle cell anaemia. Normal: Hb S: 0%; Hb F: <2%; Hb Ca: 0%	If the client has had a blood transfusion within the last 12 weeks, the results of the test may be altered.
Haematocrit (Hct)	Measures the percentage of blood cells in a volume of blood. Clients living in high altitudes may have an increased level. Normal: male: 40–54%; female: 38–47% Critical value: <15% or >60%	The client is not required to fast for the test.
Platelet count	Measures the number of platelets per cubic millilitre of blood. Normal: 150–450 × 10 {9}/L Critical level: <50 and >1000 × 10 {9}/L	Instruct the client that strenuous exercise and oral contraceptives increase platelet level. Instruct the client that aspirin, acetaminophen and sulfonamides decrease platelet level. If the client has a low platelet count, maintain digital pressure to the puncture site.
Bleeding time	Measures the length of time for a platelet plug to occlude a small puncture wound. Normal: 1–9 minutes (Ivy method) Critical value: >15 minutes	Notify the laboratory if the client is taking aspirin, anticoagulants or other medications that may affect the clotting process.

>>

Test	Explanation/normal values	Nursing responsibilities
Prothrombin time (PT, protime)	Measures the effectiveness of several blood-clotting factors. Normal: 10–13.4 seconds INR: 2.0–3.0 In the presence of anticoagulant therapy, the values should be 1½–2 times the normal value. Critical value: >20 seconds In the presence of anticoagulant therapy, the critical value should be >3 times the normal critical value.	Ensure that the blood specimen is drawn before the daily dose of warfarin (coumadin) is administered. Instruct the client that alcohol intake may increase PT and that a diet high in fat may decrease PT. Note those medications taken that may affect results: salicylates, sulfonamides and methyldopa (aldomet), as these may increase PT, whereas digitalis (digoxin) and oral contraceptives decrease the level. Instruct the client not to take any medication without notifying the prescribing doctor as medications may affect the PT level.
International normalised ratio (INR)	Normal: 0.9–1.1 Clients on anticoagulant drugs should have an INR of 2–3 (2.5–3.5 for the client with a mechanical prosthetic heart valve). The INR is more accurate than PT in monitoring warfarin (Coumadin) therapy.	The daily warfarin (Coumadin) dose should be given after blood has been drawn for the INR.
Partial thromboplastin time (PTT), also called activated partial throboplastin time (APTT)	Normal: PTT: 60–70 sec APTT: 21–35 sec In the presence of anticoagulant therapy, the normal value is 1.5–2.5 times the control value. Critical value: APTT: >70 seconds PTT: >100 seconds	If the client is receiving intermittent heparin doses, schedule the APTT to be drawn 30–60 minutes before the next heparin dose. If heparin is given continuously, the blood specimen can be drawn at any time. If PTT is greater than 100 seconds, the client is at risk for bleeding and the medical officer is notified. The antidote for heparin is protamine sulfate. Note whether the client is taking antihistamines, vitamin C or salicylates, as these prolong PTT time.
D dimer test (fragment D dimer, fibrin degradation fragment)	Measures a fibrin split product that is released when a clot breaks. Confirms the diagnosis of disseminated intravascular coagulation (DIC). Screens for deep vein thrombosis (DVT) and pulmonary emboli. Normal: <10 mg/ml	Note whether the client is on thrombolytic therapy, as the results of this test would be increased from negative to positive.

Source: Clarke, L., Gray, S., White, L., Duncan, G. & Baumle, W. (2016). *Foundations of Nursing: Enrolled Division 2 Nurses* (ANZ edition). Cengage Learning: South Melbourne, Table 25.4, pp. 610–12.

To be able to plan care, you will need to be able to recognise an altered health status – which is why anatomy and physiology is so crucial. The common diagnostic tests are great indicators of a patient's health status – and coupling this information with laboratory testing can provide a very clear indication of what processes are in place in the client who is unwell.

CASE STUDY 11.1

Analyse this!

Angela Stingel is a 34-year-old female who has been admitted to hospital with pain while urinating. She also has some lower quadrant abdominal pain. You have just commenced your shift and you complete the following observations:

- Temperature – 38.2 C (tympanic)
- Blood pressure – 160/90
- Pulse – 98 and regular
- Respiratory rate – 20

  Angela hands you a specimen container with urine in it for testing. Upon completing a ward urinalysis the results are:

- pH 6
- SG 1.010
- Leukocytes +++
- Blood ++++
- Nitrates ++
- Ketones negative.

  The urine is amber in colour and is offensive in odour.

1 From the above clinical information, what possible condition could Angela be experiencing?
2 Discuss the vital signs and any other relevant information to support your theory.

CASE STUDY 11.2

The importance of a BGL

Caitlyn Crawford is an 18-year-old female who has presented to emergency with increased thirst, hunger and increased urination. Caitlyn also complains of being incredibly tired (lethargy) for the past few days, and has not been doing 'much at all'.

Caitlyn's observations are as follows:

- Blood pressure – 140/75
- Pulse – 110 and regular
- Respiratory rate – 24
- Temperature – 37.9 C.

Caitlyn also is clammy (diaphoretic) and feels cool to touch (centrally and peripherally cool).

You have returned from your morning tea break to find Caitlyn in your cubicle. Caitlyn remains diaphoretic and is pale. Her breath smells 'funny'. Reviewing this information, and in your basic assessment of Caitlyn, you perform a blood glucose level which is 24.7 mmoLs.

1 What do you think is causing Caitlyn's symptoms?
2 What education would be required for Caitlyn?
3 What other investigations, if any, do you think need to be undertaken to ensure an accurate diagnosis is made?

Reflective practice 11.2

BGL, BGL, BGL!

I was on one of my final placements in my program and I was looking after a bed bay area of four patients with a buddy RN. I was so close to completion and in this placement I was working as the primary care nurse and managing care and time to try to be as 'real' as possible for me to prepare for graduation. It was an incredibly busy day with a medical emergency in another part of the ward that really threw my time management. I was attending and assisting with the medical emergency for at least 45 minutes. I was sent to morning tea and asked to return to my patients afterwards. During the time I was away, my worksheet was used by another nurse who was covering my patients. The BGL box looked like it was crossed, and the nurse handed over to me that

my patients were 'all up to date, nothing needs doing right now'. With this in mind, I continued on, working through my priorities. I went to Mr Calabricia's bedside to attend his wound dressing. I found him on his bed, unrousable, groaning.

Immediately I assumed that his BGL for 1000 hours had been done and was normal, so this was something unexpected. I discounted low blood sugar level initially and told the medical offers attending the medical emergency that the BGL at 1000 was within normal limits (WNL). Another nurse who arrived with the medical emergency team was very kind and said she would take it again as part of a full assessment. The reading was 1.4 mmoLs. Mr Calabricia was essentially unconscious because his BGL had dropped so far and

>>

was not detected sooner as the BGL was not done at 1000 hours.

What I took away from this situation (and yes, Mr Calabricia was fine after some glucose) was that communication and constant assessment of your patients is essential. Changes can occur at any given time. After your break, after an unexpected situation, always reassess your patients. Even if it is just to walk through and talk to them and look at how they are functioning. I have also learnt that it is more

than OK to directly ask another nurse if something, like observations, or a BGL, have been done in your absence. Often when you are relieving, you are busy managing two differing workloads, and sometimes reading someone else's worksheet is not an easy task.

Tiffany, 31, Enrolled Nurse, 6 years post-graduate

1   How do you think this will, if at all, influence your handover after relieving or after a break?
2   How do you think occurrences like this can be avoided?

11.2 Planning to address identified health status

Part of your nursing role is to develop a plan of care and determine what actions are going to be used to minimise the effect of the client's altered health status. Each body system works together to maintain homeostasis, and when external forces or factors occur, the balance is shifted. Some examples for each body system that you may encounter during your placement and career are described in **Table 11.5**.

TABLE 11.5 Example of body systems

Body system	Function and disorders	Problems that may result	Nursing actions	Skills for assessment
Integumentary system	The skin is our largest organ and is our first line of defence against infection	Once the integrity of the skin has been broken, there is an immediate portal or entry point for potential infection	Part of the nursing process and implementation of care entails assessment of skin integrity	
Musculoskeletal system	The musculoskeletal system's primary function is protect and support the body, allow movement, maintain heat production and also to produce blood cells Common disorders of the musculoskeletal system are due to trauma	A fall, an accident, a slip or a trip can be the causative factor. Bones break and muscles tear and it is dependent upon where the injury was sustained as to the treatment provided	Referral to physiotherapist Specialised tests to assess injury Specialised preparation may be required Falls risk assessment Mobility or gait assessment	

>>

Body system	Function and disorders	Problems that may result	Nursing actions	Skills for assessment
Circulatory/ cardiovascular system	One of the first signs or symptoms of disease or altered physiologic process in the circulatory system is blood pressure. Blood pressure refers to the pressure of blood on the walls of the blood vessels of the body. Many processes in the circulatory system occur as a response – for example, for volume loss or bleeding the blood pressure lowers and the heart rate increases due to a lower circulating volume. The volume loss can be a direct result of many external factors – trauma, internal bleeding, and infection – appendicitis, for example, or cardiac failure A great deal can be inferred from palpating a pulse. The pulse reflects the cardiac functioning	If blood pressure falls too far, blood flow is reduced, and perfusion of the tissues is lowered and shock can occur. Fainting is an example of this where blood flow to the brain is reduced and loss of consciousness is the result If someone is bleeding or in shock, his or her pulse is often described as 'thready'	Regular monitoring of blood pressure Specialised monitoring such as lying and standing blood pressure measurement Regular pulse monitoring ECG tests	Review the skill in Tollefson *Essential Clinical Skills* 2.10 12-lead ECG recording
Nervous system	There are two main divisions of the nervous system – the central nervous system (CNS) which includes the brain and the spinal cord, and the peripheral nervous system (PNS), which consists of the nerves that connect the CNS with the rest of the body	The most common signs and symptoms of nervous system disorders/conditions allude to level of consciousness, changes in personality, paralysis and confusion	Need to asses using the Glascow Coma scale	Review the skill in Tollefson *Essential Clinical Skills* 2.7 Neurological observation
Sensory organs	We have four special senses – taste, smell, hearing and balance, and vision	The most common disorders associated with the sensory system are deafness, blindness, injury to eye/ear, balance disturbances due to middle ear disorders, glaucoma, vertigo, tinnitus and cataracts	Falls risk assessment Visual testing	Review the skill in Tollefson *Essential Clinical Skills* 2.6 Blood glucose measurement
Endocrine system	The primary function of the endocrine system is to produce hormones. A hormone is a chemical messenger with a specialised function. Hormones regulate growth, blood sugar, metabolism, reproduction and sleep rhythm. Hormone secretion is controlled by three mechanisms – negative feedback, biorhythms and the central nervous system. Any alteration in secretions is a direct interruption to secretion	You will soon observe that diabetes mellitus is by far the most common endocrine disorder	Blood glucose monitoring and adjustment of medication and diet	

>>

Body system	Function and disorders	Problems that may result	Nursing actions	Skills for assessment
Gastrointestinal system	The gastrointestinal system is responsible for the intake and ingestion of food, the absorption of nutrients from digested food and the elimination of solid waste products	There are many altered health statuses in the gastrointestinal system. Cancers of the stomach, liver, pancreas or bowel are common. Other examples include cirrhosis of the liver or hepatitis	Faecal testing Bowel charting Using the Bristol Bowel chart Stool collection for testing	Review the skill in Tollefson *Essential Clinical Skills* 3.9 Faeces assessment and specimen collection
Urinary system	The urinary system performs many functions that are important in maintaining homeostasis. It maintains proper balance of water, salts and acids in the body fluids by removing excess fluids from the body or by re-absorbing water as needed. It constantly filters the blood to remove urea and other waste materials. Finally, it converts the waste products and excess fluids into urine in the kidneys and excretes them from the body via the urinary bladder	Some urinary disorders include dysuria, incontinence, oedema, retention of urine and changes in voiding pattern	Urinalysis Bladder scanning Incontinence charting Urine M&C 24-hour urine collections Fluid balance charting	Review the skill in Tollefson *Essential Clinical Skills* 3.8 Urine specimen collection and urinalysis
Reproductive system	The reproductive system is innately different in the male and female	The most common alteration in the reproductive system is infertility and sexually transmitted infections	Cultures of discharge for testing Preparation for inspection of vaginal cavity	
Respiratory system	Primarily the respiratory system is responsible for ventilation and respiration. Ventilation is the movement of air in and out of the lungs. Respiration is the process of gas exchange, which is the movement of oxygen from the atmosphere into the blood stream and the movement of carbon dioxide from the blood stream into the atmosphere. Signs and symptoms of respiratory disorders generally relate to breathing itself. For example, a cough can affect someone's ability to breathe effectively.	Clinical disorders include hypoxia, asthma, pneumonia, laryngitis, emphysema, lung cancer and chronic bronchitis.	Respiration rate O_2 saturation monitoring Arterial blood gases	Review the skill in Tollefson *Essential Clinical Skills* 2.5 Pulse oximetry

As you can see, the human body is a marvellous and phenomenal machine. When one system suffers damage or disease, we generally can return to our previous level of wellness. There are many diseases, infections, conditions and processes – the list is exhaustive. Above are some common examples that you are likely to encounter in your placement. The important component in all nursing care is baseline assessment. What is normal for one patient may not be for another – due to underlying disease processes. For example, a patient with chronic kidney disease is likely to have hypertension, and their treating team are 'happy' to accept a blood pressure of 180/100. For a 30-year-old person with no medical history, this blood pressure would be alarming.

Documentation

To ensure you provide holistic nursing care, you need to focus your assessment on your patient and their findings. Documenting this is also of absolute importance. Nursing care plans and clinical pathways are designed to ensure that all aspects of disease processes are covered to ensure nothing is overlooked. Remember, documenting in nursing notes any variances is essential to ensure that all health-care professionals are able to see this information.

There are many diseases, conditions and altered pathophysiologies in the human body. Experience and exposure in nursing care delivery will increase this knowledge. Remember, disease treatments change with evidence-based practice, so the notion of lifelong learning is vital in providing safe and holistic nursing care.

Review the skill in Tollefson *Essential Clinical Skills*, 7.1 Documentation

SUMMARY

- Analysing client health information assists the health-care team make decisions regarding services and supports to be implemented for the person.
- Assessment of the client's health status includes observation, physical assessment and analysis of information.
- Care planning requires a problem-solving approach to address the identified health status of the client.

SELF-TEST QUESTIONS

1 What are the normal parameters for vital signs?
2 When planning care, how does the nurse gather the information to ensure a thorough assessment of the person?
3 How does a detailed understanding of the anatomy and physiology of the body assist in identifying actual and potential problems of a client and assist in identification of relevant interventions?
4 Why is a problem-solving approach employed when deciding on service planning for a client?
5 Why should all the processes of observation, physical assessment and analysis of other information be used to assess clients?

BIBLIOGRAPHY

Clarke, L., Gray, S., White, L., Duncan, G. & Baumle, W. (2016). *Foundations of Nursing: Enrolled Division 2 Nurses* (ANZ edition). Cengage Learning: South Melbourne.

Patton, K.T., Thibodeau, G.A. & Douglas, M.M. (2012). *Essentials of Anatomy & Physiology*. Mosby Elsevier: St Louis, MO.

Rizzo, D. (2015). *Fundamentals of Anatomy and Physiology* (4th edition). Delmar Cengage Learning: Boston, MA.

Tollefson, J., Watson, G., Jelly, E. & Tambree, K. (2016). *Essential Clinical Skills: Enrolled Division 2 Nurses* (3rd edition). Cengage Learning: South Melbourne.

Tortora, G. & Grabowski, S. (2002). *Principles of Anatomy and Physiology* (10th edition). John Wiley & Sons: Brisbane.

Waugh, A. & Grant, A. (2010). *Anatomy & Physiology in Health and Illness* (11th edition). Mosby Elsevier: St Louis, MO.

World Health Organization (WHO) (2018). *Frequently asked questions*. Retrieved from http://www.who.int/suggestions/faq/en/. Accessed 19 March 2018.

Nursing care for a person with complex needs

LEARNING OUTCOMES

After reading this chapter, you should have an understanding of:

12.1 Performing nursing interventions to assist a person with complex needs

12.2 Contributing to the nursing care of people with common disorders and conditions

12.3 Using critical thinking to improve care quality

Complex nursing

I remember nursing two patients who came in on the same day with a stroke. Both were male. There was not a great deal of difference in their ages, and they both had a right-sided CVA. The first patient, Joe, had aphasia and left-sided weakness, but could still move his arm. The second patient, Tom, had no aphasia and very minimal weakness to his left side. He could still dress himself and mobilise – even with an obvious deficit. The big differences between the two – Joe had diabetes and hypertension. Tom had previously had an MI, and had no other medical conditions.

It was very interesting to see the different needs of both patients and their outcomes from a very similar occurrence. Joe required a great deal of rehabilitation, whereas Tom, from memory, went home with assistance from community nurses.

12.1 Nursing interventions to assist a person with complex needs

Complex nursing is more than just chronic disease. It is nursing clients with a significant illness or injury and the potential presence of **co-morbidities** such as ischaemic heart disease, diabetes or respiratory conditions. Each client responds differently to disease, illness, surgery or conditions such as a stroke, and complex nursing care looks at all the intricacies of our clients. Complex nursing involves the nursing process, holistic care and critical thinking.

Nursing interventions have been a fairly constant element of your learning so far. Nursing interventions are actioned after a health assessment and are often predetermined in care plans or **clinical pathways**. These clinical pathways are an essential component of the nursing process and contain a summary of care requirements, goals and specific interventions for each individual patient. Some clinical pathways are generic – for example, post-operative hip replacement. This is because, generally, most patients follow the same recovery path. Nursing care plans are usually formulated between many members of the health-care team. They are quite often evidence based and are reviewed at specified dates to ensure clinical currency.

An example of nursing interventions based on a clinical pathway would be guidelines for measurement of vital signs post-operatively. Routine management will be subject to an accurate nursing assessment of each individual patient and may vary accordingly. Nursing assessment is outlined in **Figure 12.1**.

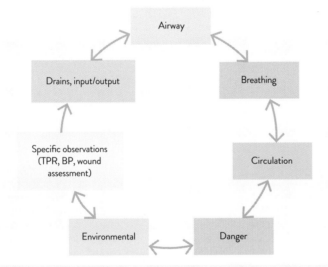

FIGURE 12.1 Nursing assessment

Some operations – for example, a femoral popliteal bypass graft – require pedal pulses checked with each set of observations to assess the patency of the graft. A carotid endarterectomy would require neurological observations performed with each set of vital signs to assess pupillary response to light and to observe any complications from reperfusion of the carotid artery. Post-caesarean section, you would need to check the fundus and any PV loss. Despite the nature of the operation, the basics of vital signs are required in all cases, with additional specified observations as the surgery deems.

Generally, vital signs (and specific observations) are performed half hourly for two hours, hourly for two hours and then every four hours until the condition of the patient is stable. The timing of this is from when the patient returns to the ward.

complex
Complicated and intricate – in health care it relates to patients who have multiple conditions or diseases that impact upon the presenting condition

co-morbidities
The presence of one or more diseases; for example, if a patient has diabetes and hypertension these are co-morbidities when they present with chest pain

clinical pathways
Standardised management plans that are evidence-based and are applicable to the multidisciplinary health-care team

So you see that there are many nursing interventions that are required for each patient regardless of their presentation or clinical condition. It becomes even more involved when there are co-morbidities (such as pre-existing heart conditions, diabetes and asthma) in planning for safe and effective nursing care. This is where working as part of a multidisciplinary team is essential!

Nursing interventions based on predetermined care plans

It is the uniqueness of patients that makes a nursing care plan or clinical pathway individualised and holistic. Holistic caring is looking at the client and providing the needs that they can't meet or need assistance with – no matter how small it may seem to you, it may be a very serious or very important concern for the patient.

Some argue that clinical pathways do not allow for this – as they are all the same. The refuting comment would be that clinical pathways are designed as guidelines and there are many spots to enter a variance or alteration in the care plan.

Nursing care plans or clinical pathways should always be adapted to the patient as an individual. They should always address the needs outlined in **Figure 12.2**.

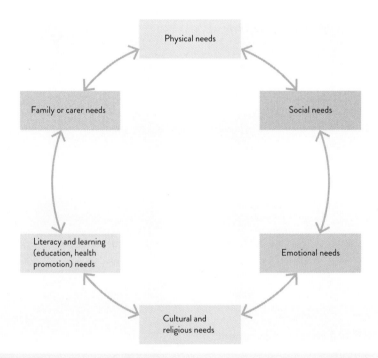

FIGURE 12.2 Holistic care planning

Nursing interventions demonstrating respect for dignity and cultural diversity

It is extremely important to maintain the dignity of the patient while performing nursing care. When talking to patients ensure that it is done in privacy. In a private room setting this is much easier, but the reality is often a four-bedded bay with only curtains for 'privacy', and this is where you need to be discreet and respectful. Unfortunately, curtains are not soundproof, and with this in mind if there is something of a particularly sensitive nature you should look at moving the patient and his/her family to a meeting room where they can feel confident in their privacy being maintained.

Some nursing interventions require exposing the patient – and this may make the patient uncomfortable, embarrassed or ashamed. Think about having to be on the receiving end of some of the caring that nurses provide and then try to take that thought with you! Administering suppositories, shaving, enemas, inserting catheters – they are all part of nursing interventions and all require exposing genital areas. Ensuring dignity is maintained as much as possible is also an underpinning notion in the framework for nursing care and delivery.

Religious, spiritual or cultural care

As discussed in Chapter 9, having an understanding of the difference in the beliefs and practices based on the client's cultural, spiritual and religious backgrounds enables you to provide appropriate care for the client. Absence of this understanding can lead to frustration and misunderstandings for the patient and the nurse.

The nurse can implement spiritual care by offering a supportive presence, facilitating the patient's practice of religion and, importantly, resolving conflicts between treatments (timing, for example) and spiritual activities.

You can do this by:

- familiarising the client with religious services within the facility
- respecting the patient's needs for privacy during prayer or spiritual activity
- arranging for the client to receive sacraments if desired
- attempting to best meet any dietary restrictions or preferences
- arranging for the priest, minister, pastor or rabbi to visit if the patient wishes.

When looking at issues related to cultural, religious and spiritual beliefs, it is important to identify what these are. For example, not all Muslims follow the same practices regarding health care. This is, in part, due to the fact that religion and culture factor heavily in our approach to health care and our beliefs. Religion is practised by so many people – but never is it identical. Therefore we must ensure that we provide culturally competent and appropriate care. It is okay to ask what is suitable or required, and there are many manuals and workbooks available in health-care facilities.

To deliver culturally competent care, the following can be of some assistance:

- Ask where your client was born and what the implications of their birthplace have on health care. (Do they have access to Medicare? Do they have private health insurance?)
- Ask what language is spoken at home. Do they use English as a second language? You may want to ascertain the level of actual versus language comprehension early in the encounter. Allowing a family or friend to accompany the client during the examination so they can translate should be a last resort – arrange a hospital-provided interpreter to ensure that the correct and full information is given to the patient and reported back to you. The family member can stay as a support person.
- Ask whether the client has a specific dietary pattern.
- Ask if the client's religion prohibits any medical treatments or interventions – for example, some religions do not allow blood products, fasting, or timing of events.

Being able to determine what support mechanisms are in place in the patient's family and carers is important to the nursing process. The patient may be a first-generation Australian, have no family support and feel quite isolated. Chronic and complex medical conditions require support of family or carers or health professionals in order to maintain health status.

Encouraging patient involvement during care interventions

There are many nursing interventions with which a patient can be encouraged to be involved, for example, a patient who is being discharged with a wound. As the nurse, you can start preparing the patient for caring for the wound themselves through education, demonstration and health promotion. If the patient can be assessed in hospital on the management of their wound, education or learning gaps can be addressed immediately to avoid any possible complications.

While it is always positive to have the patient complete their own care, the nurse is still accountable for the patient while they are in hospital. So you still need to assess and implement nursing care as required. For example, if a patient was emptying their catheter bag and not following safe and effective infection control measures you would need to address this with the patient and their caregivers.

The nursing process involves education, assessment, constant review and addressing the holistic needs of the patient. Holistically caring is ensuring that these needs are incorporated into the nursing care as they all interrelate and impact on health outcomes. A client whose emotional or psychosocial needs are not being met is at risk of being unable to meet the physical demands of the nursing interventions. For example, socially the client may have no support networks or be unable to afford the cost of the required home care after discharge. Consider the emotional needs of a client because some clients may not communicate these needs. How do you know if these needs are being met? How would you ensure that these needs are met? By taking a holistic approach and referring the client to appropriate health-care professionals is how!

Rehabilitation

Rehabilitation is a dynamic process in which an individual is helped to achieve optimal function and independence within their limitations (if any). Rehabilitation is what is involved in hospital care – after surgery, or during periods of illness, the aim of acute care provision is to rehabilitate the patient to their previous level of functioning if possible, or to assist the patient and their family to adjust to new care requirements. For example, when patient is in hospital for a hernia repair, rehabilitation will include deep breathing exercises, education regarding lifting and wound care, and nursing assessment to determine the physical status of the patient. The patient will be discharged with physical limitations for a short term. Another example that is far more complex would be that of a patient who has experienced a cerebrovascular accident or stroke (CVA). The patient may have residual deficits such as hemiparesis, aphasia or dysphagia. These conditions will require ongoing and long-term health-care intervention, assessment and management. The patient and their family will need to be supported throughout the entire process.

Rehabilitation:
- recognises the worth of the individual
- must be an integral component of care offered by the health-care facility
- offers a comprehensive plan arranged through active participation and coordination of all health-care members
- requires active participation by the individual with a disability to achieve their optimal rehabilitation potential
- should always actively involve the carers concerned with rehabilitating the individual as a whole through all five parameters of health
- aims to achieve the highest level of independence possible for the individual.

It is important to remember that when performing nursing interventions, or any nursing care, all clients' rights need to be protected.

- Be aware of the client's bill of rights.
- Respect the dignity of each client and family.
- Respect the client's right to refuse treatment.
- Listen attentively to clients and their family. Convey concerns to the registered nurse.
- Unless otherwise instructed, answer client's questions completely and provide information as would normally be provided by the health-care professional responsible.
- Respect the right to confidentiality of information.
- On admission, inform the client of facility policies, rules and regulations.
- Assist the clients to maintain their rights to freedom and to make decisions.

Activity 12.1

Assisting clients to maintain independence

Choose one of the clients you are providing support for.

1 What nursing interventions are prescribed for the client?

2 What is the goal and rationales for these nursing interventions?

3 How do the interventions assist the client to achieve independence?

Physical, emotional and psychosocial needs to consider

Every day nurses observe behaviour – of colleagues, patients and relatives. A component of nursing assessment is assessing the patient's behaviour. If the patient is aggressive or abusive this is clearly not appropriate and may mean that they are acting in this manner due to a need not being met. Never doubt the power of a simple observation in an interaction with your patient. Asking the patient how they are is often overlooked – due to many factors. As a nurse, it can be easy to fall into a 'task-oriented' approach and work towards crossing things/tasks off of your worksheet rather than listening to a patient's concerns.

From assessment of behaviours the nurse can formulate such deficits into the care plan. Using these concepts nurses can identify when their nursing interventions are satisfying an expressed need of a client. The difficult task is determining from the expressed behaviour what the actual deficits of needs are. Again, this is where a multifaceted and holistic approach to patient care is essential in ensuring all needs are met.

Underlying all nursing interventions are the professional legal and ethical standards that are our scope of practice, as discussed in Chapter 4. It is essential that all nursing staff are aware of their professional requirements as well as their specific organisational requirements. In any situation, no matter how seemingly urgent, all nurses must act within their scope of practice.

The importance of reporting and recording

It is essential that nurses report and record all responses to nursing interventions, regardless if they have been effective. It is important that these responses are noted in the daily care notes so a timeline of responses can be viewed. It is not always appropriate to document these at the end of the shift.

Review the skill in Tollefson *Essential Clinical Skills* 7.1 Documentation

For example, vital signs are documented at the time of being performed and a response to an intervention that is identified by a nurse also should, in most cases, be recorded at the time. There are many situations where responses/reactions should be reported to an RN or another appropriate person prior to commencing written records. An example of this would be if the client's pain management is not effective or the client is showing adverse medical reactions.

Effective responses are just as important to report and document as non-effective ones. For example, a patient that was going to be discharged is still nauseous. An anti-emetic is administered and the client feels better and decides that they would like to leave. The EN should report this change immediately to the RN or shift coordinator so staffing levels and occupancy levels can be adjusted if need be. You would also need to ensure that you document the effect of the anti-emetic and any education or information regarding follow-up treatment for nausea you have provided.

Additional nursing interventions may be planned for a client that may not be needed if a positive/effective response from other treatments occurs prior to these happening. Reporting and recording client responses assists in ensuring that unnecessary interventions aren't undertaken.

The EN should be aware of whom to report client responses to; this will vary between team members. For example, this can occur during verbal handover to the nursing team, the next care provider or to the RN, CN or shift coordinator.

As nursing care is provided by a team, all members of the team contribute to the sharing of all information where appropriate. In the handover you should report all care given and the responses that have significance to the client.

TIP 12.1

Nursing interventions

So much can be gained by recognising that all patients are unique and are individuals. We all have a certain way to brush our teeth or our hair, or the time of day we choose to shower. Imagine being told when to shower or when to perform oral hygiene? As a nurse, you should always remember this. Even if someone has suffered a stroke, it does not mean they have to shower when they are 'told' to. Always factor in the individual aspects of nursing care. This is definitely one of the rewarding aspects of nursing – working with a person to return them to health. Assisting them through times of illness, injury or prolonged rehabilitation. Empowering them to take part in their health care. So my only advice is always remember that that patient is a person.

Jasmine, EN, 35

Reflective practice 12.1

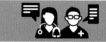

Complex diseases

You have been allocated to look after four patients on your placement. One of your patients, Ken, is a 38-year-old male who has cardiomyopathy. Ken's cardiomyopathy is related to his alcohol consumption – he has drunk excessively for many years. He has been admitted due to pulmonary oedema and other congestive cardiac failure symptoms and for management of these.

When you receive handover from the morning staff, the nurse, Rebecca, says, 'It's all his fault anyway, he has drunk himself to this state'. She further asserts that she has not provided any pain relief that he requested as it is 'his problem, and he can wait'. Complex conditions are exactly that, and Ken's condition, regardless of his alcoholic intake, needs to be treated.

1   What, if anything would you say to Rebecca?
2   What would be your first nursing intervention for Ken?
3   What observations of Ken should be performed?

12.2 Nursing care of people with common disorders and conditions

As your experience grows, you will notice that there are several chronic conditions that are common reasons for admission to hospital; examples include an exacerbation of COPD, infective bronchitis, acute or chronic renal failure, or worsening of congestive cardiac failure.

What is also evident is the notion of how disease affects each person differently. You could have four patients all with the same illness – let's say pneumonia – and if we observed the process of the illness in the patients we would be able to see a different recovery period for each. Some would take days to recover and others weeks. It is dependent upon other variables such as age, other illnesses/conditions, medications and general state of wellbeing.

Nursing care for complex conditions

There are many complex conditions that require nursing interventions and care. The list is exhaustive, and only some examples will be given here. The focus of nursing care should always be to provide holistic and individualised care through thorough client assessment and data collection.

TABLE 12.1 Complex conditions and the clinical skills associated

Description	Examples	Nursing care	Tollefson Clinical Skills
Respiratory system			
Respiratory conditions are often chronic with acute exacerbations or infective processes. Infections and other conditions can further debilitate the patient and increase their need for nursing and medical care. Pneumonia accounts for a number of deaths annually.	Chronic-Acute: COPD (chronic obstructive pulmonary disease), asthma. Acute: pneumonia, hemothorax, pleurisy, pneumothorax, trauma and cancer. Infectious: bacterial and viral infections, Legionnaires' disease and tuberculosis.	Respiratory rate O_2 saturations These are the skills required for complex nursing interventions for a person with respiratory conditions. Oxygen therapy Suctioning Tracheostomy care Isolation care These skills may be required depending on the needs of the client	2.3 Temperature, pulse and respiration (TPR) measurement 2.5 Pulse oximetry 8.1 Oxygen therapy (includes peak flow meter) 8.8 Suctioning of oral cavity 8.9 Tracheostomy care 8.13 Additional Precautions
Cardiovascular system			
The cardiac system is vital to maintaining blood circulation to the vital organs of the body. There is a close interrelationship between the cardiac system and the respiratory system. Provision of nursing care and interventions relies heavily upon the nursing process – assessment, reassessment and interpretation of data.	Myocardial ischaemia, coronary artery disease, hypertension, carotid stenosis, heart failure, pulmonary oedema, peripheral vascular disease and atherosclerosis.	TPR BP O_2 saturation 12-lead ECG	As well as all of the skills listed for Respiratory System above: 2.4 Blood pressure measurement 2.10 12-lead ECG recording

>>

Description	Examples	Nursing care	Tollefson Clinical Skills
Neurological system			
The nervous system has three essential roles: sensing, integrating and responding. The components of the nervous system responsible for performing these roles are the sensory component, the integrative component and the monitor component.	Neurological conditions are mainly classified under the following headings: Congenital: • Hydrocephalus Degenerative – movement and seizure: • epilepsy Infectious: • meningitis • tetanus • Gullain-Barre syndrome Neoplastic: • brain tumours Traumatic: • head injury, spinal cord injury Vascular: • stroke	As given for the cardiovascular system, but also the Glascow Coma Scale. The lowest score is 3, while a score of 15 is the best and indicates a fully alert, orientated client.	Glascow Coma Scale: http://www.glasgowcomascale.org/
Gastrointestinal system			
The major function of the GI system is to supply nutrients to the body cells.	GI system disorders include problems related to nutrition, malnutrition and obesity: • obesity • rickets • osteoporosis Upper and lower GI system disorders: • reflux • peptic ulcer Problems with the liver, biliary tract and pancreas: • diabetes • pancreatic cancer • cirrhosis of the liver	As above and also nasogastric tube insertion and feeding, gastric drainage and gastric tube feeding BMI measurement Stool observation Assisting the patient to eat and drink Blood glucose measurement	8.11 Nasogastric tube insertion 3.7 Assisting the patient with elimination – urinary and bowel elimination 3.9 Faeces assessment and specimen collection 3.4 Assisting the patient with eating and drinking 2.6 Blood glucose measurement
Endocrine system			
The endocrine system is responsible for hormone secretion, which is something that can affect all body cells.	Diabetes is a major disease that you will encounter. Others include hyperthyroidism, cancers, Cushing's syndrome and Addison's disease.	Blood glucose measurement These require monitoring of vital signs and also rely on blood tests.	2.6 Blood glucose measurement 6.1 Venepuncture

>>

Description	Examples	Nursing care	Tollefson Clinical Skills
Integumentary system			
The skin is the largest organ. The nursing care of skin is always focused upon restoring its integrity.	Skin can be compromised in many ways – through allergic reactions to skin cancers, ulcers and pressure area sores, and burns.	Prevention of pressure injuries. Assessment charts such as Braden, Waterlow and Norton.	 3.13 Preventing and managing pressure injuries Waterlow scale: http://www.health.vic.gov.au/__data/assets/file/0009/233667/Waterlow-scale.pdf Braden risk assessment tool: http://www.sahealth.sa.gov.au/wps/wcm/connect/b24a8480438d09be9e63dfbc736a4e18/2010maybradenrisktool.pdf?MOD=AJPERES&CACHEID=ROOTWORKSPACE-b24a8480438d09be9e63dfbc736a4e18-m08aZR- Norton scale: http://www.health.vic.gov.au/__data/assets/file/0010/233668/Norton-scale.pdf
Musculoskeletal system			
These conditions result in a dysfunction of the body's bones, joints or muscles. The effect of these can impact upon patients' ADL performance, due to reduced mobility or pain.	Some examples of conditions you could expect to provide nursing care for would be arthritis, fracture or bony injury, bursitis, gout and infection.	Assessment of the client for mobility, falls, range of motion.	 3.14 Active and passive exercises A guide to understanding balance and mobility for health staff: http://www.cec.health.nsw.gov.au/__data/assets/pdf_file/0003/327711/a-guide-to-understanding-balance-and-mobility-document-For-website-Aug-2016.pdf Falls Risk Assessment Tool (FRAT): https://www2.health.vic.gov.au/about/publications/policiesandguidelines/falls-risk-assessment-tool
Urinary/reproductive system			
The need for an indwelling catheter can be due to a reason as simple as a decreased level of consciousness, or as complex as a debilitating illness or long-standing condition.	The most common urinary and reproductive disorders are related to infectious processes; otherwise there are cancers, urinary calculi, renal failure and hormonal imbalances.	Can require the management of urinary drainage bags and the insertion of indwelling catheters	 8.6 Catheterisation (urinary)

Cardiovascular assessment is imperative and is assessed as shown in **Figure 12.3**.

Heart rate. Measured manually by palpating an artery. Remember to always note the rate, regularity and strength

Cardiac rhythm. Evaluated by recording the electrical activity of the heart using an ECG, either by 12-lead ECG or by continuous monitoring

Blood pressure. Measured non-invasively by means of a manual or an automatic cuff, or invasively using an intra-arterial line, which provides a constant blood pressure reading

FIGURE 12.3 Cardiovascular assessment

CASE STUDY 12.1

Importance of skin

Margaret Cowen is a 31-year-old female who has been hospitalised for the past four weeks post a motor vehicle accident. She sustained significant head injuries and has been in the rehabilitation unit for one week. Margaret has developed a pressure injury on her left heel. The wound is a cavity, the size of a 10-cent piece, and involves subcutaneous tissue. The wound has previously not been documented so the length of time it has existed is unknown.

1   What stage of pressure area injury does this sound like?
2   What factors could be contributing to the wound developing?
3   What would you document in regards to finding this wound?

The one-armed man

On my first placement in acute care, I was working in an orthopaedic ward. I was allocated four patients with my buddy nurse. One patient was in a car accident and he had his left arm fractured in about three places. It meant that he had only one arm to use to attend his activities of daily living (ADLs). He was 18, and was incredibly embarrassed. I remember asking him when I was assisting him with his ADLs how we could work it so he could get as much done as possible without needing someone to help or see him exposed. The solution was to put on a singlet that was slightly too big (easy to get on) and for him to wear boxer shorts as they were (coupled with his other injuries) easiest to get on. So, always ask what you can do to help the patient perform the task rather than assuming they have an injury and can't do any of it.

Scott, 42, EN.

When providing support to a person with complex needs it is necessary to assess the client on an ongoing basis. This is done pre-intervention and post-intervention. Any unusual response needs to be reported and documented and a full assessment of the client be undertaken. This could be in response to administration of a medication or the client not responding well to the intervention. At times you will need to report and document a deterioration in a client's condition. This can be an emergency situation or a time when the health-care team needs to reassess the client and the care plan.

12.3 Critical thinking to improve care quality

The nursing process provides nurses with a five interrelated step systematic method of client problem solving as shown in **Figure 12.4**. Nurses utilising the nursing process must use critical thinking and clinical reasoning skills to collect, review and validate client data, to plan, implement and then evaluate client care through evidence-based nursing practice.

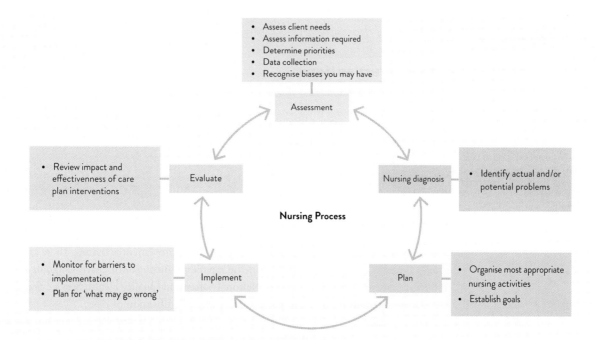

FIGURE 12.4 The nursing process and critical thinking

At any time in the care of a client, a nurse may move back and forth from one step of the process to another as new information emerges.

Nursing practice is always changing and as new knowledge becomes available professional nurses need to challenge traditional ways of doing things and discover new interventions that are the most effective and have high scientific relevance, resulting in better outcomes. The nursing process is a traditional critical thinking competency that allows nurses to make clinical judgements and take actions based on reason. A process is a series of steps or components taken to achieve a goal.

Identifying nursing interventions

While performing nursing care, and through following your nursing care plan in collaboration with the registered nurse, you will soon discover your ability to assess both forms of data – objective and subjective. With this data, you will relate it to the patient and make planned interventions and unplanned ones. For example, if a patient has low blood pressure – let's say 90/60 – you would first review the baseline observations, or previous observations to see what they have been. From here, you would question the patient – 'Are you dizzy?', 'How do you feel?' – and with this information you would formulate your next intervention/s.

Conversely, if interventions are planned for a patient that are not appropriate, you will need to communicate this clearly and effectively to the registered nurse with whom you are working collaboratively. This could include simple things such as assisting with ADLs – the client may wish to have the care completed at another time. Another example could be client refusal to comply with the intervention, which requires documentation and explanation to the multidisciplinary team.

Another component of your role will be to explain procedures and processes to your client and their carer or family. Of course, if you are unaware of the exact details then be honest – it is never frowned upon to ask for further information, and in doing so advising the client that you are 'unsure but will find out' is the best approach.

Activity 12.2

Understanding complex interventions

Select one of the complex nursing care interventions that you are required to complete. Locate the policy and procedure for this intervention.

1   Can you explain the rationale for each step of the process?
2   What evidence-based practice was this intervention and steps based on?
    You might like to refer to Tollefson's Clinical Skills if you are unable to explain the processes, or discuss this with the clinical supervisor.

Quality improvement processes

While on placement, you may be involved in quality improvement activities. These can be as simple as audits completed at the bedside on a patient's medications chart. Ongoing review and management, with a focus on the National Safety and Quality Health Service Standards (2012), are methods to maintain patient safety and identification of risks.

Some examples of audit tools can be found here: https://clinicalexcellence.qld.gov.au/resources/audit-tools-national-safety-and-quality-health-service-standards.

Audits, continuing improvement and best practice are all interlinked components in nursing. You will see with each different placement and with increasing experience that each facility will manage this process differently. The end goal is always related to improving patient safety.

There will always be change in health-care delivery. Equipment, processes and procedures will change based on evidence-based practice. An element of your role will be to remain up to date with clinical practice relevant to your area of nursing. It is quite clear that observation ranges do not alter – what alters are the methods of nursing care and interventions. Complex nursing requires the nurse to be aware of many conditions, and more importantly, their potential impact on the client and their wellbeing and recovery. By utilising a holistic approach, and through obtaining data from the client, you will be well able to assess and manage all clients with complex nursing requirements.

Activity 12.3

The nurse's role in auditing

Select one of the audit processes that the clinical area in which you are doing placement is involved in.

1   What activities are being allocated to the nursing staff?

2   What is the goal of the activity?
3   Have other activities been undertaken in this area previously? Why has the workplace chosen this activity? Is it in response to a clinical outcome?

CASE STUDY 12.2

Indwelling catheters

You have a full patient load, and one patient, Susy Kent, is a morbidly obese 40-year-old lady who is requiring frequent panning for a UTI. To put this patient on a pan requires three people – two to turn Susy, and one to place the pan. Your buddy nurse, Alice, states 'It would be just easier to stick a catheter in than doing this every hour or so'. Susy has a reduced exercise tolerance, and is unable to mobilise to the toilet 'in time' to void. She has been incontinent several times and is very embarrassed regarding this. Alice collects the equipment for an IDC and asks for you to assist her.

1 Is this a valid reason for inserting an IDC?
2 What considerations need to be made for Susy?
3 Is performing this action within ethical and respectful principles?
4 What are some alternatives to inserting an IDC?

SUMMARY

- When providing care for a person with complex needs, the nurse needs to follow the care plan and ensure that the person is supported holistically and encouraged to be as independent as possible.
- When providing support to a person with complex conditions, the nurse is responsible for monitoring the person's response to treatment and reporting any unexpected outcomes to the registered nurse.
- A person's conditions can change rapidly and the nurse needs to use critical thinking skills to identify situations where the care requires alteration in response to the person's needs.

SELF-TEST QUESTIONS

1 How can the nurse show respect for the person's dignity and cultural diversity while performing nursing interventions for a person with complex needs?
2 What strategies can the nurse employ to encourage the person with complex needs to be as independent as possible?
3 What is the responsibility of the nurse when a client's condition alters in response to their conditions or treatment regime?
4 How can the nurse contribute to quality improvement when providing care to a client with complex needs?
5 How does the nurse employ critical thinking skills when performing complex nursing interventions?

BIBLIOGRAPHY

Australian Commission on Safety and Quality in Health Care (2012). *National Safety and Quality Health Service Standards*, https://www.safetyandquality.gov.au/wp-content/uploads/2011/09/NSQHS-Standards-Sept-2012.pdf. Accessed 19 March 2018.

Clarke, L., Gray, S., White, L., Duncan, G. & Baumle, W. (2016). *Foundations of Nursing: Enrolled Division 2 Nurses* (ANZ Edition). Cengage Learning: South Melbourne.

Queensland Government (2017). *Audit Tools for National Safety and Quality Health Service Standards*. Retrieved from https://clinicalexcellence.qld.gov.au/resources/audit-tools-national-safety-and-quality-health-service-standards.

Tollefson, J., Watson, G., Jelly, E. & Tambree, K. (2016). *Essential Clinical Skills: Enrolled Division 2 Nurses* (3rd edition). Cengage Learning: South Melbourne.

Principles of wound management

LEARNING OUTCOMES

After reading this chapter, you should have an understanding of:

13.1 Applying protocols for wound assessment

13.2 Assessing the impact of a wound on a person, family or carer

13.3 Contributing to planning care for a person with a wound

13.4 Undertaking clinical nursing care in implementing wound care strategies

13.5 Applying contemporary wound management strategies to complex or challenging wounds

13.6 Assisting in evaluating outcomes of nursing actions in wound care

Pressure sores

Fresh from studying skin integrity and patient handling, I was placed on a medical ward, where Sam Chesterfield, 68-year-old man, had been admitted for cellulitis. Sam had been working in the garden when he was bitten by an insect. Sam's left arm was warm, red and swollen. Pain was significant and Sam stated it was more comfortable laying down.

Sam was hospitalised for five days for intravenous antibiotics and dressings. Due to pain and location of his wound, Sam developed a pressure injury on his left shoulder. After a case review on the ward, the general consensus was that because Sam was normally fit and healthy, he did not require 'turns' or 'pressure area care'. Sam is a prime example of just how easy it can be to gain a pressure injury in hospital. Such is the expense and the debilitating effect of pressure injuries, their prevention and management is one of the National Safety and Quality Health Service Standards – Standard 8. This Standard further highlights the importance of prevention and awareness. Standard 8 information can be found here: https://www.safetyandquality.gov.au/wp-content/uploads/2012/10/Standard8 _Oct_2012_WEB.pdf.

13.1 Applying protocols for wound assessment

The nursing process provides us with the ideal model to ensure appropriate wound management after a holistic assessment of the client. When we assess our patients holistically, we are looking at both subjective and objective data. We need to establish if there are any co-morbidities or other contributing factors that can impair the healing process. Things to consider in relation to wound care and healing are:

- age
- co-morbidities
- vascular disease
- medications
- drug and alcohol use
- obesity
- nutrition.

This information, coupled with an accurate record of the wound, including size, depth, location and description, is essential in determining wound treatment and the nature of the wound. Wound assessment requires the following to be identified:

- The nature of the wound – is it acute or chronic?
- What caused the wound?
- Is there evidence of any healing? Is there primary intention, for example?
- Is there any tissue loss?
- What exudate is there? What is the type, colour, amount, consistency and odour?
- What do the wound edges look like?
- What is the condition of the surrounding skin?
- Is there pain associated with the wound?
- Is there any evidence of infection?

Wounds can be classified in a number of ways. The terms *acute* and *chronic* are used to describe wounds in terms of onset and duration. Types of wounds include:

- surgical incision
- traumatic/lacerations/punctures
- ulcers
- burns
- avulsions
- abrasions/skin tears
- amputations
- graft and donor sites.

Wounds Australia includes a highly useful publication *Standards for Wound Prevention and Management*: http://www.woundsaustralia.com.au/2016/standards-for-wound-prevention-and-management-2016.pdf.

Members of the wound management team include nurses, medical practitioners, occupational therapists, microbiologists, pharmacists and carers. Communication and documentation of treatments and progress in healing need to be consistent and objective.

The aims of wound care are to:

- promote wound healing
- manage the wound effectively
- collaborate with the RN and multidisciplinary team members to ensure correct treatments are used
- ensure adequate analgesia is administered for dressings
- prevent infection or cross-contamination
- document, record and review the wound and its progress.

Effective assessment is essential for all types of wound management.

TIP 13.1

Wound
assessment

While you are on
placement, investigate
what documentation
is used for assessment
of wounds. Is there a
wound service at your
facility that will review
the wound and discuss
optimum treatment?
Are photographs stored
of the wound to show
healing or infection
processes? What
occurs after hours?

Make it a priority
to find this information
as you will soon see
just how many people
are hospitalised with
wounds!

Client cooperation and consent

When undertaking assessment of the client and their wound it is necessary to gain their consent and cooperation. It is important to view the wound management as part of the holistic assessment of the client. Important questions to address include:

* How does the client view the wound?
* How does it impact on their activities of daily living (ADLs)?

It is important to include the client as part of the process of planning care. Some areas that the client needs to have input into include:

* What is the cost of wound dressings?
* What features of the wound affect their ADLs? Examples may be an offensive odour or excess exudate.
* Who is going to manage the wound? For some areas of the body it will be necessary for another person to support the regime of wound management.
* When can an outside person assess the wound? For people who are required to attend work how will this be timetabled?

All of these factors will have a direct impact on the success of the wound management program and the cooperation of the client.

Maintaining client dignity and privacy

It is important to always remember that the client is the priority and not the wound. Some clients feel embarrassment if their wound has an odour or excessive exudate. It also may be that the wound is in an area of the body that they are reluctant to expose to others. By undertaking a holistic assessment and taking all factors such as cultural identity into account, the nurse will be able to institute a therapeutic relationship that will allow the client to trust the nurse to provide the necessary care for effective wound management.

It is important to ask the client what they have done in regard to wound management. Be careful to maintain a non-judgemental attitude to any disclosure, even if it is not recognised practice.

TIP 13.2

Maintaining
privacy

As a nurse you will
become accustomed to
different and complex
wounds. Always bear
in mind that this is the
first exposure for the
client. Always ensure a
private area by closing
doors or curtains
before exposing
wounds.

Documentation and reporting

When undertaking wound dressings one of the responsibilities of the nurse is to accurately report on the progress of the wound. Is it getting better?

Nurses use pre-printed checklists to document the progress of the wound. Other ways to measure how the wound is responding are:

* Is the wound getting smaller in size?
* Is the surrounding area looking healthy?
* Is there an offensive odour?
* Has the amount of pain experienced by the client decreased?
* Taking photographs at set intervals to assess the progress of wound healing.

It is always important to follow the wound management plan of care to ensure best outcomes. If you assess that the wound is not improving, it is important to document this and report it to the health-care team before implementing changes to the wound management routine.

Non-disturbance of wounds

Some wounds and wound care products require a period of time left undisturbed to enable the body's healing mechanisms to take effect. In surgical nursing the surgeon may order that the wound is left undisturbed until a certain period of time elapses. The nurse still is required to check the wound dressing but should not take off the dressing, rather just record any breakthrough ooze on the surface of the dressing and reinforce the dressing with another sterile combine. The nurse should document this and report to the RN who will contact the surgeon for further orders.

For other wound care products it is best to leave the wound undisturbed to allow moist wound healing to occur. The nurse will be able to find out if this is the case by researching the type of wound product being used.

The type of dressing that is prescribed for the wound will depend on several factors:
- cost of the dressing
- cost of staff changing the dressing
- pain experienced by the client having the dressing changed
- impact on the ADLs by having the wound dressed.

If the wound is infected

Once you have established 'what' the wound is, you need to plan your care. Some things to remember:
- Holistic assessment – you will need to consider all aspects of the patient's situation, for example, what time, if any, will they lose from work? Will they require support from a carer?
- Type of management – what wound care products will be used? Enlist a wound care specialist review regularly if necessary.
- Remaining skin integrity – this is crucial in ensuring no further breakdown or pressure injuries can occur. Patients need to be educated regarding the potential for skin breakdown or pressure injury due to inactivity.
- Document and record – ensure that you document the wound care, and all relevant interventions and observations regarding the wound.

CASE STUDY 13.1

Same wound, different outcomes

You are completing your placement in a primary health clinic, where two workmates have presented for wound care. Jason Barnett and Gary Muller have both lacerated their legs on a metal pipe that was exposed at a worksite. The wound is a perfect 'O' from the pipe end and is on the lateral aspect of their thighs at slightly different heights (due to their height differences). The wounds are not gaping, and haemostasis has been maintained by bandages applied to the wounds at the worksite. Both gentlemen have had tetanus in the past few years.

Jason is a 42-year-old male, with no significant medical history. He is obese at 132 kg and 180 cm, but is physically active and maintains a full-time labour-intensive job. Jason takes no medications.

Gary is a 54-year-old male with hypertension, diabetes and gout. Gary takes medication for high blood pressure and is currently diet-controlled for diabetes. Gary is 108kg and 189cm tall.

1. What, if any, differences in healing do you think will occur between Jason and Gary?
2. Jason maintains a diet of highly processed foods because he lives alone and works six days a week. Do you think this will have an effect on wound healing?
3. Gary presents a week later with redness and heat around his wound. What could this be?
4. Jason presents a week later with the wound clean and healing, but very slowly. What factors could be contributing to a slowed healing process? What could be done to assist Jason?

Figure 13.1 outlines some factors that affect wound healing. The skin acts as a barrier between the external environment and the body's internal environment. It assists in maintaining a stable temperature for the body and is the largest sensory organ. When the skin is not intact it becomes a considerable infection control risk.

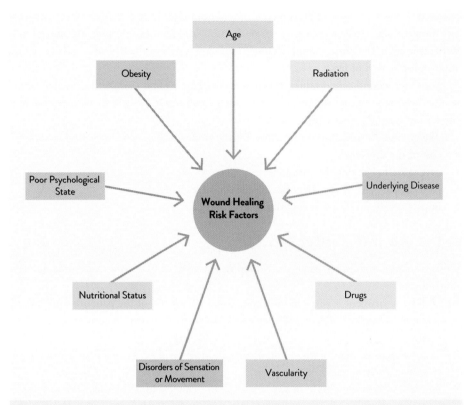

FIGURE 13.1 Factors that affect wound healing

Strategies to minimise cross-contamination and spread of infection

The nurse always needs to be aware of how infection is spread and how to implement strategies to avoid this from occurring. Good hand hygiene will prevent both cross-contamination and spread of infection. It may be necessary to employ additional measures such as the use of sterile gloves if the client is immune compromised or if the wound contains an organism that is particularly virulent or easily spread to others.

Other strategies include:

- aseptic technique or non-touch technique when undertaking wound care
- the use of secondary dressings to contain the exudate or minimise the spread of infection
- the use of isolation nursing to protect either the client or others from the invasive organism.

Aseptic non-touch technique

aseptic non-touch technique (ANNT)
Infection control practice used to prevent the transmission of pathogens

Aseptic non-touch technique (ANTT) is a framework for aseptic practice that is intended for use in a range of settings. The National Health and Medical Research Council provides an overview of ANTT at: https://www.nhmrc.gov.au/book/australian-guidelines-prevention-and-control-infection-healthcare-2010/b1-7-1-aseptic-non-touch.

ANTT principles are used throughout many aspects of nursing care delivery. They are especially important in the care of wounds and assist in prevention of cross-contamination and the spread of infection. ANTT attempts to prevent the organism from access to the health worker's hands and the possible spread of the infection to other areas of the client's body or to other people.

Cross-contamination attempts to stop the spread of infection from one area of the wound to another. This is why you have been taught to clean the wound in specific ways, such as swabbing from clean to infected areas. ANTT and aseptic principles should always be used when there is a breach in the client's defence mechanisms, such as the integrity of the skin surface.

Review the skill in Tollefson *Essential Clinical Skills*, 4.1 Aseptic technique – establishing a general or critical aseptic field

---

CASE STUDY 13.2

Wound dressings

You were on placement in an acute care facility on a medical ward. You and your buddy RN were about to commence a wound dressing on Mark Raines, a 58-year-old male, when you were called to assist in a medical emergency. You returned to the trolley you had set up approximately an hour ago. Mark's children had been visiting and the wound dressing equipment had been moved. Your buddy RN said to 'just use it, it will take too long to get all new stuff again and it is a waste'.

1 What principles here, if any, have been compromised?
2 What potential risks can using this equipment cause?
3 What would you disclose to Mark regarding his dressing?

13.2 Assessing the impact of wounds

Following on from a holistic assessment of the wound, the nurse needs to determine any potential underlying causes of the prevention of wound healing. Does the patient have any diseases that will affect or impact upon healing? Are they able to attend dressing changes? Will they attend appointments if the wound dressing becomes soiled or damaged? A component of your assessment should also consider the impact that the wound is having on the client and their family in terms of physical or emotional impact. Stress, anxiety and depression can further reduce the efficiency of the patient's immune system and thus retard healing.

Other factors that affect healing include the following:

- *Wound temperature* – for optimal wound healing to take place the wound needs to be kept at a constant body temperature of approximately 37°C. A stable wound temperature must be maintained for healing to occur.
- *Hydration of the wound* – moisture balance in wounds is also necessary for healing to occur. In a moist environment wound healing facilitates the migration of cells across the wound surface. A dry wound environment impedes this process and an excessively moist wound environment can promote bacterial growth.
- *Inappropriate wound management practices* – knowledge of the different wound care products and their mode of action is necessary to prevent poor wound management choices.
- *Pressure, shearing force and friction* – can occur as a result of restrictive dressings or clothing, inactivity and overactivity, abrasive dressings or practices. The healing wound is very fragile and needs protection from external forces and the environment. To ensure healing it is essential to promote vascularity.
- *Presence of foreign bodies* – any foreign body in a wound can prevent or slow healing. Examples of foreign bodies are:
  - dirt
  - hair
  - glass
  - cotton wool fibres
  - sutures
  - surgical implants
  - infection.

Activity 13.1

The impact of wounds

Think about the following wounds – a chronic leg ulcer that started out as a scratch from a dog, and an abdominal wound post a caesarean that has dehisced and not closed/healed. Consider the impact upon ADLs and ability to work, parent or complete normal tasks and routines. This is without factoring in pain and changes to self-care because of the wounds. The impact of wounds is significant, and factors such as recent birth or inability to perform paid employment can further create feelings of frustration, fear, lack of control and anger, to name but a few. The entire gamut of processes relating to the wound needs to be considered in order to provide holistic care. A wound will not heal quickly if, for example, a person is lifting children and babies and placing the area that is broken down under constant tension.

1   What impact do you think the impact would be on each patient in this scenario?
2   Do you think the patient could work with either wound being present?

It is essential in this process of holistic assessment that a clear understanding of the client's psychological state is gained to implement a clear plan for caring for the wound. Lack of compliance can be a major factor in delayed wound healing. Clients with chronic wounds suffer greater limitations of activity and mobility, more severe pain and increased stressors about their health. These clients can have significantly lower self-esteem as they do not feel they are contributing to their family or social circumstances due to the wound. Wounds can be totally debilitating and this should never be overlooked.

13.3 Planning care

When planning wound management care with your client, you will need to also factor in the basic principles of primary health care. Primary health care is characterised by a holistic understanding of health as wellbeing rather than the absence of disease and the focus is upon wellness. Care is based on best outcomes for the patient and how they can be achieved. The plan should involve the client, their family or significant others, their general practitioner and the wound management team.

Major complications of wound health fall into three categories:

1   *Wound dehiscence* – occurs when the wound bursts open or breaks down in sections, as shown in **Figure 13.2**.
2   *Wound infection* – occurs when bacteria is able to overcome the body's defence mechanisms. Wound infection prolongs the inflammatory stage of healing. Most wounds are colonised by some microorganism, however, acute infections require appropriate treatment. Clinical signs of infection include:
    –   inflammation: hot to the touch, painful and reddened
    –   **oedema** around the wound margin
    –   oedema around the edges of the wound
    –   increased **exudate** discharge from the wound. It can be:
        –   purulent – green, yellow or red. Green indicates a large growth of bacteria, yellow is less growth and red signifies blood
    –   offensive odour
    –   pyrexia: a higher systemic temperature as the body attempts to kill of the organism
    –   tachycardia (systemic response to infection): increased blood flow to the area brings white blood cells to fight the infection
    –   **granulation**: tissue that bleeds easily.
3   *Haemorrhage* – persistent bleeding due to dislodged clot, slipped ligature or erosion of a blood vessel. This is more common in a surgical wound.

oedema
Excessive amount of fluid trapped in the tissue of the body, generally the limbs

exudate
Fluid that is leaked or drained from a wound. It is a response to the tissue damage in the wound

granulation
Growth of new tissue on the surfaces of the wound

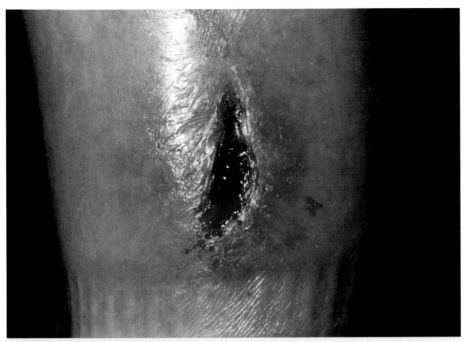

FIGURE 13.2 Wound dehiscence

Science Photo Library/Dr H.C. Robinson.

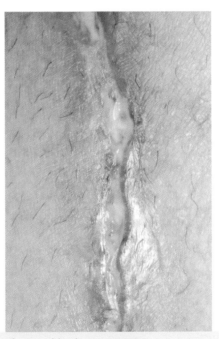

FIGURE 13.3 Images of wound bed presentation

Science Photo Library/Dr P. Marazzi.

TIP 13.3

Wound loss/
bleeding/exudate

When you assume
care of a patient,
try to review wound
dressings to see if
they are intact, dry or
oozing. For example,
if a surgical wound is
bleeding it is important
to know how much
blood loss and over
what period of time
it has occurred. Often
surgical wounds
are 'marked' with
blood loss or ooze so
they can be closely
monitored.

Review the skill in Tollefson *Essential Clinical Skills*: 4.2 Simple dry dressing using a general aseptic field, 4.3 Wound irrigation & 4.5 Packing a wound – 'wet-to-moist' dressing

13.4 Clinical nursing care of wounds

Clinical nursing care in the management of wounds requires you to become proficient in wound dressings. There are several skills you will need to undertake in the dressing and care of wounds. As we have established, no two wounds are alike, and as such, some wounds are packed, others are dry dressed, and many require bandaging for added protection (see **Figure 13.5**). It is always useful to view the wound dressings (with consent of the patient and nurse) to visualise any differences and treatment modalities. This will greatly assist with your exposure and understanding of wound care therapy.

CASE STUDY 13.3

Wound swabs

Molly Bishop is an 80-year-old female who has a chronic ulcer on her left shin. She has presented to clinics for a wound dressing. The wound generally is dressed once every three days. Molly has presented a day earlier as she feels the dressing is tight and it is 'a bit smelly'. When you remove the dressing you notice an offensive yellow exudate. You ask the RN working with you to review the wound, and he suggests a wound swab.

1 What is the primary reason for a wound swab?
2 Should antibiotics be started immediately?
3 Other than the exudate changing, what else should you review in Molly's wound?

Reflective practice 13.1

Infection control and wounds

During my first placement in a hospital there were several patients, who, after a few days, were found to have multi-resistant staphylococcus aureus (MRSA). They were then moved to a four-bed bay where all four patients had MRSA. Prior to this, they were sharing a room with other patients who were not colonised with MRSA. One patient, Kylie Templer, a 39-year-old woman, was three days post op following an open hernia repair. Kylie's wound exudate changed from serous fluid to yellow, offensive fluid. It was swabbed and found to be containing MRSA – but the results took about a day. I remember wondering how this could have occurred. And it was, most likely, the most simple of mechanisms – hand washing. Touching one patient's bed area or equipment item and then going to Kylie's bed area. It could have been any number of staff, and it could have occurred due to many 'jobs' going through the person's mind. A moment of lapse of concentration and an infection as nasty as MRSA has now been spread. I spoke with the infection control nurse and she advised me that Kylie would now have to be nursed with contact precautions until she has three 'clean' swabs. They swab all patients on admission to hospital now – I thought only wounds would be swabbed; but no, a swab of the nose and the groin are taken. I ended up presenting my clinical reflection on this patient because it really stuck with me how much hand washing, or lack of it, had changed the potential outcome for this patient. Kylie had to take antibiotics and her wound was really gross. I honestly though MRSA was just a bug you did not have to worry about. I have a mantra now in my head – 'five moments of hand washing' plays like elevator music – always there but in the background. I am so conscious of clean hands now.

Suzanne, 31, Enrolled Nurse,
Infection Control Worker

1 What are the five moments of hand hygiene?
2 Why do you think it was hand washing, or lack of it, that has contributed to the contamination of Kylie's wound?
3 How could this infection be explained to the patient?

13.5 Complex or challenging wounds

Complex, intricate and complicated wounds are generally challenging, as they often take a significant period of time to heal, and during this time can befuddle all health-care professionals involved. The cost of dressings and therapies are not inexpensive! However, evidence-based care for wounds has resulted in health improvement and cost savings (AusHSI, 2017).

There are consistent types of complex wounds – these include wounds related to diabetes, ulcers (both arterial and venous), burns and pressure injuries. Surgical wounds can become incredibly complex if they break down or if dehiscence occurs. The presence of diabetes, collagen vascular disease, (i.e. lupus, rheumatoid arthritis) arteriosclerosis and venous incompetence all complicate wound healing.

Wounds that fail to heal or periodically reopen may be associated with an underlying chronic bone infection (osteomyelitis) or the presence of a foreign body (i.e. glass or metal fragments). Additionally, the use of radiation for treating tumours can produce permanent tissue damage and diminished healing potential. Certainly, the size and mechanism of injury add to the complexity of the wound.

Chronic wounds occur as healing is interrupted at any one stage of the healing process. Healing may also be impeded by the accumulation of necrotic tissue or slough, a clinical feature of chronic wounds.

Other forms of wounds that are commonly chronic are ulcers. Chronic ulcers are generally cause by venous stasis, diabetes, pressure and arterial insufficiency. The ulcer size is determined using a number of classification scales which then assist in determining the width, depth and shape of the ulcer. Ulcers should be measured quantitatively before and after debridement and as a means of assessing progress towards closure. Ulcers are commonly caused from pressure injuries (see **Figure 13.4**).

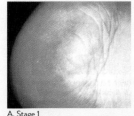 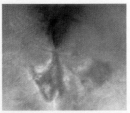 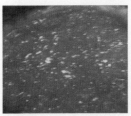 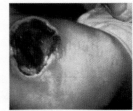

A. Stage 1   B. Stage 2   C. Stage 3   D. Stage 4

FIGURE 13.4 Stages of pressure injuries

Courtesy of Emory University Hospital, Atlanta, Georgia.

Other nursing skills you will utilise in management of wounds is removal of sutures, clips or drains – these will always be completed with a written or verbal order from the treating medical officer. Sutures, staples or clips are generally the result of surgery or an acute injury. These are removed using the principles of asepsis and the clinical steps as outlined here.

Finally, wound drains are often inserted into wounds – both surgical and complex – to assist in the removal of serum, blood and debris that if not removed could cause complications. Wound drains can be inserted for a number of reasons:

* to remove post-operative blood loss in the surgical site (abdominal cavity)
* to drain lymph
* to remove contaminants – for example, pus

Review the skill in Tollefson *Essential Clinical Skills* 4.7 Suture and staple removal

- to remove air in the pleural space and re-inflate the lung
- to prevent accumulation of secretions.

There are two types of drainage systems, open and closed. In the open system, the drainage flows freely from the drain into the dressing or a drainage bag. In closed draining systems the fluid is extracted through suction. This may be low-pressure suction connected to the wall suction unit or through a vacuum drain.

While on placement it may not be possible for you to remove a drain – there may be no patients with a drain, or it may have occurred on another shift. Familiarise yourself with the clinical skills required and if possible observe the procedure.

Review the skill in
Tollefson *Essential Clinical Skills* 4.8 Drain removal and shortening

13.6 Evaluating outcomes of nursing action in wound care

Evaluation is a key component to determining if the current wound treatment is effective. Nurses when evaluating wounds will use special charts to describe the wound in detail and also pictorial evidence such as measures or photographs to ensure the wound is healing.

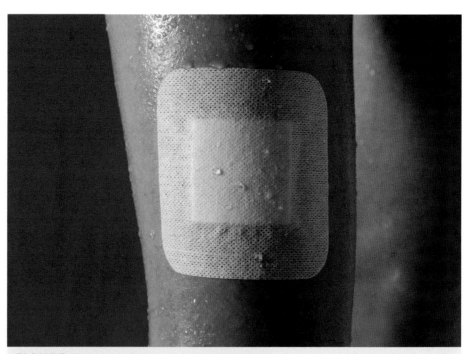

FIGURE 13.5 Protecting the wound dressing

Alamy Stock Photo/numb.

The client, as well as the wound, also requires constant reassessment and evaluation of their needs. Has the wound healed sufficiently to reduce the level of analgesia? Can the client undertake ADLs, such as showering, with the current wound management regime?

Wound review and reassessment

Wounds, as you will begin to observe, come in all shapes and sizes and can take varying amounts of time to heal. When you are documenting your wound assessment, you should try to remember that the next person to read your notes may not have seen the wound before. That person, from your notes, should be able to review the assessment and care plan and establish if the wound is healing, progressing and doing 'all the right things'.

When assessing a wound and the nature of the wound has altered, you will need to review the manner in which the wound is dressed and/or the products used to do this. For example, if a wound was moist and is now dry and crusting, then the products being used will need to be altered to ensure it is kept moist to promote healing.

Documentation

The purpose of documentation is not only to provide all members of the health-care team with the overview of wound assessments, interventions and evaluation of care, it is to communicate treatment and goals. Documentation can take the form of emails, photographs of wounds, progress notes and specialist reviews.

Review the skill in Tollefson *Essential Clinical Skills* 7.1 Documentation

Wounds are documented using protocol and assessment or care plans in many facilities. These will differ depending on the health-care facility, the type of wound and the acuity of the patient – for instance, are they an in-patient or an out-patient? Do they have any other medical conditions? It will be a unique assessment for each and every patient with a wound requiring intervention.

Due to constant research and evaluation, there are always new wound products and techniques. This information is disseminated through the specialist wound care team, so asking for assistance is never detrimental. We all have different opinions, and sometimes this can be the very undoing of wound care – many different ideas and no consistency in completing the treatment, leaving a patient with a wound that has had four different dressings on it in as many days.

SUMMARY

- When describing wounds it is necessary to use the correct terminology when documenting and reporting on wound care procedures.
- The nurse should assess both the client and the wound to deliver care that will support the client and assist them to maintain their activities of daily living.
- When planning the care for a client with a wound it is important to work as a team and access wound care experts to assist in decision making.
- Wound care will require complex nursing interventions such as specimen collection for microbiology and cytology to determine care planning procedures.
- Using an aseptic technique when undertaking wound care will assist in preventing the spread of infection.
- Evaluating the outcomes of nursing actions will require monitoring the client's response to wound management strategies and the progress of the wound healing process.

SELF-TEST QUESTIONS

1   What are the responsibilities of the nurse in relation to documentation of wound care?
2   Why is it important to maintain aseptic non-touch technique when undertaking wound care for complex and challenging wounds?
3   How does the use of contemporary assessment tools assist in the management of complex and challenging wounds?
4   Why is a holistic approach required when planning the care for a person with a complex or challenging wound?
5   What factors impact on wound healing?
6   How can the nurse minimise cross-infection during assessment and implementation of wound management strategies?

BIBLIOGRAPHY

ABC, RN Health Report (2014). *Wound care*, http://www.abc.net.au/radionational/programs/healthreport/wound-care/5391274. Accessed 21 April 2014.

AusHSI (2017). *Issues Paper: Chronic Wounds in Australia*. Retrieved from http://www.aushsi.org.au/wp-content/uploads/2017/08/Chronic-Wounds-Solutions-Forum-Issues-Paper-final.pdf.

Australian Commission on Safety and Quality in Health Care (2012). *Standard 8: Preventing and Managing Pressure Injuries: Safety and Quality Improvement Guide*. ASCQHC: Sydney.

Carville, K. (2007). *Wound Care Manual*. Silver Chain Foundation: Perth, WA.

Clarke, L., Gray, S., White, L., Duncan, G. & Baumle, W. (2016). *Foundations of Nursing: Enrolled Division 2 Nurses* (ANZ Edition). Cengage Learning: South Melbourne.

Estes, M.E.Z., Calleja, P., Theobald, K. & Harvey, T. (2016). *Health Assessment and Physical Examination* (2nd edition). Cengage Learning: South Melbourne.

Hand Hygiene Australia (n.d.). *5 moments for hand hygiene*, http://www.hha.org.au/home/5-moments-for-hand-hygiene.aspx. Accessed 19 March 2018.

Hand Hygiene Australia (2018). *The national hand hygiene initiative*, http://www.hha.org.au.

National Health and Medical Research Council (NHMRC) (2010). 'B1.7.1 Aseptic non-touch technique (ANTT)', in *Australian Guidelines for the Prevention & Control of Infection in Healthcare*. Retrieved from https://www.nhmrc.gov.au/book/australian-guidelines-prevention-and-control-infection-healthcare-2010/b1-7-1-aseptic-non-touch.

Satterfield, K. (June 2006). 'Diabetes watch! A guide to understanding the various wound classification systems', *Podiatry Today*, 19(6): 20–7.

Tollefson, J., Watson, G., Jelly, E. & Tambree, K. (2016). *Essential Clinical Skills: Enrolled Division 2 Nurses* (3rd edition). Cengage Learning: South Melbourne.

Wounds Australia (2016). *Standards for Wound Prevention and Management* (3rd edition). Cambridge Media: Osborne Park, WA.

Nursing care plans

LEARNING OUTCOMES

After reading this chapter, you should have an understanding of:

14.1 Preparing a person for care procedures

14.2 Implementing care procedures to meet identified needs

14.3 Monitoring a person's identified care needs

14.4 Evaluating outcomes of care provided

Planning care

I was excited to be undertaking clinical placement. It was a little daunting to know what exactly I had to complete and I found that I needed to write down everything in a list to make sure I did not forget a task. I was very focused on completing all the tasks allocated to me.

I had practised all the tasks in the clinical lab but was a bit apprehensive about doing these in the clinical workplace. I found that most of the clients I was assisting were so grateful for my help, but there was one that was very demanding and bossy. It did not seem to matter what I did, she did not appear to be happy with me. This made me feel very inadequate and as a result I tried to avoid her as much as I could. I relayed this information at debrief time and the clinical supervisor told me to do further research on the client. I found that the client had suffered from polio as a child and consequently had spent long periods of time in hospitals. The client was now elderly and the condition had returned.

I was allocated to this client each day and one of the strategies I put into place was spending additional time when attending to her personal hygiene needs and to converse with her. Initially the client was closed off and mainly directed me to her needs. After a few days she started to relax and appeared to enjoy the conversations we had. She told me that she was frightened that she would not be able to return home and was very sad about this.

At the end of the placement I found that I had really enjoyed implementing nursing care procedures and had managed to gain a better understanding of the feelings and emotions of the clients I was performing care for.

14.1 Preparing a person for care procedures

Planning and implementing nursing care is a challenging and rewarding experience when one sees the high-quality client care provided as a result. Each care plan is individualised to the client's needs. The **care plan** takes into account all the collected data from the admission assessment, the client history, the current diagnostic data and the input from the client as to what their concerns and goals are.

Education is a fundamental task in preparing the client for the procedures outlined in their care plan. Many clients undergoing medical or diagnostic procedures are familiar with the actual procedures, related terminology used by the health professionals and any associated side effects. Clients that understand what is being done and why are less anxious and more empowered. Therefore, education is an important role that the enrolled nurse can undertake.

Wherever possible clients need to be provided with a full explanation of both the procedures and the preparation required. Clients may not understand the medical terminology being used and such terminology needs to be explained in lay terms, and respect given to the level of the client's knowledge of the procedures. The nurse may be required to provide rationales for preparations and ensure that the client understands the importance of them.

It is much easier nowadays to locate information. 'Dr Google' is an ever-present phenomenon in health care with patients seeking 'medical' advice online before attending hospital. As with any education or health-care promotion, your role will be to holistically review your client's needs and ensure that the information you are providing is at a level easily understandable to your patients and their family.

Consent

Consent must be obtained from your clients for all interventions. Consent can be written, implied or verbal (Clarke et al., 2016). It is essential that you seek consent when performing nursing interventions prior to commencing them. Examples are as follows:

- **Implied consent** – when a patient holds their arm out and elevated for you to complete their blood pressure.
- **Verbal consent** – 'Mr Owens, is it OK if I check your BGL?' 'Sure, that is fine.'
- **Written consent** – specific for an invasive procedure, research participation or for a person who is unable to make the determination of consent themselves (intellectual impairment, child, mental health legislation). See **Figure 14.1**.

You can imagine the confusion of a patient if you are performing interventions and they have no idea why you are doing them, what they are for, and have not agreed to them.

Documentation

Documenting the preparation related to procedures or investigations is important, especially when the preparation continues over a shift change. This allows other health-team members to know what has been completed and what still needs to be completed. Documentation should reflect any anxieties or non-compliance of the client.

Many health-care facilities have standard documentation for some procedures that are included on the clinical pathway. For example, on the clinical pathway for a colonoscopy there would be a section dedicated to the preparation of the client.

---

care plan
An individualised document outlining relevant interventions and planned care for the client. It is a communication tool and incorporates the needs of the client

Review the skill in Tollefson *Essential Clinical Skills* 7.5 Health teaching

---

TIP 14.1

Dr Google

Many patients will Google their signs and symptoms and arrive at a diagnosis before they present to hospital! While it is a good thing that patients are interested in understanding their health, it can also be incredibly difficult to try and persuade a patient that they don't have the rare disease that Google has identified! Be mindful of maintaining a professional image, and use the opportunity to provide health education.

---

consent
Permission or agreement to be allowed to take action or perform some type of care

implied consent
When consent is given implicitly, such as by a person's actions or lack of actions, rather than expressly (such as verbally or written)

verbal consent
When a person expressly grants consent verbally

written consent
When a person expressly grants consent in writing

Review the skill in Tollefson *Essential Clinical Skills* 7.1 Documentation

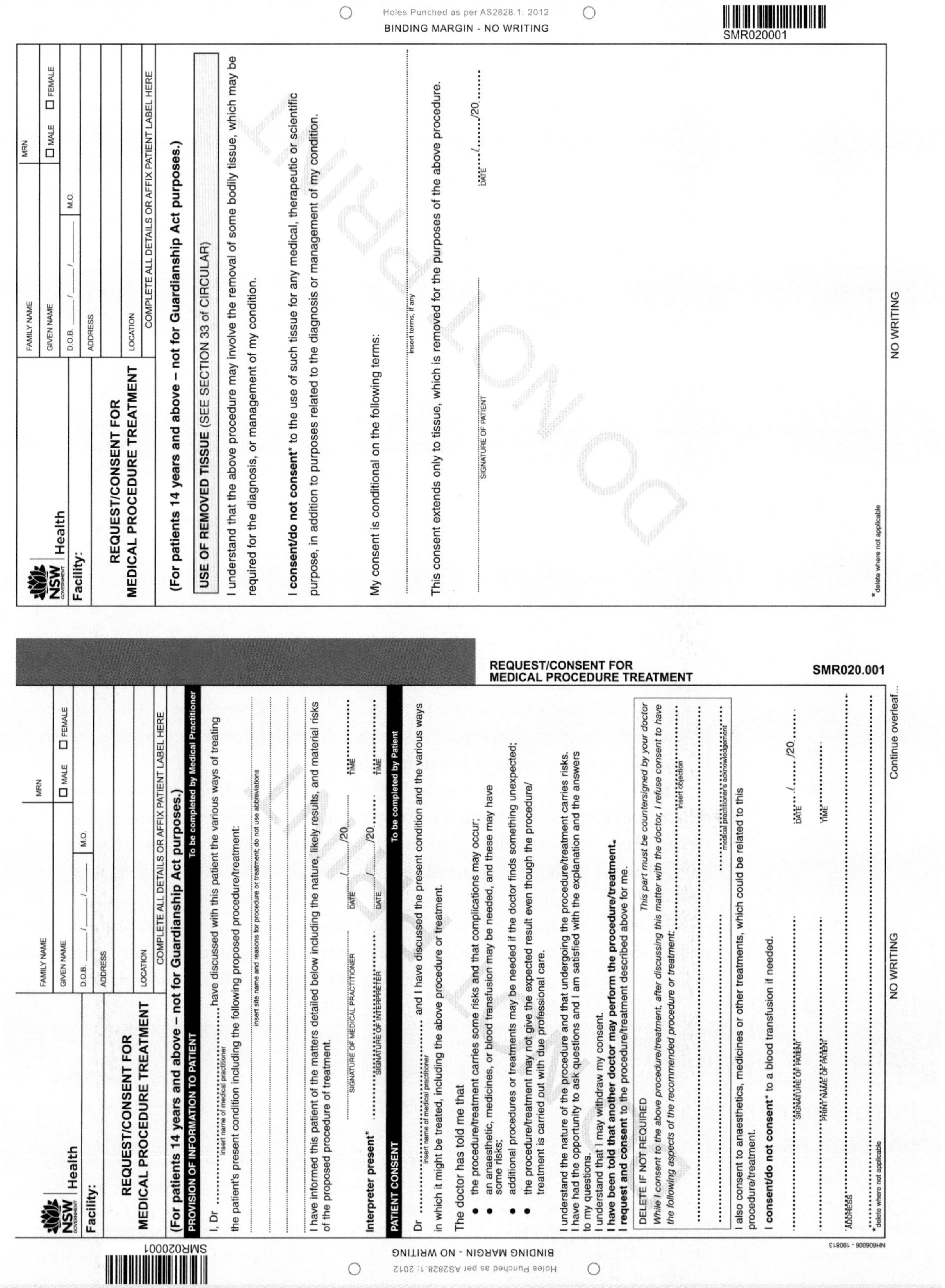

NSW Health

Facility:

REQUEST/CONSENT FOR MEDICAL PROCEDURE TREATMENT

FAMILY NAME | MRN
GIVEN NAME | ☐ MALE ☐ FEMALE
D.O.B. ____/____/____ M.O.
ADDRESS
LOCATION
COMPLETE ALL DETAILS OR AFFIX PATIENT LABEL HERE

(For patients 14 years and above – not for Guardianship Act purposes.)

PROVISION OF INFORMATION TO PATIENT — To be completed by Medical Practitioner

I, Dr ………………………… (insert name of medical practitioner) have discussed with this patient the various ways of treating the patient's present condition including the following proposed procedure/treatment:

………………………… (insert site name and reasons for procedure or treatment; do not use abbreviations)

I have informed this patient of the matters detailed below including the nature, likely results, and material risks of the proposed procedure of treatment.

SIGNATURE OF MEDICAL PRACTITIONER ……… DATE …/…/20… TIME ………

Interpreter present* ……… SIGNATURE OF INTERPRETER ……… DATE …/…/20… TIME ………

PATIENT CONSENT — To be completed by Patient

Dr ………………………… (insert name of medical practitioner) and I have discussed the present condition and the various ways in which it might be treated, including the above procedure or treatment.

The doctor has told me that

- the procedure/treatment carries some risks and that complications may occur;
- an anaesthetic, medicines, or blood transfusion may be needed, and these may have some risks;
- additional procedures or treatments may be needed if the doctor finds something unexpected;
- the procedure/treatment may not give the expected result even though the procedure/treatment is carried out with due professional care.

I understand the nature of the procedure and that undergoing the procedure/treatment carries risks.
I have had the opportunity to ask questions and I am satisfied with the explanation and the answers to my questions.
I understand that I may withdraw my consent.
I have been told that another doctor may perform the procedure/treatment.
I request and consent to the procedure/treatment described above for me.

DELETE IF NOT REQUIRED — *This part must be countersigned by your doctor*
While I consent to the above procedure/treatment, after discussing this matter with the doctor, I refuse consent to have the following aspects of the recommended procedure or treatment: ……… (insert objection)
……… (medical practitioner's acknowledgement)

I also consent to anaesthetics, medicines or other treatments, which could be related to this procedure/treatment.

I **consent/do not consent*** to a blood transfusion if needed.

……… SIGNATURE OF PATIENT ……… DATE …/…/20…
……… PRINT NAME OF PATIENT ……… TIME ………
……… ADDRESS
*delete where not applicable

NO WRITING — Continue overleaf...

REQUEST/CONSENT FOR MEDICAL PROCEDURE TREATMENT — SMR020.001

SMR020001 — Holes Punched as per AS2828.1: 2012 — BINDING MARGIN - NO WRITING — NH606006 - 190813

NSW Health

Facility:

REQUEST/CONSENT FOR MEDICAL PROCEDURE TREATMENT

FAMILY NAME | MRN
GIVEN NAME | ☐ MALE ☐ FEMALE
D.O.B. ____/____/____ M.O.
ADDRESS
LOCATION
COMPLETE ALL DETAILS OR AFFIX PATIENT LABEL HERE

(For patients 14 years and above – not for Guardianship Act purposes.)

USE OF REMOVED TISSUE (SEE SECTION 33 of CIRCULAR)

I understand that the above procedure may involve the removal of some bodily tissue, which may be required for the diagnosis, or management of my condition.

I **consent/do not consent*** to the use of such tissue for any medical, therapeutic or scientific purpose, in addition to purposes related to the diagnosis or management of my condition.

My consent is conditional on the following terms:

……… (insert terms, if any)

This consent extends only to tissue, which is removed for the purposes of the above procedure.

……… SIGNATURE OF PATIENT ……… DATE …/…/20…

*delete where not applicable

NO WRITING

Holes Punched as per AS2828.1: 2012 — BINDING MARGIN - NO WRITING — SMR020001

DO NOT PRINT

FIGURE 14.1 Example of consent form

Source: Ministry of Health, NSW, https://www1.health.nsw.gov.au/pds/ActivePDSDocuments/PD2005_406.pdf. © State of New South Wales NSW Ministry of Health. For current information go to www.health.nsw.gov.au. Creative Commons BY 4.0 www.creativecommons.org/licenses/by/4.0/.

Clinical pathways are comprehensive, pre-printed interdisciplinary standard plans of care. They reflect the ideal course of treatment for the average client with a given diagnosis or procedure. The goal for clinical pathways is to improve efficiency and quality of client care (Clarke et al., p. 204, 2016). Examples of clinical pathways can be found at the Queensland Government Clinical Excellence Division site: https://clinicalexcellence.qld.gov.au/resources/clinical-pathways.

During your clinical placement, you will have the opportunity to utilise various documentation forms. Get familiar with them because many are standardised across the health-care system. Practise using them because it can take time to get used to plotting observations on the ADDS charts.

Review the skill in Tollefson *Essential Clinical Skills* 7.1 Documentation

---

Activity 14.1

Gaining consent

Your patient, Margaret Murphy, has told you to 'go away' several times today when you have attempted to complete her observations. You have tried explaining to her the reason you want to record the observations, but she remains adamant that her observations not be taken.

1   What would you document in this instance?

2   What are some communication strategies you might utilise to attempt to gain Margaret's consent?

Margaret is normally mobile, and is often seen walking around the unit after she has had her wound dressing attended to. Today she is lethargic, and remains in bed. Her respiratory rate is 28 breaths per minute. When you ask her if you can take her observations she does not answer you, just keeps staring at you.

3   Is it appropriate to take Margaret's observations?

Dignity

It is extremely important, as with all nursing care, to maintain the privacy and dignity of the client while explaining or performing procedures or interventions. When explaining a procedure to the client, you should ensure that this is done in privacy. Simply drawing the bedside curtains is not enough to maintain privacy.

The concepts of education, privacy and dignity are fundamental and paramount in nursing care delivery. Ensuring you act as a patient advocate and provide care that is holistic and patient centred is essential in promoting health and educating your patient on interventions and procedures.

Review the concepts of client advocacy in Chapter 4 and culturally competent care in Chapter 9.

The delivery of nursing care to your client is derived from a nursing care plan and through utilising the nursing process. A large component of the nursing process is assessing each patient individually; which is where cultural competency is required in health-care delivery.

Reflective practice 14.1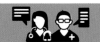

Providing care to a person with burns

You are allocated the care of Christine Newton, a 49-year-old woman who has burns to 50% of her body. She has been hospitalised for several months and is in the burns unit for ongoing dressings. This is your first day of placement and you did not receive a handover on Christine because the nurse was too busy and said, 'I will handover later; she just needs a dressing change'. After completing the dressing you document the relevant findings and details. After you have

completed this your buddy nurse Cheryl provides you with handover as follows:

'Christine is a 49 year old who has 50% burns post being after her partner doused her in petrol and set her alight.'

1   Does this change the way in which you would speak to Christine? Would you perform anything any differently?

Consider the following – instead of being set alight by her partner, consider Christine's injuries as self-inflicted.

2   Does this change the way in which you would speak to or perform cares on Christine?

Activity 14.2

Multicultural resources

When delivering nursing care it is important that the care is person centred and that consent is obtained before commencing the nursing interventions. For clients where language is a barrier, hospital is a confusing place where people want to do things that they do not understand. Locate the multicultural resources in the health-care facility. If this situation occurs, identify the actions that you could implement.

1   Do you need to contact a designated person?
2   Are there readily available interpreters?
3   Could you locate information regarding care of the deceased person of a particular culture?

14.2 Implementing care procedures to meet identified needs

A *nursing intervention* is any treatment that a nurse performs on a client in response to a nursing diagnosis to reach a projected outcome. All nursing interventions must be explained to the client in a manner they can understand. The client has the right to refuse any intervention, which is why it is imperative that the client is involved in the planning for interventions to ensure they are aware of the interventions. Types of nursing interventions include:

- *Nurse-initiated* – actions performed by nurses without a doctor's order
- *Doctor-initiated* – actions initiated by the doctor in response to a medical diagnosis but carried out by nursing staff
- *Collaborative* – treatments carried out by nurses initiated by other providers, such as a dietician or a physiotherapist.

    Examples of nursing interventions include:
- hygiene and grooming
- physical comfort
- oral/dental care
- wound care
- toileting
- pressure area care
- fluid balance maintenance
- nutrition/feeding
- care of drains and invasive lines
- application of prosthesis
- health education.

    Implementation begins after the care plan or clinical pathway has been developed and the planned care is in action. These interventions will be delegated to you from the nursing care plan by the registered nurse.

    When dealing with clients on a busy ward, it is sometimes easy as nurses to lose sight of their needs due to the pressure of a busy workload and time constraints. However, it is sometimes small things that nurses don't always see as important that can make a major difference to the client. For example, when responding to a call bell and you are not able to carry out the desired task immediately – set a timeframe so that the client can see that their needs are warranted and important and will be dealt with as soon as possible. Sometimes, all the patient needs is reassurance and the acknowledgement of their needs being met.

Personal hygiene

Personal hygiene is necessary to stay clean and comfortable. For many people it is also necessary to preserve a sense of dignity. The importance of grooming and hygiene in achieving health outcomes relates very much to our personal perceptions; for example, when we feel clean and refreshed and well presented our self-esteem is improved and our attitude becomes more positive. The frequency of bathing varies widely according to cultural and individual variances. As a person ages, their skin often becomes thinner and drier and the need for bathing may change.

There are many health reasons why bathing is important:

- it restores cleanliness by removing dirt and body odours
- it removes bacteria and germs from the skin
- it cools and refreshes the skin
- it promotes good skin integrity
- it stimulates circulation
- it provides movement and exercise
- it provides the nurse an opportunity to check the client for changes, abnormalities and skin integrity
- it feels good and helps the client to relax.

Bathing allows a fantastic opportunity for you to assess the client's physical status, such as skin integrity and ability to self-care. It also provides an excellent opportunity for the nurse to establish and extend a therapeutic relationship.

An important thing to remember when assisting the client with their hygiene needs is to obtain their consent beforehand. This is easily obtained through effective, open and honest communication. Imagine being a patient in a hospital and a nurse came at you with a bowl and some water and just started washing you – no explanation, no interaction! Think about how you would feel if you were reliant on someone to complete your activities of daily living (ADLs) – with this in mind, communicate your intended practice to your patient prior to commencing.

Despite it becoming an everyday routine for nurses, you must remember that this is a major intrusion for the client. Some clients try to avoid the process at all costs, even going to the extremes of telling you that they have already been bathed by another staff member.

Hygiene needs are always a priority in nursing care – remember, the skin is the largest organ and the first line of defence against infection. It needs to be clean and dry to maintain integrity.

Skin integrity

As we have established, skin is the largest organ, and our biggest protective barrier in terms of infection control. Helping to maintain the integrity of a clients' skin is crucial in ensuring that they do not develop pressure injuries, which are essentially preventable. Nursing interventions you can expect to perform for maintaining skin integrity are:

- pressure area care
- maintaining hygiene
- skin assessment
- identification of any risk factors that could impact upon skin integrity such as age, general condition, and mobility status.

Refer to Chapter 13 for more information regarding wound management.

Review the skill in Tollefson *Essential Clinical Skills* 3.5 Assisting the patient to maintain personal hygiene and grooming needs – sponge (bed bath) with oral hygiene, hair wash in bed, eye and nasal care & 3.6 Assisting the patient to maintain personal hygiene and grooming – assisted shower (chair or trolley), undressing/dressing, shaving, hair and nail care

---

TIP 14.2

Bathing

I will never forget the first showers and bed baths I performed. I think I was more embarrassed than the patient! I was worried that the water was not right, that they were cold, that it was not being done the right way. Then I was buddied with a nurse who, after we had performed a bed bath together, spoke to me. She told me that no matter what, the patient is always going to be grateful for a freshen up. To feel slightly less 'sick' and clean is always going to be a positive thing. Her advice was to gauge the situation, talk if the patient wants to, and always wash someone like it was your own skin. Her advice helped me a great deal, because now I see it as more than just a bed bath or shower. It is a chance for that person to feel better, more human, and that they are more than just a bed number, that their hair is brushed, their teeth are clean and they can focus on getting better.

Lorelei, 24, EN.

Explore the theory in *Foundations of Nursing*, Chapter 19: Safety/hygiene

Nutritional needs

Nutrition is a large component of health and wellness. As a nurse, you will be answering questions at some stage regarding diet for your client. Nutrition is reliant upon several factors including:

- co-morbidities – disease processes such as hypertension, heart disease or diabetes
- age
- mobility.

Involvement of the multidisciplinary team – including a dietician – should be considered when the client's diet is inadequate or there are illness-related concerns from poor nutrition, be that excessive or insufficient calorie intake. Nutritional needs have an impact upon the healing process, so diet and nutrition are important factors in holistic patient care and nursing interventions.

CASE STUDY 14.1

Health education

Mark Benson is a 31-year-old who is day two post an inguinal hernia repair. He has been asked by the physiotherapist to perform 'deep breathing exercises' with this 'thing with balls in it'. He is asking for assistance from you, as he is unsure what he is supposed to do, or why.

1   What are deep breathing exercises used for?
2   Why would Mark be instructed to complete them?
3   How could you explain the process to Mark?

Respiratory function

Usually we do not focus on our breathing as it is an automatic function. However, when our respiratory system is not working well due to infection, trauma or other problems from interrelated systems breathing becomes a focused activity.

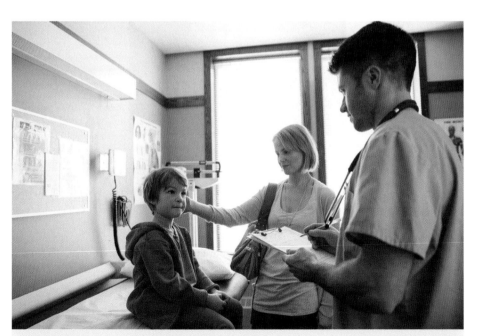

FIGURE 14.2 Pre-operative care

Source: Alamy Stock Photo/Hero Images Inc.

Review the skill in Tollefson *Essential Clinical Skills*, 8.2 Pre-operative care

Review the skill in Tollefson *Essential Clinical Skills* 3.14 Active and passive exercises

As nurses we can assist the respiratory function of the people we are providing care for by demonstrating the techniques of deep breathing and coughing. This education may also be given to clients who will be undergoing surgery where their normal respiratory function is interrupted by the anaesthesia.

Encouraging the person to contribute to their own independence and mobility

All clients need to be encouraged to mobilise as much as possible either in bed or through ambulation. If the client is unresponsive or confined to bed, the nurse needs to educate the client on moving the joints appropriately through range of motion exercises or perform this for the client. By doing this the nurse will assist the client to:

* increase independence
* prevent contractures
* prevent complications such as deep vein thrombosis by stimulating the circulatory system through movement and the application of anti-embolic aids such as TED stockings (see **Figure 14.3**).

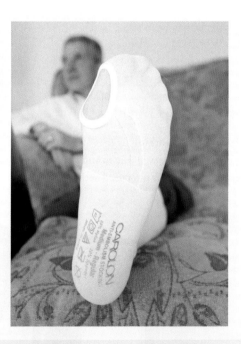

FIGURE 14.3 Using TED stockings

Source: Science Photo Library/Ashley Cooper.

Comfort, rest and sleep

Generally, people find it easy to rest and sleep, but at times changes occur that affect these patterns. These changes can include:

* a change in routine – getting up earlier than usual, going to bed later, reduction in exercise
* environment – noise, quiet, new house, hospital
* emotional state – depression, stress, anxiety
* medication – certain medications
* position – if you injure part of your body and you cannot lie as you normally would

- equipment – old lumpy pillows, mattresses, temperature
- pain
- nursing interventions – disruptions due to medications dispensing, observations or dressings
- visitors – can intensify stress, for example, a mother in hospital with young children at home.

As well as promoting emotional wellbeing and enhancing various physiologic processes, the benefits of 'good' sleep can include reducing fatigue, stabilising mood, improving blood flow to the brain, increasing protein synthesis, maintaining the immune system, promoting cellular growth and repair, and improving learning and memory storage.

Sleep duration and quality vary among individuals of all age groups. One person may feel adequately rested after four hours of sleep, while another person may require 10 hours. Generally, the need for sleep decreases from birth to adulthood.

Explore the theory in *Foundations of Nursing*, Chapter 18: Rest and sleep

Dealing with emergencies

All staff working in health-care facilities have an obligation towards the implementation and maintenance of safe working practices as discussed in Chapter 1. Such practices include the use of personal protective equipment (PPE), correct manual handling procedures, implementing standard precautions and following procedures related to the cleaning, decontamination and storage of equipment (again the focus is on WHS and infection control).

Another safe practice principle is being aware of the guidelines and procedures involved in an actual or imminent emergency. Emergencies can happen at any time in any type of workplace. The types of emergencies to plan for include fire, injuries, rescues, incidents with hazardous substances, bomb threats, armed confrontations and natural disasters. Emergencies that occur on-site are often referred to as 'internal emergencies'. All health-care facilities should have an 'Internal Emergency Response Plan' that guides and instructs staff on what to do in the event of an internal emergency.

Before you undertake your first clinical placement you will be required to complete a first-aid course. First-aid in a hospital can differ to that within the community. In hospitals, life-saving equipment and medications are more readily available. However, you must also remember that most of the clients are there because they are unwell – they may have underlying conditions and specific circumstances that predispose them to requiring first-aid and emergency care.

A medical emergency is an injury or illness that is acute and poses an immediate risk to a person's life or long-term health (Clarke et al., 2016). Some of the most common emergency situations nurses face include:
- choking/aspiration
- burns and scalds
- allergic reactions
- cardiac arrest.

Nurses, every day, face the probability that their clients may experience emergency and/or life-threatening situations. It is the nurse's responsibility to ensure their own knowledge and skill level is up to date in regard to the interventions required to safely recognise and manage these situations.

In an emergency you need to act fast. Therefore, it is extremely important that you are aware of any clients who elect not to be resuscitated. Can you imagine the legal (not to mention ethical) ramifications if a client has a *NO CPR* order and CPR is commenced? Of course, if the status is not known you cannot get into any trouble for starting CPR.

14.3 Monitoring a person's identified care needs

Nurses often see the client more than any other care provider. Therefore, nurses are in the best position to monitor the client's progress, spot problems early and judge what care is needed to solve the problem or situation. To do these things, the nurse must use every opportunity to assess the client through visual assessment, diagnostic tools, communication with the client and nursing observations. All changes in baseline data or client condition need to be documented and reported to the RN.

Ongoing assessment through observation, monitoring equipment and devices

It is the responsibility of the enrolled nurse to ensure that all data collected is documented and variations from normal are acted upon immediately. Ongoing observations are needed to ensure nursing care is meeting the client's needs.

As outlined in Chapter 5 and Chapter 21, the following principles should be used to evaluate and monitor progress:

*   observe the client (colour, warmth, demeanour etc.).
*   talk to the client.
*   gather supportive and objective data (observations).
*   check equipment is working properly.
*   check that all devices attached to the client are patent and working (oxygen, surgical drains etc.).
*   ensure that care is evaluated whenever possible (if pain is treated then patient's pain level should be re-evaluated post the dose of analgesia).

Re-evaluation of nursing care is the core of the nursing process. All interventions must be reviewed and re-evaluated for effectiveness. Nursing interventions must be prioritised if the patient's condition deteriorates or improves, and the ongoing cycle of data collection and analysis continues!

Risks associated with hospitalisation

Clients are admitted to health-care facilities for a variety of reasons. It could be a planned or unplanned admission, or an emergency or non-emergency situation. Clients may be admitted for as little as a few hours to more long-term or even permanent care. No matter the reason or the length of stay, there are still risks or potential risks that can be associated with hospitalisation and medical treatment.

Some risks may include:

*   adverse reactions – medications, wound dressings or even hospital food
*   shock/haemorrhage – especially post-surgical intervention
*   deep vein thrombosis (DVT)/pulmonary embolism (PE) – due to lack of activity and/or underlying condition
*   health-care acquired infection (HAI)
*   constipation – due to decreased activity, change in oral intake, medication etc.
*   loss of muscle tone – due to reduced activity
*   slips and falls
*   social isolation
*   sleep deprivation.

So how can these risks be prevented? And what can you, as an EN, do?

First and foremost, the best risk prevention strategy is to monitor your client. This includes obtaining both *objective data* (such as vital signs, BGLs, fluid balance monitoring etc.) and *subjective data* (listen to what the client is telling you and, more importantly, what they are not).

Reporting and recording changes

Any change to a patient's condition, whether it be to their overall condition or only one element (such as pain or behaviour), needs to be reported to the RN/doctor. Any such change may reflect minor or serious changes to the patient's wellbeing, and needs to be assessed, documented and acted upon appropriately to ensure the best possible outcome for the patient.

Documenting not only vital signs but also pain scores is essential in monitoring your patient's progression and response to treatments or procedures. Always document pain scores and describe the pain as the patient has described it to you. Giving analgesia is simple enough, but reassessing its effectiveness is essential! As with any intervention, you need to evaluate its effectiveness and look at methods to ensure the patient is pain free.

Review the skill in Tollefson *Essential Clinical Skills* 7.1 Documentation

14.4 Evaluating outcomes of care provided

Evaluation of care requires the nurse to think about client responses to determine the effectiveness of their intervention. It requires you, the nurse, to have knowledge that is current, specific and evidence based. Client education and evaluation of their progress are integral components of the nursing care plan. Also, bear in mind that all patients have different requirements; for example, some will understand post-operative instructions, while others will require your time and educational skills to enable them to comprehend what is going on.

Consulting and collaborating with the interdisciplinary health-care team

You are required to constantly evaluate, communicate and discuss the patient's progress with other health-care professionals. This can be in the form of clinical handovers, referrals to other services (dieticians, social workers, occupational therapists, wound care nurses etc.) or team meetings.

This consultation and collaboration is an ongoing process as the person moves towards achieving their goals. The progress of the person is important to evaluate as the care plan may need to be changed in response to their progress. At times, interventions may not have achieved what was first planned or may have given rise to unexpected or undesired outcomes.

Evaluating outcomes and changing care plans

Evaluation is about reviewing the effectiveness of the care that has been given and it serves two purposes. First, the nurse is able to ascertain whether the desired outcomes for the client have been achieved, and second, evaluation acts as an opportunity to review the entire process and determine whether the assessment was accurate and complete, the diagnosis correct, the goals realistic and achievable or the proscribed actions were appropriate.

As discussed previously, the planned interventions may cause an undesired response or reaction in the client that prevents them from achieving their goals. The nursing care process, as shown in **Figure 7.4** in Chapter 7, is a cyclical one that is undertaken by nursing staff on each shift. This will require reassessment of the problem, diagnosis, goal and intervention. In some instances it could be that the problem was not correctly identified or a potential problem arose during the client's stay. **Figure 14.4** provides an example.

Goal
Client will be able to independently perform
ADLs without discomfort in 2 days

Evaluation Measures
Ask client about pain levels pre and post attending to ADLs
Monitor vital signs pre and post attending to ADLs

Expected Outcomes
Client will report a pain scale of <3 (out of 10) within 2 days
Client will initiate bathing and ADLs within 2 days

Client Response
Client rates severe right-sided abdominal pain
as 5/10 while attempting bathing on day 2

Evaluation Findings
Client's condition still indicates a problem
Continued therapy with possibly new care measures required

FIGURE 14.4 The nursing care process

CASE STUDY 14.2

Assessing outcomes

Sam Owen is a 37-year-old-male who is day one post-operative following a laparoscopic hernia repair. Sam has mobilised but has reported pain in his shoulder.

1   How would you ask Sam to rate his pain?
2   How would you document his pain in the care plan and in his notes?

You have administered 5 mg of oral Endone. It is 30 minutes since you administered this and you return to reassess Sam's pain. He is now rating his pain as 1/10 and is able to mobilise.

3   How would you evaluate your nursing interventions?

Once the nursing care has been evaluated, the nursing care plan can then be modified based on the data obtained. While you are on placement, take the time to review care plans or clinical pathways to see the varieties out there and also to become familiar with completing them. It is also a good idea to look at the differences between two patients who may be on the same clinical pathway.

If the plan of care requires changing then you need to collaborate with the RN and other members of the health-care team. At times research may be required to apply a different intervention to meet the client's needs. This research may include the following:

- computer research for best practice guidelines
- discussion with other specialists and team members.

Review the skill in Tollefson *Essential Clinical Skills* 7.1 Documentation

Documentation

If the care plan is changed, this needs to be reflected in all documentation that relates to the client. This can include the following:

- care plan
- client file
- handover sheet
- administration documentation (if a new diagnosis is made).

By updating all the documentation the team will be able to work towards the new goals. It is important to follow the rules of documentation and include the date and time of the change and the rationale for implementing the new interventions.

Discharge planning

Discharge planning is an important process that impacts directly on health outcomes. The current trend in the health-care environment is to encourage early discharge. In most cases this is a positive action that sees the client returning to their own environment to complete the recuperation process. It also limits the exposure to hospital-acquired infections and conditions associated with reduced activity.

When beginning the discharge process it is recommended to assess both the client and family preferences early to incorporate them into the discharge plan. It is essential that clients are assessed carefully, especially with early discharge, to ensure they are well enough to meet those tasks, or have someone at home who is able to assist them.

The discharge plan should consist of safety considerations, living environment and provision of service, as well as transitional care planning.

TIP 14.3

Evaluation

When I was on my first placement I recall thinking that I would never be able to handover patient care as well as the other nurses were. I was always worried that I would lack the skills to evaluate what I was doing in terms of patient outcomes. So many factors, different patient needs and, of course, different types of nursing interventions were needed. I then started reviewing the care plans in detail – looking for common findings, looking at patient recovery as a whole, and, more importantly, realising that every patient is unique. A care plan will not fit all patients. Once I realised this and started assessing and managing every patient individually I felt far more confident in my abilities of assessment and documentation. I used to be petrified of handing over any work I had not yet completed – like something non-urgent – because I saw it as a failure on my part. Now, I realise that nursing is 24 hours a day, and that you can be an excellent nurse and still not get everything done on your time planner. You need to review and evaluate your patients, your workload and your priorities and you will get used to doing this as you progress. Use your practical time wisely.

Jason, 22, Enrolled Nurse

Review the skill in Tollefson *Essential Clinical Skills* 7.4 Admission, discharge and patient transfer

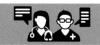

Reflective practice 14.2

Planning for discharge

There is a saying in health care, 'discharge planning begins on admission'. This is to ensure that all the variables are considered for the patient and interventions necessary are planned for, and discharge needs are communicated early on to relevant health-care team members – think of all the allied health staff. Consider the following two patients:

Aletta Knicks is a 59-year-old female who lives independently on acreage with livestock. She has been

hospitalised after being involved in a motor vehicle accident.

Megan Strong is a 72-year-old female who has been hospitalised due to the same motor vehicle accident. Megan lives with her husband and is his primary carer. She was independent in all her ADLs prior to hospitalisation.

1   What discharge planning would be necessary for each patient?
2   How would you discuss discharge planning with Megan and Aletta?

Discharge planning should include the following information to assist with anxiety and unnecessary stress on the client and their family:

- medications
- self-care required
- any relevant information of the health condition/s
- follow-up appointments and referrals
- when to seek medical assistance
- contact details of the hospital if the patient has questions post discharge
- information about services and programs available in the community following discharge if a referral has not already been made.

Information and provision of available community-based services is likely to assist in the recovery and maintenance of the patient's health and wellbeing when returning home or to a community setting.

SUMMARY

- Nursing care plans contain discharge planning and ongoing assessment, evaluation and recording of any variances.
- Nursing evaluation is an ongoing assessment and analysis of planned or unplanned interventions. It will require you to review both objective and subjective data and collate this information, then document it and report it to your colleagues.
- In no time you will soon become adept in the process of analysing your client's response to interventions, and identifying the factors that have contributed to the response – be it successful or unsuccessful – and finally, in planning for further nursing intervention/s.
- In order to prepare a person for care procedures the nurse must explain the procedure, preparation required and time frame involved before informed consent to the intervention can be obtained.
- When implementing care procedures to meet identified needs, the nurse needs to address the activities of daily living and also monitor for emergency situations that may arise.
- When monitoring a person's care needs, the nurse will prioritise work activities according to the urgency of the needs.
- The health-care team will evaluate the person's progress towards planned outcomes and adjust the care plan in response to their progress.

SELF-TEST QUESTIONS

1   How can the nurse obtain informed consent for nursing interventions?
2   What strategies can the nurse implement to ensure the privacy and dignity of the client?
3   What activities of daily living does the nurse need to assess in formulating a care plan?
4   How can the nurse monitor the response of clients to planned interventions?
5   Why is it important to document changes to the care plan?

BIBLIOGRAPHY

Clarke, L., Gray, S., White, L., Duncan, G. & Baumle, W. (2016). *Foundations of Nursing: Enrolled Division 2 Nurses* (ANZ edition). Cengage Learning: South Melbourne, pp. 85, 204.

Queensland Government Clinical Excellence Division (2018). *Clinical pathways.* Retrieved from https://clinicalexcellence.qld.gov.au/resources/clinical-pathways.

Tollefson, J., Watson, G., Jelly, E. & Tambree, K. (2016). *Essential Clinical Skills: Enrolled Division 2 Nurses* (3rd edition). Cengage Learning: South Melbourne.

Improving professional practice

LEARNING OUTCOMES

After reading this chapter, you should have an understanding of:

15.1 What it means to reflect on your own practice

15.2 How you can enhance your own practice

15.3 The importance of facilitating ongoing professional development

Reflective practice

On my first placement I felt overwhelmed and extremely tired at the end of each day. I was anxious not to hurt the residents and found it quite challenging to complete all the work that was required. I was so busy I did not have time to think. At night scenarios from the day went round and round in my head. My clinical supervisor suggested that we keep a journal and document not only what we did but also how we felt about the activities and interactions we were involved in.

I found this to be a very useful thing to do. I was able to write down all the activities and interactions and examine how I felt about them. Did I do the interventions well, or was there something I did not know or could improve upon?

At the end of the first week I had a one-on-one interview with my clinical supervisor who went through some of the things I had documented. I found that by using this tool and feedback on my performance from the clinical educator I had a plan of action that I could use to research or practise to improve my skills and knowledge.

The clinical supervisor also assisted me in identifying some of my strong points and I felt a sense of achievement at the end of the placement.

15.1 Reflecting on your own practice

While you are on placement, you will notice that nursing involves many situations that can be emotionally draining. You will be dealing with death, disability, loss and a myriad of feelings in between. Reflection is an incredibly effective method of dealing with this barrage of emotions and can assist in ensuring you are effectively debriefing and aware of your responses to clinical situations.

You may not be aware, but reflective practice is something that we actively participate in every day. Think of most things that we do from day to day – we look back upon our actions for the day, or think 'next time I will do it this way' or 'if only I remembered to take the bin out'. Small things like this form our reflective practice. This carries on to our working arena in nursing – with verbal reflective tools evident through patient handover, documentation and referrals to other health-care providers. Intertwined in reflection is our ability to critically think – this is the logical sequence of analysing the information we are reflecting upon.

TIP 15.1

Journaling

Using a journal in your placements is a fantastic way to debrief, analyse and review your experiences. A journal is also a great tool for seeing your progression and consolidation of knowledge. Most clinical log books require you to reflect upon your practice and keeping a journal will ensure that you have all this information available should you need it.

While on placement time goes quickly. It can be helpful to jot down in point form what you did and how you felt about it. Later at home these points will assist in remembering the activity and how you felt about it.

Reflective practice 15.1

Improving practice through reflection

Reflection is an essential element of learning; it is the careful consideration and examination of issues of concern related to an experience (McClure, n.d.). Reflective practice does not need to be a negative experience and should in fact be a positive one. Upon reflection of an experience or event you may discover the experience went well. From each piece of reflection you are able to identify what you have learnt from the experience and how this relates to the nursing theory or practice that you have been taught or researched.

Reflective practice is a key skill for nurses. It is a conscious, dynamic process of thinking, analysing and learning from a clinical experience (Asselin, 2011). The outcome of this process enables the nurse to gain insight into themselves and also their clinical practice. This insight allows them to then make changes, if required, for future clinical situations.

There are many benefits of self-reflection and the integration of reflective practice, both to the individual and the profession as a whole. They are:

- improves practice by promoting greater self-awareness
- enhances critical thinking and decision making in complex and uncertain situations
- increases learning from experience
- improves self-esteem and confidence
- promotes continual professional growth and professional responsibility
- empowers practitioners
- increases social and political emancipation.

There are many ways that you can evaluate your clinical practice. Some common ways that can be used are:

- discussions with a colleague, mentor or preceptors
- peer review
- client feedback
- clinical supervisor feedback.

Barriers to reflective practice

Although reflective practice has many positive outcomes, it is important to look at barriers that may inhibit the use of reflective practice. When engaging in reflective practice with colleagues or educators, for example, we must be willing to be open with others for the experience to be successful.

Time is often identified as a barrier to reflective practice. The novice learner in the beginning of reflective practice may struggle with motivation and commitment. To alleviate these barriers, set aside time in your workday for reflective practice. Setting aside time while you are on placement can be of benefit. Where do you reflect? During a noisy train or bus trip on way home from work? Or at home with interruptions and other chores vying for your attention? Setting aside time on a routine basis will assist in decreasing these barriers.

Psychological barriers can also hinder reflective practice. Fear of judgement or criticism or being closed to feedback can impede a person's ability and willingness to reflect on a situation. If reflecting creates anxiety, pain and/or discomfort, we are less likely to reflect.

Models of reflective practice

Reflective practice is more than 'thinking about an event'. It involves a critical review of an incident to identify methods to improve practice and deliver high-quality care. There are multiple models of reflective practice and the model each individual nurse chooses to implement in practice comes down to individual preference. An example is Gibbs reflective cycle, shown in **Figure 15.1**, which encourages a clear description of the elements.

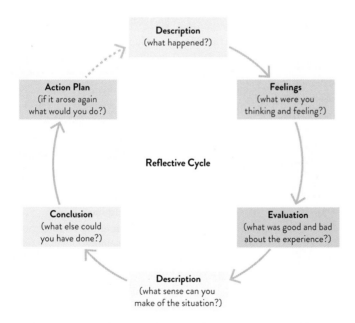

FIGURE 15.1 The Gibbs reflective cycle

Source: Gibbs, G. (1988). *Learning by Doing: A Guide to Teaching and Learning Methods*. Further Education Unit, Oxford Polytechnic: Oxford.

Aspects of reflective practice may already be incorporated into your life before you began nursing. Now you will need to develop and think about these reflective skills more as your ability to utilise reflective practice can affect patient care and outcomes. Part of living is drawing meaning from our experiences and interactions within society. As a nurse the same process occurs but is refined by the nursing framework in which we operate. **Figure 15.2** outlines some different reflective practice models that a person may choose to use.

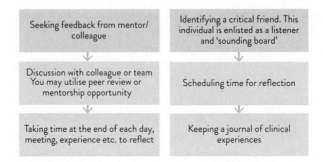

FIGURE 15.2 Methods of reflective practice

As nurses we are educated to be competent in performing skills and we have knowledge and theory to form a basis for our practice. Through reflective practice nurses can establish a meaningful connection or 'bridge' between theory and practice.

Utilising the reflective process can also help nurses critique personal performance and assess compliance with standards of practice. It is a process that helps make sense out of an experience and facilitates the incorporation of the experience into one's view of oneself as a professional.

Reflective practice 15.2

Journal for self-reflection

When I first started my diploma, an educator said to our class we should all 'keep a journal, particularly on placement'. I had a book that I took with me and I started writing an entry every day. Some days there were pages of information, other days, not so much. What I have observed is my progression from novice to developing practitioner. It is quite amazing reading back on the first time I inserted an indwelling catheter or removed a drain. All these 'milestones' in my education were reached with equal parts of fear and nervousness. Skills that I know now I give very little thought to as they are so well practised. Measuring blood pressure I used to struggle with, now I can perform it quickly and accurately. Whenever I am

worried that I am not progressing, or I don't know 'enough' I will read my book again and really see where I have been! I can also review incidents with more critical eyes, and hindsight review of some incidents has left me understanding exactly why events occurred. Some incidents I will never forget, and others are examples of how one small aspect overlooked in checking something can result in dire consequences.

Angela, Enrolled Nurse

1   What do you think the benefit of hindsight is in reviewing critical incidents?
2   How do you think re-reading your journal would be beneficial to your practice?
3   Do you think journaling is sufficient for reflective practice?

Actively seeking feedback from others

Reflective practice is not just dwelling on what occurred but learning from the experience. Perhaps one of the tasks you undertook did not go according to plan. Reflecting on the activity and outcome will assist you in identifying a plan of action for future interventions.

Obtaining feedback from different sources is also useful. Feedback can be obtained from clients, supervisors or work colleagues. Often with feedback it is surprising to hear the good things we have done. Usually we focus on the negative aspects. Reflecting on the positive is also a way to improve our clinical practice. It may be daunting to hear feedback from supervisors or work colleagues as you are aware that they hold a greater balance of power, but they can provide valuable insight into your clinical practice. It is important to remember that we all started at some point.

Feedback is an ongoing process that you will use daily, not just in nursing. Think of a conversation with a friend, or any acquaintance where you were not sure your message had been received and you sought feedback in the form of confirmation or clarification.

Activity 15.1

Feedback from your buddy

Organise for your buddy to watch you undertake a task. Prepare them beforehand by telling them that you would appreciate feedback and supply them with associated checklists for the activity.

Ask them to provide comments.

Now review your own practice and then compare them. Are they the same?

CASE STUDY 15.1

Professional feedback

Sam is a student nurse on his final placement. He has been allocated a full patient workload. His buddy nurse, Aletta, has gone to assist another colleague, leaving Sam with the patient cares. Sam has performed all observations and finds one patient's blood pressure to be elevated. The reading is 170/90, but on review of the patient's observation baseline, this is not an unusual or concerning finding, and the observation form has modifications in place for blood pressure. Another nurse takes the monitoring equipment away to use it to perform observations on her patients. She notes the high blood pressure and walks back to Sam and says, 'What do they teach you? This blood pressure must be reported. What are you doing just standing there?' The patient hears this also, and Sam is trying to explain the situation. At this moment, Aletta returns to the four-bed bay and is trying to determine what is going on.

1 What type of feedback has the nurse provided here?
2 What could Sam do to explain his clinical judgement?
3 How could this situation have been handled more professionally?

15.2 Enhancing your own practice

As students you are already engaging in the process of enhancing your own practice. This is completed through attending classes and labs, practising your skills and undergoing assessment procedures that allow you to identify areas for improvement.

Review the skill in Tollefson *Essential Clinical Skills* 7.6 Nursing informatics

Support networks

As a nurse there are a number of support networks, both internal and external to the workplace, that can be accessed to improve skills and knowledge.

The governing bodies of nursing also recommend this process of professional development. They review and audit the activities that registered nurses undertake each year to maintain industry currency and professional standards.

Some of the networks that nurses can use are:

* conferences
* nursing memberships such as the Australian College of Nursing
* the Australian Nursing Federation
* focus groups that specialise in specific areas, for example, the continence nurse group
* focus groups that operate within the workplace, such as WHS or infection control
* work colleagues.

Activity 15.2

Research support groups

Research different support groups that nurses use. Ask your buddy which ones they find helpful and why. Also review the clinical education program that is run by the facility.

Self-care and support

It can be daunting and frightening to be in a situation that you feel underprepared for. It is important to follow the decision-making framework and let your clinical supervisor know you need additional support on clinical placement if this is the case.

At times things can go wrong or evoke a negative emotion. A client may die or a mistake may occur. It is important to realise that negative emotions may be quite normal but if they continue and affect your own ADLs you should seek assistance in dealing with them.

Some behaviours of concern that require assistance include:

- crying
- being unable to sleep
- loss of appetite
- loss of interest in social activities.

Some ways that nurses can access **self-care** and support is through:

- debriefing
- talking about situations with colleagues and friends
- ensuring good dietary, exercise and rest patterns.

If your work situation has progressed to the point that there is a negative impact, you should inform the clinical supervisor who will organise some counselling through the school you attend. If you feel unable to discuss this with your supervisor, contacting your local GP is another option.

Nurses are often the 'constant' with the patient. Nurses provide comfort, support and are a source of information for patients and families alike. Patients will ask you for advice, they will ask you what you would do or what you think – be prepared for this and ensure that you are answering professionally and with honesty. If you don't know – ask! There is no harm in seeking information to ensure you are providing correct and appropriate information to your patients and their families.

Examples of who you could seek advice from include:

- clinical facilitator
- buddy nurse
- nurse unit manager
- nurse educator
- specialty nurse – for example, wound care specialist.

Recognising the need for self-development

Journaling, reflection and critical thinking all lead you to self-development. You can establish clearly with your ongoing review any shortcomings or areas of particular interest. A good example would be if you have just completed placement in an emergency department short-stay unit and would like to find out more information about the process of returning patients

self-care
Learnt behaviour and a deliberate action in response to a need

to nursing homes, what communication occurs, how does the patient get back to the nursing home and what handover, if any, occurs. You would identify that this is something that you are unsure of, and work out how to develop and acquire this knowledge.

On placement and during the first few years of your career there will be many areas of clinical practice that you are not familiar with – recognising this and working towards improving your knowledge, skills and awareness is a step towards accountable practice.

When you gain employment, you will need to complete a professional development plan – and this will outline the learning goals you may have, which might be generic or very specific. Your employer needs to work with you to support these goals, especially if they are relevant to clinical practice in your role.

15.3 Facilitating ongoing professional development

As nurses it is important to always undertake professional development. This will assist you to provide the best practice for your clients. If you refer to the Enrolled Nurse Standards for Practice (NMBA, 2016), you will notice that ongoing professional development is required. In fact, for registration with the Australian Health Practitioner Regulation Agency (AHPRA) annually, nurses must complete 20 hours of continuing professional development (CPD).

Professional development

To practise nursing in Australia you must hold a current registration from the AHPRA. It is the responsibility of each individual nurse to ensure his/her registration is current. To ensure registration continues, the nurse must ensure that fees are paid and demonstrate that he/she is indeed fit for practice. AHPRA requires the following in order to maintain registration:
- continuing professional development
- criminal history check
- professional conduct – Australian Nursing and Midwifery Council (ANMC) code of conduct for nurses
- recent evidence of practice.

It is ultimately the nurse, as a professional, who holds the accountability for ensuring he/she meets their annual CPD requirements. However, the employer also holds some responsibility in this area by making available the opportunity for nurses to access CPD activities. Continuous professional development is not only a mandate but also an essential component in ensuring our skill and knowledge is current, relevant and is based on the latest evidence and best practice standards to be well equipped to provide quality health care to clients.

While you are on placement, take any opportunity to participate in in-services or in-house education as you can include this in your CPD portfolio.

Confirming own practice against ethical and legal requirements

The most common barrier to professional development activities is access. It can be difficult to find the learning activity that will meet your learning needs by being delivered in a format that you are able to access. A general consensus is to undertake CPD that you are interested in – it will add to your skills and also ensure you are compliant with your registration requirements. For example, even if you currently work in the operating room, you can undertake professional development in emergency nursing.

TIP 15.3

Specific goals

Prior to placement, think about specific goals you want to achieve – do you want to become more proficient in taking a manual blood pressure? Or in interviewing and assessing patients on admission? Think about areas that you feel you need more practice in and see if you can convert this into achievable goals. You can work towards these goals over the duration of your placement and you will find a great sense of achievement in completing them.

Nursing is constantly evolving and what might have been considered best practice five years ago is now not the standard of care expected from a registered nurse. Legal and ethical requirements also change with developments in the health-care environment. An example of this is the use of restraint. At one time it was considered ethically and legally right – this has now changed.

Activity 15.3

Restraint policy and procedure

Access the policy and procedure on the use of restraint in the health-care facility. What actions are required by staff and how is restraint used?

Performance review

Health-care facilities are obligated to provide their employees with a yearly performance review. Your performance review is an opportunity for you to receive feedback on your performance against the job description and professional framework of the ANMC. To prepare for attending your review with your manager/supervisor, you can complete a personal copy of the review form as a reflective exercise to assist you to develop education goals for the upcoming year.

The Enrolled Nurse Standards for Practice (NMBA, 2016) set the core competency standards by which the health-care facility you are employed by will evaluate your performance. All enrolled nurses in all health-care facilities must meet this standard to maintain registration in Australia.

Performance review is a planned, structured process aiming to highlight areas of professional development opportunity; for example, if you identified to your manager that you would like to undertake learning opportunities in a specific area relating to your employment, you would both 'map out' a process for this to occur. It is also a forum to provide feedback to your manager about how you think you could improve, increase your responsibilities or possibly look at increasing your role within your area. Performance review is not a negative tool. It is a positive tool aimed at empowering staff to find ways to achieve professional satisfaction. It is also great to hear positive and encouraging feedback from your manager who you may not work closely with.

Review processes

When on placement you will notice that on certain days there is in-service education and other forms of in-house learning. This can be as simple as information regarding new equipment, a new product or an audit that needs to be completed in line with continuous improvement. While you are on placement, and as a student, it does not preclude you from providing an in-service or reviewing a procedure or process that is occurring. Using reflective and analytical practice you can proved feedback on an intervention or a procedure to staff and enhance their awareness. The beauty of nursing lies in the sharing of information and experience, and through sharing ideas, knowledge and learning outcomes you will be benefiting other staff and colleagues.

Reflecting upon your practice is a tool you can begin using now; in fact, you are most likely already using reflective practice. It is an ongoing mechanism for reviewing your own practice and receiving feedback and insight into your practice. Learning can only benefit from this and learning needs can be clearly identified when you review your practices and analyse them.

TIP 15.4

Performance review

Performance review is not something you can 'get out of'. As a student you will obtain a performance review and you will receive feedback on how and where, if at all, your practice needs to improve. When you are employed as an enrolled nurse, you will be required to complete an annual professional review. Use this time to discuss any learning goals you may have and maintain a professional portfolio to keep track of professional activities that you have undertaken.

SUMMARY

- To reflect on practice involves self-evaluation with others. It involves assessing your own values, beliefs and behaviour and reflecting on feedback from others.
- To enhance practice the nurse should identify what additional learning activities are required to be taken. It is important that nurses evaluate their own feelings and emotions and take adequate self-care or seek specialist assistance.
- Professional development is an ongoing activity that nurses undertake to provide the best care to clients. This can be as a result of reflection and feedback from others that identify new learning objectives.

SELF-TEST QUESTIONS

1 How can I undertake self-evaluation activities to improve my clinical practice?
2 How do I handle feedback from others?
3 What supports do I need from others to ensure self-care?
4 How can I ensure my practice meets legal and ethical requirements in the fast paced and changing health-care environment?

BIBLIOGRAPHY

ANMC (2016). *Information and guidelines*. Retrieved from http://www.nursingmidwiferyboard.gov.au/Codes-Guidelines-Statements/Professional-standards/enrolled-nurse-standards-for-practice.aspx. Accessed 18 March 2018.

Asselin, M.E. (2011). *Using reflection strategies to link course knowledge to clinical practice: The RN-to-BSN student experience*. Retrieved from https://www.ncbi.nlm.nih.gov/pubmed/21210605. Accessed 18 March 2018.

Caldwell, L. & Grobbel, C. (2013). The importance of reflective practice in nursing, *International Journal of Caring Sciences*, 6(3): 319–26.

Chabeli, M.M. (2007). Facilitating critical thinking within the nursing process framework: A literature review, *Health SA Gesondheid*, 12(4): 71–88.

Craven, R.F. & Himle, C.J. (2008). *Fundamentals of Nursing* (6th edition). Wolters Kluwer/Lippincott, Williams & Wilkins: Sydney.

Dolphin, S. (2013). How nursing students can be empowered by reflective practice, *Mental Health Practice*, 16(9): 20–3.

Gibbs, G. (1988). *Learning by Doing: A Guide to Teaching and Learning Methods*. Further Education Unit, Oxford Polytechnic: Oxford.

Huckabay, L.M. (2009). Clinical reasoned judgement and the nursing process, *Nursing Forum*, 44(2): 72–8.

Jasper, M. (2003). *Beginning Reflective Practice – Foundations in Nursing and Health Care*, Nelson Thornes: Cheltenham.

McClure, P, (n.d.). *Reflection on practice*. A resource commissioned by the Making Practice-based Learning Work project, an educational development project. Retrieved from http://cw.routledge.com/textbooks/9780415537902/data/learning/8_Reflection%20in%20Practice.pdf. Accessed 18 March 2018.

Mgbekem, M., Ojong, I., Odey, L., Lukpata, F., Uka, V., Ojong-Alasia, M. & Chiotu, C. (2016). Knowledge and application of reflective practice: A tool for meaningful nursing practice among nurses in University of Calabar Teaching Hospital, Cross River state Nigeria, *International Journal of Nursing, Midwife and Health Related Cases*, 2(2): 26–38.

Nursing and Midwifery Board of Australia (NMBA) (2016). *Enrolled Nurses Standards for Practice*. Retrieved from http://www.nursingmidwiferyboard.gov.au/Codes-Guidelines-Statements/Professional-standards/enrolled-nurse-standards-for-practice.aspx. Accessed 18 March 2018.

Philosophy – Critical Thinking Web (n.d.). *What is critical thinking*. Retrieved from http://philosophy.hku.hk/think/critical/ct.php. Accessed 18 March 2018.

Ruth-Sahd, L.A. (2003). Reflective practice: A critical analysis of data-based studies and implications for nursing education, *Journal of Nursing Education*, 42(11): 488–97.

Willingham, D.T. (2007). Critical thinking, why is it so hard to teach?, *American Educator*, Summer: 8–20.

Care for a person with chronic health problems

LEARNING OUTCOMES

After reading this chapter, you should have an understanding of:

16.1   Identifying the impacts of chronic health conditions on a person, family or carer

16.2   Contributing to a coordinated service approach

Chronic health conditions

I was shocked at how a chronic disease could severely impact on the life of the person. When we learnt about diabetes I was interested in the A&P and pathophysiology of the disease as I felt distressed when I saw its long-term effects. I had thought chronic diseases only applied to old people. When I went on the rehabilitation ward I was confronted by people not much older than myself, who had had an amputation of their lower limbs, due to diabetes. The dressings were horrific to see and I felt sorry that they could not be as carefree as myself. It was really confronting to go to some of the allied health service departments, especially physiotherapy, and see clients who were trying to regain a level of independence as they confronted the ravages of chronic disease. One of the areas that the hospital specialised in was the treatment of clients who suffered from cardiac disease. I had not thought that this could affect people in their early thirties.

16.1 Identifying the impacts of chronic health conditions

Chronic health conditions, such as heart disease, stroke, cancer and diabetes, can limit participation in community activities, prevent freedom of lifestyle choices and cause suffering and anxiety in all affected. The World Health Organization has identified that heart disease, stroke, cancer, chronic respiratory diseases and diabetes are the leading causes of mortality in the world accounting for 60% of all deaths. Chronic health conditions affect the family and carer as well as the individual. They can limit the physical capacity to do everyday activities, lead to social isolation and cause fear, anxiety and distress due to their impact on life or the possible outcomes of the disorder for both the person and the carer.

Chronic health problems and possible impacts

Chronic disease is a disease that persists for six months or longer and has a persistent effect on the person's wellbeing. Chronic disease can affect an individual in many ways. Initially the disease will be restricted to the organ system in which it begins and the person may progress to develop other symptoms and disease states due to other organ systems being affected. An example of this is cardiac failure that affects the person's respiratory system.

The person will have difficulty in meeting their activities of daily living (ADLs) and may become severely disabled and progress to death from either the disease, a complication of the disease or the effects on another organ system of the body. Chronic disease is usually slow in the initial stages and at times the individual will not feel the effects of the disease. This period of time is usually called **remission**. At other times the disease symptoms will reappear and this is called **exacerbation**.

Figure 16.1 shows the chronic disease continuum. The first two categories 'Not at risk' and 'At risk' will benefit from prevention strategies to maintain and improve their health. The next two categories 'Previously undiagnosed' and 'Diagnosed without co-morbidity' will need intervention to first detect and delay effects of the disease to improve the individual's health. The 'Diagnosed with co-morbidity' category requires interventions to diagnose other disease states and support the person with the disease often till the time of their death.

remission
The period of time that the person does not suffer the symptoms of the disease

exacerbation
The time when the symptoms reappear

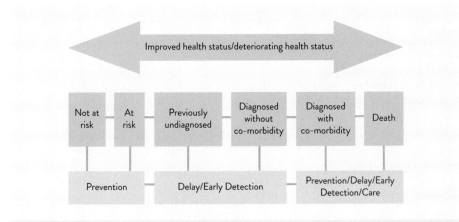

FIGURE 16.1 The chronic disease continuum

Explore the theory in *Foundations of Nursing* 2e, Gray et al., Page 540, Chapter 23: Chronic health conditions

Source: Grant, J.F. et al. (2006). The North West Adelaide Health Study: Detailed methods and baseline segmentation of a cohort for selected chronic diseases, *Epidemiologic Perspectives & Innovations*. Retrieved from https://openi.nlm.nih.gov/detailedresult.php?img=PMC1462963_1742-5573-3-4-1&req=4.

Table 16.1 lists some of the common chronic diseases and symptoms that you may come across in clinical placement.

TABLE 16.1 Body systems, chronic disease states and symptoms

Human body	Diseases	Symptoms	Tollefson Clinical Skill
Heart and blood vessels	Coronary artery disease, stroke and heart failure are diseases usually caused by **atherosclerosis**. This deposit stops the flow of blood from reaching the tissues.	Chest pain (angina) due to temporary cessation of blood to the heart muscle. Shortness of breath as the heart cannot pump enough blood to areas of the body. Heart attack – central chest pain, and pain in shoulder, arm or neck that is not relieved by rest.	2.3 Temperature, pulse and respiration (TPR) measurement 2.4 Blood pressure measurement 2.10 12-lead ECG recording Explore the theory in *Foundations of Nursing* 2e, Gray et al., Page 541, Chapter 23: Chronic health conditions
Cells	Cancer is a collection of abnormal cells that grow and multiply and attack other areas of the body. These cells can develop but stay in the place they arise and cause little problems for the person, but some cells will migrate to other areas of the body and cause the body to react in response causing a disease process to occur.	No specific symptoms. If cancer spreads to other areas of the body it may put pressure on those organs or affect the normal functioning of the organ it has invaded; for example, lung cancer may cause a persistent cough or a change in voice. Other signs are non-specific such as: • tiredness • weight loss • fever.	
Renal system	Chronic renal disease occurs when the filters of the kidneys are damaged or the functioning of the kidneys is reduced for a period of three months.	90% of kidney function can be lost before symptoms appear. Altered renal function is detected by blood tests.	
	Incontinence is the inability to prevent passing urine, faeces or flatulence (wind) consciously. It involves losing control of sphincters usually under voluntary control. The types of incontinence are: • stress incontinence • urge incontinence • incontinence associated with chronic retention • functional incontinence • faecal incontinence		3.7 Assisting the patient with elimination – urinary and bowel elimination

>>

See next spread, Definitions *Continued*

>>

Human body	Diseases	Symptoms	Tollefson Clinical Skill
Renal system (cont.)	Stress incontinence is the leaking of small amounts of urine during activities that increase pressure in the abdomen and press down on the bladder. Women are more at risk due to childbirth and at menopause when levels of oestrogen decline.	Small amounts of urine that is leaked during certain activities such as sneezing, laughing, walking, lifting or playing sport.	Review the skill in Tollefson *Essential Clinical Skills* 3.7 Assisting the patient with elimination – urinary and bowel elimination
	Urge incontinence is the sudden and strong urge to urinate.	Passing of usual amount of urine. Often not able to hold onto urine.	
	Incontinence associated with chronic retention may be caused by: • pressure of a full bladder on the urethra • enlarged prostate • prolapse of pelvic organs • nerve damage that controls the bladder • diabetes, multiple sclerosis, stroke, Parkinson's disease • medications	Straining to pass urine Weak or slow urine stream Not feeling as though bladder empties fully No warning of the need to empty your bladder Passing urine while asleep Frequent urinary tract infections Dribbling urine after going to the toilet	3.7 Assisting the patient with elimination – urinary and bowel elimination
	Functional incontinence may occur with: • dementia • poor eyesight • poor mobility • poor dexterity • mental health illnesses • environmental factors such as poor lighting, difficulty in getting out of chairs	Inappropriate passing of urine	
	Faecal incontinence may be due to weak pelvic muscles, constipation or diarrhoea. Other diseases can cause this to occur, such as: • irritable bowel syndrome • Crohn's Disease • ulcerative colitis	Difficulty in controlling bowel movements.	
Endocrine system	Diabetes – three types – whereby the person cannot maintain a healthy blood glucose level. Include: • type 1 due to an auto immune • type 2 associated with lifestyle factors • gestational diabetes – higher than normal BGL in pregnancy.	Increased thirst Passing more urine Tiredness Feeling hungry Slow to heal cuts Blurred vision	2.6 Blood glucose measurement

>>

Human body	Diseases	Symptoms	Tollefson Clinical Skill
Muscular system	Arthritis, such as: • osteoarthritis, which produces wear and tear on joints leading to destruction of the cartilage • rheumatoid arthritis, which is an auto immune disease leading to chronic inflammation of the joints	Loss of function of joints Stiffness Pain Swelling of joints	2.9 Pain assessment 3.14 Active and passive exercises
Skeletal system	Osteoporosis is the progressive loss of bone density	Increased fractures of bones Pain Change in posture	3.14 Active and passive exercises
Respiratory system	Asthma inflammatory disease of the airways Chronic obstructive pulmonary disease limits the amount of air taken into the lungs Hay fever and allergies affect the nasal passages and sinuses	Shortness of breath Increased respiration Hypoxia 'Runny' nose and itchy eyes, sneezing	2.5 Pulse oximetry
Nervous system	Chronic pain is pain that lasts longer than three months. Changes occur to the nerves which keeps them firing and signalling **pain** Chronic pain is pain that persists for an extended period of time Long-term unconsciousness	Mild to severe pain that does not go away Pain that may be described as shooting, burning, aching or electrical Discomfort, soreness, tightness or stiffness	2.9 Pain assessment
	Motor neurone disease is a condition in which the muscles that control movement of specific muscles slows and becomes extinct	Early symptoms: • stumbling due to leg weakness • inability to hold objects • slurring of speech and swallowing difficulties • cramps and muscle twitching Later symptoms: • breathing difficulties • fatigue • insomnia • changes in cognition • dementia • excessive laughing or crying • pain and discomfort	2.7 Neurological observation
	Neurological injury – trauma to the brain produces an injury that results in a physiological change. The four types are: • penetrating injuries • **anoxic** injuries • toxic injuries • closed head injuries		
	Penetrating injuries can be any of the following: • Open fractures of skull where the completeness of bony covering is broken. • Gunshot wounds – a bullet entering skull and causing damage to brain's tissues. • A foreign object such as a pair of scissors entering brain through the skull.	• Reduced ability to respond to stimuli • Changes in muscle tone • Difficulties in respiration and other vital functions • Increased intra-cranial pressure of fluid build-up.	

>>

Human body	Diseases	Symptoms	Tollefson Clinical Skill
Nervous system (cont.)	Anoxic injuries, whereby a lack of oxygen to assist the metabolism of cells causes the cell to die.		
	Toxic injuries result from exposure to poisons and poisonous substances that can affect the brain and cause damage to brain's cells.		
	Closed head injuries occur when the brain is injured by the pressure of the tissue against the bony inside of the skull		

Source: Cancer Council Australia (2016). *What is cancer?* Retrieved from https://www.cancer.org.au/about-cancer/what-is-cancer/; Continence Foundation of Australia (2017). *What is incontinence?* Retrieved from https://www.continence.org.au/pages/what-is-incontinence.html; Australian Pain Management Association (n.d.). *What is chronic pain?* Retrieved from https://www.painmanagement.org.au/resources/about-pain/what-is-chronic-pain.html; Neurologic Rehabilitation Institute at Brookhaven Hospital (n.d.). *Frequently asked questions about brain injury.* Retrieved from http://www.traumaticbraininjury.net/faqs/.

Activity 16.1

Identifying nursing problems

For one of the disease states identified in **Table 16.1**, complete the nursing process to identify three actual problems and three potential problems the person may experience. For each nursing diagnosis identify two nursing interventions and a method that you can use to evaluate the person's physical status.

The person's and their carer's understanding of the disease process

A therapeutic relationship will allow the nurse to explore with the person their understanding of the disease process, identify any knowledge gaps about the disease and also identify barriers to fully understanding the disease process.

Often the carer will have important information to contribute to the assessment process. Carers can give their impressions of how the disease is affecting the person and their ability to maintain their normal activities of daily living. At times the person may reveal more to the carer, with whom they have a strong tie, than with the health-care team, who they may not know before admission. It is important that the person gives consent to the carer discussing and knowing about their health status.

Understanding the disease process

The nurse needs to know about the presentation of the disease and the likely progression of the disease in order to care for the person. The nurse may research the disease and access information from other members of the health-care team to update their knowledge base of the disease.

If it is the person's first admission with the problem they may have significant knowledge deficits. This can include risk factors that trigger an exacerbation of the disease and how the disease impacts on the ADLs.

Writing

atherosclerosis
Where the artery wall narrows due to a build-up of a hard substance that adheres to the surface of the artery wall. Usually consisting of fat, cholesterol and other body substances that bond together

pain
Unpleasant sensations perceived by the individual

anoxic
Lack of oxygen

The amount of knowledge about the disease and treatment is increasing due to the availability of information on the Internet. Many young people will have already looked up their symptoms but will still require education, which may need to be 'chunked', that is, given in manageable amounts. It is important that the nurse times the education session appropriately – when the person's symptoms are managed and they are not distracted by other issues, such as a need to urinate.

Reflective practice 16.1

Education for chronic diseases

1 When delivering education on health conditions why should the nurse give both written and verbal material?

2 Why is it important to have the person explain the objectives of the education system to you in their own words?

Explore the theory in *Foundations of Nursing* 2e, Gray et al., Chapter 9: Client education

Review the skill in Tollefson *Essential Clinical Skills* 7.5 Health teaching

Identifying knowledge gaps

After an education session, as shown in **Figure 16.2**, the person may not retain all of the information given to them. You can check the person's understanding by questioning techniques and observation. This can be an informal observation; an example might be a person who is suffering from shortness of breath, and who has been given education on the correct postures to ease breathing – are they performing this action correctly? As depicted in **Figure 16.2**, you may observe how the person uses a medical aid and provide education or reinforce the use of correct techniques. At times observation may be direct, for example, observing the person using their inhaler or taking their BGL measurement. At all times that you interact with the person, checking their knowledge is an important nursing action in identifying their educational needs relating to managing their condition.

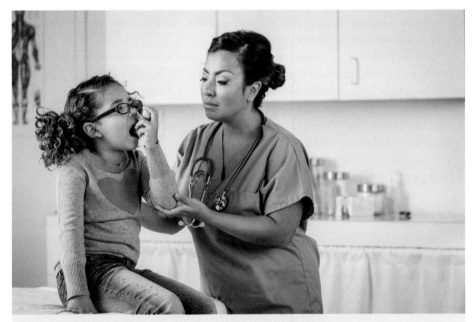

FIGURE 16.2 Education on how to use medical devices

Getty Images/Terry Vine

Barriers to education

There are many reasons why education is not successful immediately and may need to be continuously reinforced, including physical, emotional and psychological barriers.

Physical barriers

A person who is in pain or discomfort will not be able to pay attention to the education session fully. The nurse must attend to these issues before commencing to give the education.

Other disabilities relating to vision and hearing should also be assessed. Does the person wear glasses or a hearing aid? Are these present and do they work? For the person with a hearing problem is the education in a quiet area where surrounding noise does not interfere with the information? For the person with a visual problem is the education in a well-lit room where the person can see the nurse demonstrate techniques?

For the person with a disability has the education been adjusted to accommodate the disability? An example may be the person with arthritis who is unable to grasp or perform an action with their fingers due to their condition.

Emotional barriers

A person can experience a range of emotions upon diagnosis of their disease and during its exacerbation. The nurse needs to allow the person to communicate how they are feeling. Some examples of common emotions experienced by the person can be anger, 'Why did this happen to me?' or denial, 'This is not happening'.

Psychological barriers

Education will vary in accordance with the person's motivation to change. See **Table 16.2** for the stages involved in the motivation to change.

TABLE 16.2 Motivation to change

Stage	What is occurring at each stage	Need for education
Precontemplation	In this stage the person is unaware of how their behaviour may affect the disease process and be unaware of the need to change any aspects of their life.	The person needs to be given information on the disease, how it can affect the person and the changes that are required.
Contemplation	The person is aware that aspects of their life are impacting on their health. They make a decision to change.	At this point consolidation of the general information is required.
Preparation	They start to plan how to make the change; they will be researching and evaluating different approaches.	Assist with evaluation and implementing a plan. This may need review and readjusting. Information on new skills.
Action	At this point the person commences new behaviours and takes on new skills and knowledge.	Education will focus on the maintenance of the new skills and knowledge.
Maintenance	Established new behaviours and control over their life.	Education is given to monitor progress.
Relapse	The person goes back to previous behaviour.	It's important to give education on what to do if this occurs. The person needs support and new motivation to persevere with the new behaviours and skills.
Termination	Achieved a lifestyle change that is healthier and automatically completes the desired behaviours.	Ongoing information and support to maintain the desired behaviours and lifestyle.

Activity 16.2

Stage of change and acquisition of new behaviours and skills

Choose one of the clients you are caring for and identify what stage of change that person is at. Does this relate to the interventions that have been planned for this individual? Describe the behaviours the person is adopting in this stage of change. What emotions/feelings does the person have in relation to changing their behaviours? What is the motivation for the change in behaviour? Has the person set short- and long-term goals and rewards?

Reading, analysing

Current treatments

There are a number of different strategies, techniques and equipment available to assist the person with a chronic disease to manage symptoms and improve their quality of life. The nurse or a member of the allied health-care team will be able to identify service providers within the local community who will be able to assist the person. Refer to **Table 16.3** for a sample of some of the services, techniques and equipment that a person with a chronic health-care problem may find useful.

TABLE 16.3 Strategies, techniques and equipment for management of chronic diseases

Service/strategy	Techniques and equipment	
Physiotherapy	Physiotherapy is the treating of disease and injury through manipulation of the body. An example is applying heat to increase circulation. Australian Physiotherapy Association, https://www.physiotherapy.asn.au	*Science Photo Library/Phanie/Burger*
Occupational therapy	Assists people to adapt to their environment or provides aids to assist the client. Occupational Therapy Australia, https://www.otaus.com.au	*Getty Images/kali9*
Hydrotherapy	Physical manipulation of the body in heated water. What is hydrotherapy? http://www.rehabcorp.com.au/other-services/hydrotherapy	*Getty Images/Image Source*

>>

Service/strategy	Techniques and equipment	
Pilates	A specialised set of exercise that aims to strengthen the core muscles of the body to build strength, flexibility and improve muscle tone. What is pilates? http://www.pfiwa.com.au/start/what-is-pilates	Getty Images/Marc Romanelli
Massage	Manipulation of body parts and muscles to improve wellbeing. Northwestern Health Sciences University, https://www.nwhealth.edu	Getty Images/Per Magnus Persson
Art and music therapy	An approach to improve wellbeing through expression in art or music. Art and music therapy have been used successfully in people with dementia or mental health issues. Australian and New Zealand Arts Therapy Association, https://www.anzata.org/About-Arts-Therapy Australian Music Therapy Association, http://www.austmta.org.au	Getty Images/AMELIE-BENOIST/BSIP
Mobility devices	There are many varied types of mobility devices to enable the individual to mobilise at home or in the community. Aids can be used to support clients with physical disabilities to move within their environment. Yooralla, http://www.yooralla.com.au	Alamy Stock Photo/Peter Titmuss
Prosthetics	An artificial body part. The Australian Orthotic Prosthetic Association, https://www.aopa.org.au	Getty Images/ERproductions Ltd

Activity 16.3

Choosing equipment to assist the person with a disability

Visit the Yooralla online service (https://ilcaustralia.org.au/search_category_paths) and choose three different equipment devices and explain how they could assist the person with a chronic disorder. You will need to identify the disorder and how they will be of particular value in assisting the person to undertake activities of daily living.

Reading

Community-based care services

The aim of chronic disease management is to provide a person-centred approach to care that will improve health outcomes and quality of life for the person. The aims are:

- to prevent the condition of the person from deteriorating
- to assist the person to be able to access assistance
- to give the freedom of choice and control back to the person and their carer
- to use existing resources effectively in the management of chronic diseases (https://www2.health.vic.gov.au).

In the previous sections it has been identified that there are a variety of strategies that may be used in the management of chronic disease. These can include appropriate therapies, aids, education and behaviour modifications. These different techniques and equipment/aids can be accessed in the community to assist the person with managing the disease without the need for hospital admission, and allow more independence and fuller participation in the community. However, not all strategies, therapies or equipment will be suitable for everyone with a common chronic disease. Some individuals may need to try a variety of strategies or techniques before finding one that is the most suitable.

TIP 16.1

Using equipment

Before using equipment ensure that it is in good working order. It is often helpful to have a staff member run through how the equipment is operated before using it with an individual.

Activity 16.4

Community resources

Often when a person is discharged from hospital they will need ongoing care. Make a list of all of the community resources in the local community and how they can assist the person or the family/carer with a chronic health condition.

Involving the person

The person who is living with the disease or disability is central to the care that is given. It is important that the person actively takes on the strategies, techniques or uses the equipment correctly so that they can improve their quality of life. It is important that the person can see the benefit of using the equipment or strategy and is motivated to assume the responsibility for their health.

Reflective practice 16.2

Person-centred care

Identify how the care plan that has been implemented for one of the clients that you are caring for incorporates a person-centred approach. Why is this approach important?

16.2 Contributing to a coordinated service approach

When providing support to a person with a chronic disease there are often a variety of providers or health services that are involved. To make effective use of services it is important that a central person is responsible for the coordination of the supports. This is initially organised by the general practitioner in the community but will require review by the health team when the person is admitted to hospital.

At other times the person may indicate a need for increased supports and may have a case manager assigned to assist with this process. The case manager may be attached to the local council or local hospital.

Other supports available

Health-care agencies and professionals work together to support the individual. This involves good communication between all agencies to enable a more effective case management approach. In all instances where a person needs a referral to another service the individual must give consent to pass on his/her personal information.

In today's technological environment the person may research other techniques or strategies to address the chronic disease independently. It is important that the nurse is aware of what the person is using because a lot of alternative treatments may be dangerous if combined with Western treatments. There have been adverse events as a result of natural medicine combined with Western medicine, such as herbal supplements and traditional medicine being taken at the same time.

The nurse may become aware of other needs of the person, and early referral or identification of areas of need may prevent other problems for the individual and their family/carer from arising. The person may require support such as counselling or intervention by a social worker if financial or personal issues arise. The nurse needs to alert the other members of the health-care team to these needs through documentation and verbal reporting.

Support of the family or carer

The family and/or carer may be faced with a number of challenging issues while giving support to the individual and they also require support. They may face a change in the economic structure of the household and the roles that family members held may change in response to the chronic disease. It is the family member or carer who needs to support the person and often they will witness the challenges, disappointments and successes that the individual has while undertaking treatment for the disease. The family or carer is often the person who sees the person at times of crisis and is critical in assisting the person to access treatments and services. It is important to remember that the chronic disease affecting the individual also affects the lives of the family or carer.

TIP 16.2

Advocating for clients
Ensure that any issues that the individual raises with you are fully documented and reported to the person in charge. This is the best way, initially, that you can ensure that you advocate for the people that you are caring for.

Verbal communication, documentation

Reflective practice 16.3

Families and carers

Often the family and carer are very protective of the person you are caring for. Describe three ways that you can include the family or carer into the care of the person with a chronic disease.

Role and responsibilities for communication and reporting

The nurse is often the person most in contact with the patient and their family or carer. The role that the nurse plays in caring for this individual will be varied. At times they will need to provide ongoing education or reinforce the education that has been given by specialist members of the health-care team. At other times they will need to offer support and encouragement to the person to continue with different treatments.

At times the nurse will be the person that the individual will talk to and confide in. This can arise as a result of the therapeutic relationship that has developed between the nurse and the person. It is important for the nurse to respect the person's privacy and confidentiality and at times this can cause conflict for the nurse if they become aware that the individual is not keeping to the goals and objectives of the treatment plan. The nurse must act in line with enrolled nursing standards. Being open and honest with the person and informing them that they need to pass on information to other members of the health-care team is important as it maintains the honesty of the relationship. At other times the nurse may be required to act as the **advocate** for the person.

The nurse must ensure that they document accurately any issues that arise with the plan of care in the case file and also verbally report this to their supervisor.

advocate
A person who speaks up for or acts on behalf of the patient

CASE STUDY 16.1

Caring for a person with diabetes

Rosa is an 89-year-old woman with dementia, who has recently been admitted into the facility where you are working for stabilisation of her type 2 diabetes and wound management. She came directly from a local nursing home, where her daughter is encouraged to continue as her prime carer. She also receives community support services from the Greek community.

Recently she has been diagnosed with type 2 diabetes which has caused her to suffer from peripheral vascular disease and occurrence of chronic leg ulcers. Her prognosis is poor. She has also suffered cerebrovascular accidents (strokes) in the last 10 years. She has hypertension, osteoarthritis and cataracts.

At present her pain appears to be under control, but staff need to monitor this carefully because the trajectory of the disease may change quickly, and if her diabetes is not kept under control it could lead to an amputation of her lower limb.

Sometimes Rosa has difficulty with communication and when she becomes stressed she often speaks in Greek, which is her first language. She is extremely expressive and requires patience and encouragement from staff to understand her communications. Rosa also uses precise body language for gestures. Her long-term memory fluctuates; during lucid times she likes to speak about her life and her family.

She requires full assistance with all aspects of her ADLs. Rosa is a much adored mother and grandmother. She has two daughters and one son, all married with teenage children. Rosa's husband died over 25 years ago and they were married for over 40 years.

Rosa is very frail and is now restricted to resting in bed or in a wheelchair. She sometimes overreaches and is at danger of falling. She is also incontinent of both urine and faeces and wears a pad at all times. Rosa was extremely close to her mother. She misses her mother terribly and spends a lot of time looking at photographs of her and when confused insists that she must leave to go home as her mother will be worried.

1 When arriving at the health-care facility Rosa is extremely distressed and disorientated. Discuss six nursing interventions you can use to assist her orientation and to calm her.

2 Identify the professionals of the multidisciplinary aged care team who will contribute to the care of Rosa and explain each of their roles.

Variations in the person's needs and the response of the health-care team

The individual will progress through different stages and needs when diagnosed with a chronic disease. Dr Kubler-Ross's stages of grief can be applied to the different needs of the person with a chronic disease. These stages give rise to the need for different support. For example, if a client is in the stage of denial it would be ineffective to commence education programs (Patricelli, n.d.).

Activity 16.5

Stages of acceptance

Choose one of the individuals that you are caring for that is exhibiting a challenging behaviour due to their condition.

1   Identify what stage of the grieving process this person may be in with their chronic disease and its impact on their life.

2   What resources may be helpful for this person to move on to the stage of acceptance?

Health education and the role of the health-care team

As discussed earlier in the chapter, education regarding the disease, treatments and interventions are an important aspect of care for the person with a chronic disease. The nurse may be the person giving the education or may support the education given by other members of the health-care team and reinforce the learning or behaviour modification of the person. An example of this is the person with diabetes and the self-monitoring of blood glucose measurements and self-administration of insulin. The nurse may prompt the person to do specific actions when completing these tasks, such as wiping the finger with water before obtaining the drop of blood for testing, and providing positive feedback to the person on completion of the task.

When a person is learning new skills and behaviour the amount of information can be overwhelming. Providing written information may address knowledge gaps that the person may have after an education session. Have you ever been to the doctor and on leaving the surgery not been able to recall all the instructions that the doctor gave? At all times it is important to give information in a manner that the person can understand. This may mean using everyday language or using an interpreter to ensure the person is receiving the verbal communication correctly.

Checking the person's understanding of the education is important. The nurse can do this by asking questions, observing the individual and monitoring the person's condition.

Review the skill in Tollefson *Essential Clinical Skills* 7.5 Health teaching

Verbal communication documentation

CASE STUDY 16.2

Providing education

Sarah is a 19-year-old woman admitted to the health-care facility after having a severe episode of asthma during which she required an emergency tracheostomy. The health-care team has been trying to get Sarah to adhere to a preventative care plan that would identify when she was most at risk of suffering another severe attack of asthma.

When speaking with Sarah, she appears to have all of the medical language under control but you notice that she constantly makes mistakes in the recording of her peak flow measures.

After going through the procedure with Sarah on two more occasions you note that Sarah still makes errors with recording these levels in her personal diary. You report this to the supervisor and ensure that it is documented in the case file.

Later that week you learn that Sarah was assessed and found to be dyslexic. The team has now brought in a learning professional to work with Sarah to assist her.

1   What other issues (identify at least two) may cause an individual to have difficulty in adhering to a learning strategy?

2   Identify two strategies that may be used to ensure that health education is successful.

SUMMARY

- Chronic diseases are complex conditions to address. The needs of a person are varied and often require specialised services and support.
- Due to the individualised nature of the effect of chronic disease a person-centred approach to services and support is required. This can be time consuming and a waste of resources if the same type of supports are implemented by different health-care team members. A coordinated approach with a case manager is often the most effective way to provide services and supports to the person with a chronic disease.
- Education of the person and carer is an important aspect for management of the disease condition. The nurse is an essential part of the health-care team that is involved with this aspect of support.
- Chronic disease not only affects the person with the condition but will also affect the person's family or carer. It is important that care and support is also given to the family and carer as part of the care plan.

SELF-TEST QUESTIONS

1   What skills do you need to identify the disease, the impact of the chronic disease and the supports required by the person, family or carer?
2   Identify three members of the health-care team that may be involved in the education of patients with a chronic disease and outline their specialist input.
3   How does the nurse contribute to a coordinated service approach?
4   Describe the role of the nurse in the education of chronic disease.
5   What support can the family offer the person with a chronic disease?

BIBLIOGRAPHY

Australian Music Therapy Association (n.d.). Retrieved from http://www.austmta.org.au. Retrieved 9 April 2017.

Australian Pain Management Association (n.d.). *What is chronic pain?* Retrieved from https://www.painmanagement.org.au/resources/about-pain/what-is-chronic-pain.html. Accessed 5 April 2017.

Australian Physiotherapy Association (n.d.). Retrieved from https://www.physiotherapy.asn.au. Retrieved 9 April 2017.

Cancer Council Australia (2016). *What is cancer?*. Retrieved from https://www.cancer.org.au/about-cancer/what-is-cancer/

Continence Foundation of Australia (2017). *What is incontinence?* Retrieved from https://www.continence.org.au/pages/what-is-incontinence.html. Accessed 9 April 2017.

Grant, J.F., Chittleborough, C.R., Taylor, A.W., Dal Grande, E., Wilson, D.H., Phillips, P.J., ... Ruffin, R.E. (2006). The North West Adelaide Health Study: Detailed methods and baseline segmentation of a cohort for selected chronic diseases, *Epidemiologic Perspectives & Innovations*. Retrieved from https://openi.nlm.nih.gov/detailedresult.php?img=PMC1462963_1742-5573-3-4-1&req=4.

Health.vic (2018), *Integrated chronic disease managemernt*. Retrieved from https://www2.health.vic.gov.au/primary-and-community-health/primary-care/integrated-care/integrated-chronic-disease-management

MND Australia (n.d.). *Symptoms*. Retrieved from https://www.mndaust.asn.au/Get-informed/What-is-MND/Symptoms.aspx. Accessed 9 April 2017.

Neurologic Rehabilitation Institute at Brookhaven Hospital (n.d.). *Frequently asked questions about brain injury*. Retrieved from http://www.traumaticbraininjury.net/faqs/. Accessed 5 April 2017.

North Western Health Sciences University (n.d.). Retrieved from https://www.nwhealth.edu. Accessed 5 April 2017.

Nursing and Midwifery Board of Australia (2016). Enrolled nurse standards for practice. Retrieved from http://www.nursingmidwiferyboard.gov.au/Codes-Guidelines-Statements/Professional-standards/enrolled-nurse-standards-for-practice.aspx.

Occupational Therapy Australia (n.d.). Retrieved from https://www.otaus.com.au. Accessed 5 April 2017.

Patricelli, K. (n.d.). *Stages of Grief Models: Kubler-Ross*. AMHC. Retrieved from https://www.amhc.org/58-grief-bereavement-issues/article/8444-stage-of-grief-models-kubler-ross.

Pilates Fitness Institute (n.d.). *What is Pilates?* Retrieved from http://www.pfiwa.com.au/start/what-is-pilates. Accessed 5 April 2017.

Rehabcorp physiotherapy (n.d.). *What is hydrotherapy?* Retrieved from http://www.rehabcorp.com.au/other-services/hydrotherapy. Accessed 5 April 2017.

RN Central, Notes from the Nurses' Station (2012). *What Exactly Is Patient Advocacy?* Retrieved from http://www.rncentral.com/blog/2012/what-exactly-is-patient-advocacy/. Accessed 17 April 2017.

The Australian Orthotic Prosthetic Association (n.d.). Retrieved from https://www.aopa.org.au. Retrieved 9 April 2017.

The Professional Association for Arts Therapy in Australia, New Zealand and Singapore (n.d.). *About art therapy*. Retrieved from https://www.anzata.org/About-Arts-Therapy. Accessed 9 April 2017.

Yooralla (n.d). Retrieved from http://www.yooralla.com.au. Accessed 9 April 2017.

Researching and applying evidence to practice

LEARNING OUTCOMES

After reading this chapter, you should have an understanding of:

17.1 Planning information-gathering activities

17.2 The processes involved in gathering information

17.3 The steps involved in analysing information

17.4 Using information in practice

Nursing and research

I chose to study nursing because I had a strong desire to help people in a practical, hands-on manner. During the course I studied anatomy and physiology, which I found challenging but could relate this to the wellbeing of the person. I really enjoyed the practical labs and skill development sessions and looked forward to putting these into practice. I was not looking forward to the research subject as it brought up images of people in white coats in sterile environments, far removed from the bedside. When the class started the unit I was surprised to find that research, especially evidenced-based research, was practically based and formed the basis for current best practice in nursing care.

17.1 Planning information-gathering activities

The way nursing works and the tasks nurses are required to do are constantly changing to keep up with new technology and treatment. You will need to research these products or processes to understand the rationale behind using either the product or a new way of completing a task, and to provide information that is accurate for the person you are caring for.

In the clinical area you will come across situations where a person may need a new care strategy to meet identified needs. Perhaps they have not responded well to the current care strategy or there may be a range of different reasons to identify alternate methods of care such as cost of treatment, ease of providing the treatment, and priority of care.

Cost of treatments, such as those involved with wound care, may place a burden on a client's financial resources. It may be necessary to research alternate methods of wound-care products to identify a cost-effective product. How the product or care is delivered is another factor that you may need to consider. Will the treatment impact on other activities that the person needs to undertake such as employment? Priority of care may also dictate a need for research; for example, if mobilisation of a person is the prime objective a wound product that is flexible, waterproof and self-adhering might be the deciding factor in product selection.

Another reason that you may need to undertake research activities includes the need to maintain currency of knowledge within the clinical workplace. Are there better ways of caring for people? Often new products and processes have evolved to provide better outcomes for clients and health-care workers. An example of this is 'No Lift' processes of manual handling that aim to provide a more comfortable and less harmful approach for manual handling for both clients and health-care workers.

How research can support and improve work practice

evidence-based practice
The application of the best available empirical evidence, including recent research findings, to clinical practice in order to aid clinical decision making

Evidence-based practice is one of the main approaches that impact on nursing practice as it is used to support clinical decision making. To support clinical decision making or evidence-based practice, a variety of information is sourced from the following:

- tradition
- authority
- experience
- trial and error
- logic or reason
- nursing research.

The evidence from nursing research is scientifically accountable, that is, it follows the rules of evidence, and includes:

- clinical judgement
- patient preferences
- systematic review
- clinical practice guidelines
- case reports.

At times a variety of different conclusions may be drawn from the research. When this happens clinical judgement is the determining factor in reaching a conclusion. Why are there no clear-cut decisions? When dealing with people there are a large number of variables or factors that need to be considered and evaluated. These differences can lead to many different outcomes or have an impact on the type of intervention that is chosen.

The main focus of nursing is the patient. Sharing views and honest communication as part of the therapeutic relationship and builds trust between the nurse and client. This adds credibility and reliability to evidence-based practice.

For more on this topic, read the article 'What counts as evidence in evidence-based practice' (Fitzgerald, 2007) https://www.asrn.org/journal-nursing/258-what-counts-as-evidence-in-evidence-based-practice.html.

Reflective practice 17.1

Quality improvement and reflective practice

Consider the types of treatment that are undertaken in your work area. Identify one type of treatment or nursing practice that has evolved over time.

1   How did the change in practice occur?
2   What types of activities in quality improvement occurred to assist in the change?

In contrast to evidence-based research, *quality improvement* is a systematic approach to obtain measurable improvements in health care, and is part of the health-care facility's delivery approach and systems of care.

Current trends

Research is used to study, validate or refine knowledge. By continually undertaking research, nursing care aims to base practice on evidence rather than tradition. As stated above, things are constantly changing and the nurse needs to constantly read and review current research to provide best practice for the people they care for.

Nursing research is applicable to all aspects of nursing from education and practice to administration. Some of the current trends in nursing research include:

- wide qualitative research – a form of scientific research that stems from philosophy and human sciences
- health promotion research – a more specific focus on wellness and maintaining health
- evidence – informed decision-making consideration of the best available evidence to provide care.

> **TIP 17.1**
>
> **Research and the student**
>
> As a student it is important that you follow your supervisor's direction, and the organisation's policies and procedures, and work within your scope of practice. Even though you might be keen to commence evidence gathering with people you are providing care for, you need to obtain permission to do this activity.

Activity 17.1

Current research trends

Identify a nursing process or product that you are using on your placement. How long has this process been in place? Locate the origin of the policy and procedure this relates to.

Research objectives

There are many different reasons for undertaking research as shown in **Table 17.1**. Once you know why you wish to undertake research and decide on the type of research that is required it will become easier to set research objectives.

TABLE 17.1 Reasons for undertaking research

Type of research	Reasons
Comparison	At times you may want to compare different products to determine: • cost effectiveness of product • time (in wound care how often the product needs to be reapplied) • effectiveness of product • what other benefits one product has over another, e.g. a wound dressing product that does not adhere to skin or wound bed.
Hypothesis testing	To test whether your hypothesis is true or not. For example, if diuretic medication is given earlier in the day it will prevent falls in elderly patients.
Trend identification	To determine if there is a pattern. Most health-care facilities collate all fall information to determine if there is a common thread such as time of day that clients fall.
Knowledge extension	You may not be familiar with new products or treatments and want to ensure that you have all the information required before putting a new product or intervention in place.
Quality of practice	You want to give the best and most current care to people you are caring for. There have been incidents where poor-quality practice has resulted in poor health outcomes for clients.

A research objective is a statement that defines what is to be studied. This is important as it lets the researcher decide the methodology to apply and the type of data that will be collected. This is usually stated in the form of a hypothesis.

A research study is quite lengthy and the objectives break it into smaller segments. They are normally written in the following SMART format:

- S – specific
- M – measurable
- A – achievable
- R – realistic
- T – timely.

How to decide on a research objective

Initially it may be difficult to define the objective or even the type of research you want to undertake. You may want to study palliative care and when you search the Internet there are thousands of articles. How do you know what research article you need?

A good way to start is to make a concept map. This involves starting with a broad subject such as palliative care. Place this in the middle and then write down all items that relate to it. This step can be completed as many times as you want to allow you to refine the issue you wish to research. You can then set your own research objective.

Activity 17.2

Objectives of the study

Identify an activity that your workplace is undertaking. It may relate to accreditation or continuous improvement. What is the objective of this activity? If it is not expressed using the SMART format, try to reframe it in this way.

Credible sources of data and evidence

Writing

When researching a particular topic it is important to read relevant literature to gain a broad perspective of the issue. With the emergence of the Internet there is an immense amount of literature available. The problem is that not all of it is credible. Some questions that you can ask yourself when selecting literature are:

- Who is the author?
- Where did it come from?
- Is it true or not?
- How long has it been online?
- Is it likely to change soon?

Books and journal articles that are credible undergo a rigorous checking process before a university accepts them as being valid or before they are published. One of the most important checking processes that occurs is a peer review, where experts in the area review and approve the article.

Credible sources of research literature will also provide the details of the cultural and ethical considerations that were applied in the research activity.

Cultural and ethical considerations for research

Ethics in research is essential, and approval must be obtained. The National Health and Medical Research Council (NHMRC) is Australia's peak body that governs medical research.

NHMRC gives detailed information on how culture can affect the considerations of research planning when conducting research with Aboriginal and/or Torres Strait Islander people. It specifies that the research undertaken must:

- respect the shared values of these cultures
- be relevant to people of that culture
- have a long-term ethical relationship between all people involved in the research, and
- incorporate best practice ethical standards as part of the research design (NHMRC, 2016).

When undertaking any research activity, the health, safety and wellbeing of participants must be protected.

The NHMRC standards incorporate the following points:

- honesty and integrity
- respect for human research participants, animals and the environment
- responsible use of resources
- acknowledgement of all involved in the research
- responsible communication of research results
- protection of human rights
- informed consent
- a balance of risks and benefits of the study (NHMRC, 2015).

Explore the theory in *Foundations of Nursing* 2e, Gray et al., Chapter 2: Research

Reading

Activity 17.3

Credibility in nursing research

Select a recent nursing research article. Using the criteria discussed, is this literature a credible source? What mechanisms were in place to ensure its credibility? Read the literature and determine if approval was required to undertake this research activity.

CASE STUDY 17.1

How to plan information-gathering activities

Rosa was on her last clinical placement before the completion of her Diploma of Nursing. Rosa had been allocated to a medical ward, with a special focus on oncology. One of the patients that Rosa was caring for was Mrs Whately, who had been admitted with terminal cancer of the breast. Mrs Whately had undergone a radical mastectomy four years ago and a treatment regime of chemotherapy. Until the last six months Mrs Whately had been in remission. Six months ago she developed a sore on the outside area of the scar on the left side of her chest from her radical mastectomy. After investigation tests revealed that the cancer had returned and was aggressively targeting not only her chest but other internal organs as scans had revealed metastases in lung, bladder, bone and brain. The sore had progressively worsened over the last three months till it became a fungating lesion.

Mrs Whately had been treated palliatively at home by the Royal District Nursing Service, but required admission to manage the lesion. It was painful to dress, and there was copious exudate that was very offensive.

Rosa was very keen to follow the care that the wound management nurse ordered, but the dressing was one that she was not familiar with. Rosa contacted her supervisor who advised that best practice dictated that a nurse should not apply a product or undertake a procedure unless they were fully informed about it. Rosa had two days to research the new wound product till the wound specialist nurse returned to re-dress the wound. Rosa found the wound product in the steri-room and obtained the product information leaflet. Rosa then used the Internet to research articles that were related to the product. Rosa also contacted the wound management nurse for further information.

Rosa found that the product was relatively new and fairly expensive. It had been found through clinical trials to be most effective in lessening the pain from wounds, absorption of exudate and controlling odours from exudating wounds. The cost of the product was covered by the hospital, which would supply patients free of charge who qualified for it.

Rosa was glad that she understood the rationale behind using such a new product and felt pleased that she could provide the required information to Mrs Whately and her family. The wound management nurse on her review was also very pleased to see that the product had addressed the objectives set out for its use.

Mrs Whately was discharged the next week, with palliative care services at home. Mrs Whately was very happy to return to her home and family.

1   What benefits did Rosa obtain through undertaking research on the new wound product?
2   What was the current trend for this type of wound in a palliative care patient?
3   What would the research objectives be for this scenario if it was part of a study?
4   What types of credible data and evidence could Rosa access in this scenario?

17.2 Gathering information

Gathering information sounds easy doesn't it? All you have to do is search the Internet and voila, a huge amount of information appears. If only it was that simple. How often have you surfed the Internet to find that you have spent three hours and achieved nothing? Researching online is not the only way information is obtained. You might want to interview people (see **Figure 17.1**) or give out a questionnaire. What questions are you going to ask? Who are you going to interview?

It is important to have a plan for gathering information.

Selecting and evaluating information

Once the framework for the research activity is in place, the next step is to gather information regarding the topic. If you were researching to assess how reliable the evidence for a particular topic is, you may search for literature outlining studies that have replicated the original study. If you are interested in a particular aspect of care, such as wound products, you might do a search for literature based on the product.

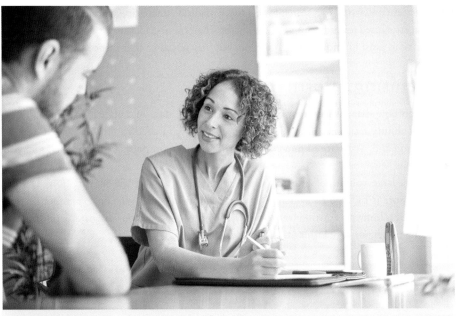

FIGURE 17.1 Gather information through patient interviews

Getty Images/sturti.

When you find a piece of information that you think is relevant, you need to evaluate the information before you include it. As discussed above, in credible sources of literature there are specific criteria to consider before accepting information.

One of the most important questions to ask is 'Does this evidence support or contradict my objective?' This will assist you in deciding how to use the evidence and assist in decision making.

Activity 17.4

Using literature to support an argument

Choose a work practice that you are undertaking on placement. Identify the key words to use for a search. Select two different articles published at around the same time. Read and analyse the information. Do they both support or draw the same conclusions? Summarise these articles together to support a point of view.

A systematic approach

As discussed it is easy to get off track and waste time when searching for evidence. To ensure that you have a systematic approach you need to have good time-management skills and a plan. Document this plan either electronically or in hard copy and continually review it to ensure that you are keeping up to date with tasks that are required.

At times the whole idea of research can seem daunting. Making a plan with successive steps that you can check off can assist you in completing all tasks required by the project in the most efficient way.

Relevance of research

To ensure that you are gathering the most relevant research, always keep the following in mind:
- Why are you researching this area?
- How will it contribute to the activities you undertake as part of your work role?

Literature uncovered in a search for evidence might be interesting and relevant to the topic but more structured towards the role of the doctor. This type of evidence is good as supplementary material or to assist in knowledge acquisition, but may not assist in evidence-based nursing.

Organising information

It is important that all information about the author, date of publication and publisher are meticulously recorded. This will save time later if you need to go back and review the information and, as discussed previously, it is an integral component for referencing in your own review.

With a large volume of information it is important to sort the information. The first way is to sort it by type of evidence. Is it a replication of a study, an experiment, a case report? This is known as sorting by theme. Then within these categories, sort the information according to date or conclusions of the study.

Reflective practice 17.2

Planning your approach

Think about one of your assignments. What type of planning process did you use to identify your sources of information? Was this approach successful? What else would you do next time?

CASE STUDY 17.2

Gathering information

The experience Rosa had with managing the wound care for Mrs Whately really ignited Rosa's interest in providing best practice in wound care for her clients. Rosa not only wanted to have up-to-date information on wound care in palliative areas of nursing but also the different types of wound care that related to different areas of nursing practice. Rosa had been very impressed with the wound management nurse and felt that eventually she would like to work in this area.

One of the assignments that Rosa needed to complete for her studies was a literature review. Rosa had already decided that she would complete a literature review on the current practice of moist wound healing. On looking up the literature online Rosa found many articles on this topic and knew it would be impossible to use them all. Rosa decided to narrow the topic of her literature review and, after talking to her teacher, made a concept map of all types of wounds that use moist wound healing. Rosa eventually decided to focus on moist wound healing for ulcers that were not infected.

Rosa allocated a substantial portion of time just to deciding what type of information she would like to use in her literature review. Rosa decided to review literature that both supported this method of wound management and also articles that proposed another method of wound management. Rosa then decided that she would further narrow the scope of her search to only include the pivotal foundation studies and then only current literature from the last three years. Rosa still found that this yielded a large amount of literature and decided to only include articles that dealt with people over the age of 65.

Rosa was careful to keep all the details of the studies so that she could easily reference the material she wanted to use. Rosa decided that she would download the articles and keep them on her laptop and iPad, as she was more comfortable reading and using material online. Rosa found some areas of interest but also found she had accomplished little. She decided that she needed to be more focused when searching for literature or this task would never end.

1   What methods did Rosa use to evaluate and select ways of gathering information?
2   Describe the systematic approach that Rosa took in the gathering of information.
3   How could Rosa establish the relevance of the information according to her work requirements?

17.3 Analysing information

Once you have collected the information, you need to analyse it by asking the following questions:

- How critical is this information?
- Is the information similar to other information or different?
- How strong is the information?
- How relevant is the information?
- How reliable is the evidence?
- When was the study conducted or evidence obtained?

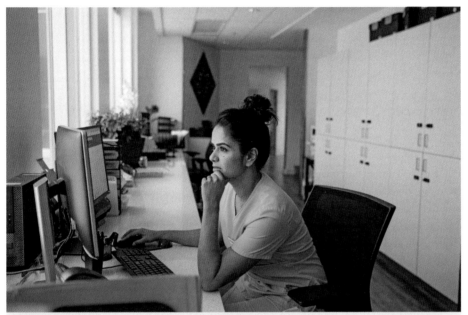

FIGURE 17.2 After your initial information search, analyse and prioritise the information

Getty Images/Hero Images.

Prioritising information

By prioritising the information you are determining its relevance to your own research. You need to identify the argument that you are researching and provide a summary of the different types of information collected and the evidence they provide. At this point you will be able to identify any areas not covered and highlight how your research activity will assist in either meeting this gap or contributing to a better knowledge base in one of the areas identified.

Comparing and contrasting information

When writing a literature review of previous evidence or studies it is important to present the evidence from two sides – examples that support each other and the research activity, and examples that refute it or have a different conclusion. **Table 17.2** shows different ways of using information. By sorting your information into themes and summarising it, you can present the findings in a concise manner.

TABLE 17.2 Ways to use information in research

Method	Explanation of method
Comparing	Analysing two pieces of work and noting the similarities and differences between each.
Contrasting	Using the information to emphasise the differences.
Challenging	Using the information to question if something is true or legal.
Reflecting	Thinking about what has happened to see if anything else can be learnt from a situation.
Distinguishing relevant from irrelevant	Deciding what is important from what is not: • identify the main topic • determine which supporting ideas are relevant to the topic • identify ideas not relevant to the main topic.
Interdisciplinary connections	Combining or involving two or more academic disciplines or fields of study.

Strength, relevance, reliability and currency

The *strength* or *validity* of evidence will decide the truth of the research findings. There are two things to evaluate: what was measured and how reliable was the measurement. Did the instruments or processes used in the research activity actually measure what they were supposed to measure? Or did they measure something else? In nursing, one difficulty experienced in research is the many variables (things that are different) that people have. While these variables may apply to the activity you undertook can you apply them to a larger audience?

Reliability is the ability to replicate the activity and obtain the same result. The instruments, if used, should also be reliable. If a person took the same test twice would they obtain the same score?

Relevance is a critical measure. Research activity as discussed under 'Cultural and ethical considerations for research' should only be undertaken with people if there is a benefit. You could also obtain results that are reliable but not valid and relevant. You might have measured some other variable, rather than the one you set out to measure.

Currency is important because there are so many advances in the medical and health field that the study might be out of date if new products or processes come into being. In this case the study will also not be relevant or reliable. An example of this is how nursing care for people has changed over time in the surgical area. At one time having the removal of a gall bladder was a major procedure involving a large incision, drain tubes and a lengthy stay in hospital. With the advent of keyhole surgery gall bladder removal only requires a minimal incision, no drain tubes and a one-night stay in hospital, if all goes well.

Feasibility, benefits and risks

Before commencing a research activity, you also need to consider the feasibility of the study and the risks and benefits of undertaking the activity (discussed earlier under 'Cultural and ethical considerations for research', p. 243). The *feasibility* is referring to the ability to undertake the activity. How difficult will it be? What resources will be required? Funding may be required to undertake a research activity. The government and other private institutions make grants available if the research is shown to have a beneficial outcome. Pharmaceutical companies often fund research activity as the benefits will provide a financial return to the company as well as a new treatment regime that will assist the person.

Activity 17.5

Feasibility of conducting the research activity

Select an article that you located previously. What resources were involved in undertaking the study?

How much time and effort would it take to replicate or extend this study? Is it still a viable study to undertake? What will the benefits of doing further research in this area achieve? What risks are there in doing the study?

Conclusions

After you have gathered all the information, checked that it is credible and sorted the information, it is time to reach some conclusions. When doing a literature review it is customary to present your argument. You should not just present the literature article by article but rather you should summarise the information into groups of similar findings and present these to support your argument.

The conclusion of research involves presenting evidence to support or negate your hypothesis. This can either be presented by numerical statistics or descriptive statistics. As nursing research involves people, descriptive statistics are useful to describe the findings. A mixture of both may be used to assess if the evidence is significant. It is useful to have a grasp of basic numerical statistics such as the mean, method and mode to understand the conclusions that are drawn. The *mean* is simply the average, the *median* the middle value and the *mode* is the most commonly occurring result.

CASE STUDY 17.3

Analysing information

Rosa felt quite optimistic when she had gathered a number of articles for her literature review. 'This should be quite easy', she thought. Rosa allocated some time on the weekend to start writing her literature review. After a couple of hours, she shut down the computer and decided to go for a walk. What she thought would be the easiest stage of the process was rapidly turning into the task from hell. 'There must be a better way', thought Rosa.

On Sunday, after a good night's sleep, thoughts of the articles had revolved around and around in her head. Rosa was determined to get on top of this task. She decided that she would attack the task in a logical step-by-step manner. Rosa then spent the next few hours summarising each article. Luckily, Sunday was a cold, wet day and Rosa had no desire to venture outside.

She decided to break for lunch and review what she had completed after the break. On return, initially Rosa was quite happy. 'I have written around 3000 words. I knew it just required me to sit and work through it methodically', she thought. But her elation soon disappeared. Rosa found that her literature review was just disjointed accounts of studies undertaken. Rosa texted her friend Josie. 'Oh Josie, I don't seem to be getting any closer to finishing this task', said Rosa.

'Look I'll come over, two heads are better than one', said Josie.

When Josie saw the effort Rosa had put in, she reassured her that it just required a different approach to the task. 'You already have done the hard part', said Josie. 'Rather than just putting one after the other, why don't we group the articles into similar themes?' 'Great', said Rosa.

After an hour of sorting the material, Rosa was left with two distinct types of information: one that supported moist wound healing and one that didn't. Rosa thanked Josie for her help. 'You saved me a lot of grief', said Rosa, who then summarised the information from each group and was able to come up with a comparison and to draw conclusions to support her hypothesis.

1. What mistake did Rosa make in prioritising her information?
2. What could you do to make different types of information support your research objectives?
3. Describe the features of the information that Rosa should analyse?
4. What method would you recommend to Rosa to facilitate analysis of the information?
5. What risks and benefits are there with different types of information?
6. How should Rosa, using the literature, develop her conclusion?

17.4 Using information in practice

All nursing care is based on evidence obtained from research. At times only part of the research may be required. An example of this is a study where it was found that antibiotics given to mothers before caesarean birth prevented an infection occurring in the incision line. Other components of the research, such as the method and the type of infecting organism, may not be required to change the nursing practice.

At times part of a research study may be used to support different aspects of nursing practice. A method used to obtain information from clients may be of value rather than the whole study.

Identifying potential areas for change and further research

Throughout history nursing has used research to change processes. An example of this is the different work practices that have been used, such as task orientation to total patient care. With rapid changes in technology and treatments there is a never-ending source of areas for nursing to explore through research.

Activity 17.6

Potential areas for change

Review current and new processes, materials and technology in your workplace. Has nursing research been conducted on these? Do a literature search on one of the new products, technologies or processes to determine if there is a gap in the nursing knowledge that would benefit from a research activity.

Further research and evaluation may also be used to assess if the changes implemented are achieving the outcomes predicted. This is useful as it can demonstrate other areas that may be contributing to outcomes and identify further areas to explore.

One area is that of clinical placement for nurses. Currently simulation is being used more than ever before. This practice has been found to be extremely useful to prepare students for placement, and at times when the task is difficult simulation can be used to assist the student to experience the situation in a controlled environment.

Activity 17.7

Further research

Using the information from the previous activity try to locate the most current literature on the process, product or technology that was undertaken. Can you replicate this activity for the new area you want to research?

Actions to address outcomes of research

When we obtain an outcome from research, it is not appropriate to immediately adopt the change in practice. If it is extremely important, critical to saving lives or critical to preventing harm, then the change will be implemented as quickly as possible. To effect a change in practice there are a number of issues to consider. Some general ones are:

- What training will be required by staff?
- Is there any required equipment to undertake the task?
- What process will be required?
- What policy changes need to be made?

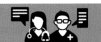

Reflective practice 17.3

Changing landscapes

Consider your placement. Imagine on day four that the objectives were changed and you were just told to meet these in order to be successful.

1 How do you think you would feel if you were put in this situation?
2 Do you think it would be difficult to be successful in the placement? Why/why not?

CASE STUDY 17.4

Using research in practice

Rosa was extremely happy that her literature review and received a competent rating. 'It was the most difficult task, but also the most rewarding one', Rosa told Josie. Rosa was also pleased that her literature review was chosen to be used as part of the teaching process for the next class. 'I also gave them some great tips, I hope they follow them or else they might find themselves in the same situation I did', said Rosa.

Rosa completed her studies and was thrilled to obtain her first employment at an aged care facility close to her home. Rosa soon became confident in her role as an enrolled nurse and team leader. One of the tasks assigned to Rosa was the wound management of the residents. Rosa really enjoyed this task and wanted to assist the residents to the best of her ability.

Mr Jacobs was an elderly resident, who had a long history of type 2 diabetes. Mr Jacobs also suffered from a chronic leg ulcer. Rosa approached the registered nurse in charge of the facility and asked if it would be possible to arrange for a review of the wound management technique for Mr Jacobs. 'You know that the wound will not fully heal', said the nurse. 'I know, but Mr Jacobs appears to have a lot of pain when the dressing is due to be changed', said Rosa. An appointment was made with

the consulting wound management nurse. The doctor for Mr Jacobs felt that this was a positive aspect to his care and sent off a wound swab to check there was no infection present.

The consultant also felt a change in dressing product would assist Mr Jacobs. The consultant provided a few samples of different products from a variety of price ranges. 'Even though some of the dressings are more expensive, they do provide better comfort for the patient, and with moist wound healing it is best to leave the dressing undisturbed as long as there is no infection', said the consultant.

Mr Jacobs was very happy with the change and the registered nurse complimented Rosa on her nursing practice. The registered nurse asked Rosa if she could develop a learning resource on moist wound healing for other staff to access.

1 How did Rosa use the information she obtained from her literature review?
2 What changes to the current treatment benefited the client?
3 What other issues might Rosa decide to use to extend her research activity?
4 Describe some actions that would be required to initiate the change in nursing care for Mr Jacobs.

SUMMARY

- After completing this unit and undertaking the reflective practice and workplace activities you will be able to meet the objectives of planning, gathering information, analysing information and translating the information into practice.
- Planning the research activity is pivotal to success in research. The research plan is like a summary in point form of how to identify a topic, the time frame for each stage of the activity, a description of how the research will be carried out and provide credible sources of information on which to base the activity.
- Gathering information in a controlled and analytical fashion will ensure you have relevant literature to use to support your own activity. This task requires arranging the information in a way that will facilitate your ability to write your literature review in an organised manner.
- Analysing information is critical; do you understand what the literature is saying? This may seem simple but it can be a complex task, as different variables or factors may influence the findings of a study. It may be necessary to use different techniques to fully utilise the information, such as comparing or contrasting information.
- Finally, the main objective is to use the information to change or better understand nursing practice.

SELF-TEST QUESTIONS

1   Why is planning critical to the research activity?
2   What resources are available to gather information that is relevant and contemporary?
3   What strategies can you use to analyse the information that you gather for research activities?
4   How can you use the information that you gather to develop actions in the clinical environment?
5   What other benefits can be gained by gathering information for research activities?

BIBLIOGRAPHY

American Society of Registered Nurses (ASRN) (2008). 'What counts as evidence in evidence-based practice?', *The Journal of Nursing*. Retrieved from www.asrn.org/journal-nursing/258-what-counts-as-evidence-in-evidence-based-practice.html. Accessed 20 June 2017.

Australian Government, National Health and Medical Research Council (NHMRC) (2016). https://www.nhmrc.gov.au/_files_nhmrc/file/publications/national-statement-2018.pdf; https://www.safetyandquality.gov.au/wp-content/uploads/2012/01/measurement-for-Improvement-toolkit-a.pdf. Accessed 27 June 2017.

Australian Government, National Health and Medical Research Council (NHMRC) (2015). *National statement on ethical conduct in human research 2007*. Retrieved from, https://www.nhmrc.gov.au/_files_nhmrc/publications/attachments/e72_national_statement_may_2015_150514_a.pdf. Accessed 27 June 2017.

Clarke, L., Gray, S., White, L., Duncan, G. & Baumle, W. (2016). *Foundations of Nursing: Enrolled Division 2 Nurses* (ANZ Edition). Cengage Learning: South Melbourne.

Fitzgerald, J. (2007). 'Finding the research for evidence-based practice', *Nursing Times*, 103(17). Retrieved from https://www.nursingtimes.net/roles/nurse-managers/finding-the-research-for-evidence-based-practice-part-two-selecting-credible-evidence/201888.article. Accessed 19 March 2017.

Gray, S., Ferris, L., White, L., Duncan, G. & Baumle, W. (2018). *Fundamentals of Nursing* (2nd edition). Cengage Learning: South Melbourne.

Health Resources and Services Administration (2017). https://www.hrsa.gov/public-health/guidelines/quality-improvement.html.

Naylor, W. (2002). 'Malignant wounds: Aetiology and principles of management', *Nursing Standard*, 16(52): 45–53. Retrieved from https://search.proquest.com/openview/9a35ece632f53eb932b6ac237aa68fdf/1?pq-origsite=gscholar&cbl=30130.

Sanjiv, S. (2014). 'Current trends in nursing research', *International Journal of Nursing Research and Practice*, 1(1). Retrieved from http://www.uphtr.com/issue_files/2%20Shobhi%20mam%201(1).pdf.

Titler, M.G. (2008). Chapter 7: 'The Evidence for Evidence-Based Practice Implementation' in R.G. Hughes (ed.) *Patient Safety and Quality: An Evidence-Based Handbook for Nurses*. Agency for Healthcare Research and Quality: Rockville, MD, https://www.ncbi.nlm.nih.gov/books/NBK2659/.

University of California Office of Research (n.d.). *Required elements of informed consent*. Retrieved from http://www.research.uci.edu/compliance/human-research-protections/irb-members/required-elements-of-informed-consent.html.

World Medical Association (2013). *Declaration of Helsinki*. Retrieved from www.wma.net/what-we-do/medical-ethics/declaration-of-helsinki. Accessed 3 July 2017.

Care for a person with diabetes

LEARNING OUTCOMES

After reading this chapter, you should have an understanding of:

18.1 The types of diabetes care services available in the Australian health-care sector

18.2 Assessing the needs of a person with diabetes

18.3 Complex nursing interventions that assist a person to achieve and maintain optimal diabetes health

18.4 Evaluating the care plan for a person with diabetes, and supporting self-management.

Diabetes

After completing the initial semester and having placement in an aged care facility I was keen to learn about the chronic disease of diabetes. A number of people that I provided care for in the aged care environment had this disease as one of their diagnoses. I was shocked that so many people suffered from this condition.

As part of the lectures we learnt about the two types of diabetes. I was surprised to learn that type 1 diabetics developed the disease as part of an immune response. I had heard about lifestyle factors playing a role in the development of type 2 diabetes, but had always thought that this was a condition that was not so serious. I had always thought that this person could safely manage the disease with modification of diet, exercise and lifestyle changes. I was shocked when I learnt about the serious consequences of this disease on the body.

On the next placement I was in the rehabilitation wards and a number of patients I was caring for had type 2 diabetes. They required rehabilitation for cardiac problems, amputations or stroke, all conditions that had a predisposing factor of diabetes.

 This chapter is cross referenced to Gray et al., *Foundations of Nursing* 2e, Chapter 22.

18.1 Diabetes care services

Diabetes is a chronic disease that requires lifelong management. If not managed correctly a person's wellbeing and state of health can be compromised. There are a number of organisations that provide assistance, support and education to people diagnosed with diabetes. Linking the person into services can assist the person with diabetes to have more control and management of their condition.

Information on diabetes care and sources of funding for related services

Table 18.1 provides a listing of some of the support services and organisations that are available for the person with diabetes or health-care workers to access for information about the disease.

Being able to access accurate and current information on the disease, current research and services is important for the enrolled nurse to ensure current knowledge for themselves and also to provide it to others.

Diabetes is a chronic disease that incurs a cost for management and treatment. Accessing relevant services or organisations that can supply funding or equipment is very important to the person or carer of the person with this disease.

TABLE 18.1 Organisations that provide services and information on diabetes management in Australia

	Types of information
The National Diabetes Services Scheme	Provides education, research and products to manage diabetes. It will provide information on: • Self-management • Programs designed for healthy living • Support groups • Fact sheets on diabetes • Subsidised products to people under 21 years of age.
JDRF	Provides support to people with Type 1 diabetes. Targeted for children is an information pack that includes: • A parent's manual • A teddy bear to assist the child with education for injecting Targeted to adults is: • A guide book written by people who have the condition • A sick day kit • Education on diet • Blood glucose testing equipment.
RDNS, now known as Bolton Clarke	• Management of diabetes that is patient centred • Education on the disease and living with the condition • Blood glucose monitoring • Management of medication for diabetes • Support programs.
Primary Care, Diabetes society of Australia (PCDSAS)	• Works with individuals and the community across the lifespan • Education for health professionals • Research in the area of diabetes • Encourages a team approach to the management of diabetes.

Specialist services and complementary roles of organisations

Diabetes is a complex disease process that requires specialist interventions. If one facet of the disease is not monitored and kept in balance, the person with diabetes can become extremely unwell very quickly.

People with diabetes are usually monitored by a team of specialist health-care workers to provide holistic care of the person with this disorder. **Table 18.2** provides a list of some of the health-care workers that are involved with the care of a person with diabetes.

TABLE 18.2 Specialist health-care workers for diabetes management

Specialist role	Service or care provided
Endocrinologists	Diagnose and treat hormone imbalances in the body to try to restore normal hormone balance.
Diabetes educators	A credentialed health professional who educates and supports people affected by diabetes to understand and manage their condition.
Dieticians	Help the person with diabetes create an individual eating plan Assist in losing weight Advise on foods to choose to prevent swings in blood glucose level Help track carbohydrates in food to keep blood glucose levels stable Educate on how to read food labels to assist in healthy food choices Devise strategies to monitor progress – how to keep a food diary.
Podiatrists	Health-care professionals that check the feet of people with diabetes Can detect problems early to prevent ulcers and other complications such as neuropathy and lack of circulation.
Psychologists	Help people change behaviours to improve eating habits, activity levels and positive attitudes Assist people to learn strategies to take on new behaviours for monitoring blood glucose levels and taking medication.

Activity 18.1

Diabetes health-care workers

Select one of the diabetic clients you are caring for and make a list of the different health-care workers involved in assisting the person to manage their condition.

Liaising with referring agencies and community organisations

As an enrolled nurse, one of the interventions that you will be involved in is the referral of people to community organisations and agencies that will provide ongoing care and services to a person with diabetes. It is important for the workplace to have clear processes in place to assist in the referral process.

The type of service you will choose will depend on a variety of factors. These can include:
- financial issues – are the services government-funded or will the person be required to pay out-of-pocket costs?
- private health insurance – what services the person is covered for in their private health insurance
- other types of benefits the person is eligible to access such as Veterans' Affairs
- the type of services required by the person with diabetes
- access to the service
- barriers for the client such as language barriers.

18.2 Assessing the needs of a person with diabetes

Each person is unique and so are their health-care needs. For the person with diabetes the type of services they require will vary greatly, some require more education, while others will need more information on different types of treatment. Though there are type 1 and type 2 diabetics, the way in which the disease affects the person will also vary. One person may experience good control while another will experience unstable control, yet both have the same condition and treatment. These differences require the nurse to assess the person's needs on an individual basis.

Pathophysiology of diabetes

The nurse should have an accurate understanding of the pathophysiology of diabetes in order to predict potential problems and to identify nursing interventions for actual problems the person with diabetes experiences.

Diabetes is a disorder or imbalance of hormone levels in the body required to maintain a stable level of blood glucose. Glucose is the body's preferred source of energy for all metabolic processes (see Figure 18.1).

Insulin is a hormone that acts as a key to allow glucose to enter cells for cell metabolism. Insulin:
- promotes the utilisation of glucose in the cells
- facilitates fatty acid transport and fat deposition into cells
- promotes amino acid transport into cells
- facilitates protein synthesis.

The pancreas is the organ responsible for the production of insulin. The pancreas has two types of cells, beta cells and alpha cells. Insulin is produced by the beta cells of the islets of Langerhans. Alpha cells secret the hormone glucagon. The function of glucagon is to increase the level of glucose in the bloodstream by stimulating the conversion of liver glycogen to glucose (Scott & Fong, 2017). This is achieved by a negative feedback mechanism. The body seeks to maintain a balanced environment and reacts to changes that are detected by receptors and the message is relayed to the brain. Refer to **Figure 18.1** for a pictorial representation of glucose storage and conversion in the liver.

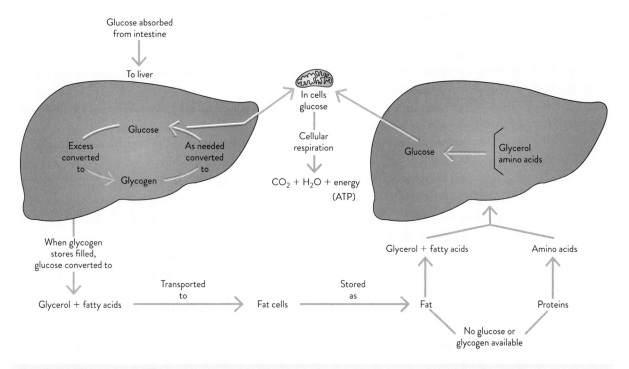

FIGURE 18.1 Glucose storage and conversion in the liver as a source of energy for the body

Source: Rizzo, D. (2015). *Fundamentals of Anatomy and Physiology* (4th edition). Delmar Cengage Learning: USA, Figure 12-7, p. 291.

There are three types of diabetes that a person may present with: type 1 diabetes, type 2 diabetes, and gestational diabetes. **Table 18.3** provides a summary of type 1 and type 2 diabetes.

TABLE 18.3 Type 1 and type 2 diabetes

Type 1 diabetes	Type 2 diabetes
Usually develops between the ages of 11–13 years but can develop as late as 30 years.	Usually develops in middle age, after 40 years.
Auto immune disorder in which the cells of the pancreas are destroyed.	Often related to lifestyle factors such as: • overweight • lack of exercise • poor diet
No insulin is produced by the pancreas.	Insulin is produced but is either insufficient quantiles for the body to maintain glucose levels within normal levels. Not as effective in allowing glucose into the cell.

Gestational diabetes is a condition that affects women during pregnancy. It usually occurs around the middle of pregnancy and disappears after birth. There is a risk of women who have had gestational diabetes developing type 2 diabetes.

Symptoms of diabetes

The symptoms of diabetes are the same for all types but are more severe for the type 1 diabetic. Both types of diabetic patients will show an:

- elevated blood glucose level (BGL). This is call hyperglycaemia. The normal range is 3.5mmol/L to 7.8mmol/L
- polyuria – excess production of urine as additional fluid is required to transport the large glucose molecules
- polydipsia – increased thirst as the body tries to restore the large amount of fluid lost in urine
- polyphagia – increased hunger as the body searches for an alternate food source as the cells cannot access the glucose in the blood.

When providing care for the person with diabetes it is important to understand and recognise some of the symptoms the person may exhibit. **Table 18.4** summarises some of the conditions and symptoms the person may demonstrate when BGLs go outside the normal range. **Table 18.4** also identifies some of the nursing actions that are required to manage this situation.

TABLE 18.4 Diabetic conditions, symptoms and nursing actions

Diabetic conditions	Symptoms	Nursing actions
Hypoglycaemia: BGL is lower than 3.5.	• Paleness • Excessive sweating • Confusion • Anxiety • Changes in behaviour – the person may appear to be drunk • Drowsiness • Hunger • Tachycardia • Nausea • Slurred speech • Tiredness or weakness	• Do a BGL level on the patient • Report to supervisor • Give oral glucose if awake • Repeat BGL 15 minutes later • Follow glucose with a complex carbohydrate such as a sandwich • Document • Report to doctor • Monitor the patient
Hyperglycaemia: BGL is higher than normal level.	• Increased thirst • Decreased concentration • Blurred vision • Polyuria • Fatigue • Weight loss • Headaches	• Report to doctor • Monitor BGL levels frequently • Give medication as ordered • Give regular diet • Additional insulin may be ordered and given as per doctors orders

>>

Diabetic conditions	Symptoms	Nursing actions
Ketoacidosis	• Thirst and dehydration • Polyuria • High BGL level • Presence of ketones in the urine If not treated: • Nausea, vomiting • Abdominal pain • Flushed skin • Dry skin • Fruity odour to breath • Difficulty breathing • Confusion	• Report to doctor • Document • BGL measurement (usually will only give HI reading on monitors) 2.6 Blood glucose measurement • Urine testing 3.8 Urinalysis and urine specimen collection • Vital signs 2.3 Temperature, pulse and respiration (TPR) measurement Medical treatment includes: • Correction of fluid loss with intravenous fluids (IV) • Correction of hyperglycaemia with insulin • Correction of electrolyte imbalance, especially potassium • Correction of acid-base balance • Treatment of infection if present This treatment is delivered in intensive care units (ICU) in Australia.
Hyperglycaemic Hyperosmolar Nonketotic Coma (HONK)	Very high BGL in type 2 diabetics. Symptoms: • Extreme thirst • Frequent need to urinate • Disorientation • Nausea Causes: • Undiagnosed type 2 diabetes • Medication for diabetes not taken • Illness	Medical treatment: • IV fluids and electrolytes • IV insulin Nursing treatment: • Same for person with hyperglycaemia • Requires more monitoring • Will need ICU till insulin infusion ceased

Holistic nursing assessment

As with any other patient you provide care for, the fundamental steps of the nursing process is undertaken to identify patient needs, nursing actions and evaluation. The steps of the nursing process are shown in **Figure 7.4** in Chapter 7.

When undertaking the admission and forming the care plan for a client with diabetes, it is important to not just focus on the disease process but also to assess the person holistically. This will involve assessing and reviewing the person's history, current situation and treatment regimes.

When assessing the diabetic patient it is important to document their usual medication regime and monitoring process. Any changes to the regime can result in their diabetes going out of normal controls. On admission, if the patient has not brought in their monitor and insulin pen, it is important that these are collected by family and next of kin because part of the treatment will be to assess the patient's techniques for self-management and to assess if their BGL monitor is working accurately.

Review the skill in Tollefson *Essential Clinical Skills* 7.4 Admission, discharge and patient transfer

TIP 18.1

Assessment

Always gather all documentation required for the assessment. All health-care facilities have pre-printed forms that cover all aspects of the assessment. This will assist you in performing a comprehensive assessment without trying to remember all aspects.

TIP 18.2

Taking a BGL
It is always important to wipe the patient's finger or part of the body before taking a drop of blood from them. This will remove any glucose from the body surface that may cause an inaccurate reading. Do not use alcohol swabs as they will cause thickening of the skin and may interfere with accurate results.

Determining the person's understanding of their condition, self-management strategies and medications

The diabetic patient needs to be empowered to undertake self-management of their condition. Self-management is a lifelong activity that they can do to prevent complications and enjoy the best quality of life possible. This involves assessing the person's current level of education and the strategies they employ to manage their condition as part of their lifestyle. The nurse needs to provide a supportive environment and establish a therapeutic relationship with the patient to comprehensively assess the person, encourage sharing of information and develop interventions that will address their needs.

For the person with diabetes, the nurse needs specific information on their diet, exercise and lifestyle factors, such as work stress and alcohol intake, to gain a picture of how their diabetes is being managed. The nurse should encourage the patient to demonstrate how they monitor their BGLs and administer their medication to ensure their techniques are accurate.

Activity 18.2

Self-management strategies

Identify and list the types of self-management strategies that a diabetic you are caring for uses to manage the disease. Are these strategies successful for this person?

Review the skill in Tollefson *Essential Clinical Skills* 7.4 Admission, discharge and patient transfer

Possible factors impacting the person's health

As discussed above, at times the person's BGL will deviate from normal. Some reasons for this include:

* excessive exercise
* missing meals
* infection
* poor monitoring of BGLs
* poor medication administration
* lack of exercise
* progression of disease and emergence of complications of diabetes.

Table 18.5 provides some examples of the complications of diabetes.

TABLE 18.5 Complications of diabetes and their symptoms

Complications	Symptoms
Peripheral neuropathy	Damage to the peripheral nerves of the body. This can result in numbness and may lead to ulcer formation if the patient is unable to feel the damage occurring.
	This in turn can lead to infection and possibly amputation.
Nephropathy	Damage to the fine blood vessels in the nephron, the functional unit of the kidney. This can progress to renal failure.
Retinopathy	Damage to the retina that may result in blindness.
Cardiovascular disease	High blood pressure, high cholesterol and high blood glucose can lead to: • Angina – chest pain • Peripheral artery disease – reduced blood flow to limbs • Congestive heart failure – heart weakness that causes fluid build-up and ineffective pumping of blood • Myocardial infarction – heart attack, death of the myocardium.
Periodontitis	Inflammation of the gums that can lead to: • Tooth loss • Cardiovascular disease.

The family or carer's understanding of and involvement in the person's diabetes care

Assessment of the family's or carer's involvement in the management of the disease is also very important. Does the patient self-manage their condition or does another person provide management of the disorder? In some circumstances another person may be responsible for food shopping and meal preparation. In other situations a carer or family member may be responsible for storing and administering medications. These situations need to be identified so education regarding management strategies can be delivered to all parties.

CASE STUDY 18.1

Diabetic assessment

Charlene was admitted to the ICU after collapsing at her local school sports day. Charlene was 15 years old and was diagnosed with type 1 diabetes two years ago. After stabilising her condition, Charlene was moved from the ICU unit to the medical unit of the hospital. Nan, one of the enrolled nurses on the unit, was assigned to care for Charlene.

Nan reviewed Charlene's history and found that initially Charlene had been well controlled with insulin injections, but over the last four months her blood tests had shown poor control of her condition. Nan completed a thorough physical examination of Charlene on her admission to the ward and found that she was currently well controlled after her treatment in the ICU.

After a couple of days, Nan and Charlene had developed a good relationship. Nan found that Charlene had an excellent knowledge of the pathophysiology of her disease, through her own research on the Internet and the education that she had received after her diagnosis. 'How did you become unwell?' asked Nan. Charlene just shrugged and said she didn't know what had happened. Nan decided not to push her on the topic and moved on to another topic, what Charlene wanted to do after leaving school. 'I think that I want to go to university and study to become an architect', said Charlene. 'What does your mother think of this? Won't you need to leave home to study in the city?' said Nan. 'Well, I can't stay home all my life', replied Charlene.

After a while Nan noticed that Charlene was not eating all of her diet. 'Don't you like the food? You can always get your mother to bring in other food if you would prefer that', said Nan. 'No, it's OK, I am just not hungry', replied Charlene. 'You know that it is important to eat properly with your medication and this condition,' said

Nan. Nan noted that Charlene was very slim, bordering on being underweight. Nan decided that she would weigh and measure Charlene to obtain her body mass index (BMI). Nan found that Charlene was on the lower end of weight for her height. Charlene's mother said that Charlene was very fussy about her food and it had worsened over the last four months. Charlene's mother, while not obese, was slightly plump.

Nan was becoming worried about Charlene's dietary habits, despite Charlene having a good diabetes education. Nan wrote down her concerns and voiced them to the registered nurse. The nurse was also concerned as over the last two days after discharge from ICU Charlene's BGL measurements were not as stable as they had been. They informed the doctor and a referral was made to the psychologist and the dietician.

Nan found out from these professionals that Charlene was preoccupied with her weight and had revealed that she tried to remain thin by reducing her insulin levels. The dietician was working with the family as well as Charlene to assist in better food choices for the family and a healthy eating plan for Charlene. The psychologist had referred Charlene to a counsellor in her local area for ongoing counselling around her body image perceptions.

1 What is the pathophysiology underlying the type 1 diabetes condition?
2 What information does a BMI give?
3 List the common blood tests that can give information about control of the disease.
4 Why did Charlene's dietary habits and medication management affect her condition?
5 Explain how educating Charlene's mother will assist Charlene in the management of her condition.

Refer to Tollefson et al. (2018) and Clark et al. (2016).

18.3 Complex nursing interventions to achieve and maintain optimal diabetes health

When trying to assist a person achieve and maintain optimal diabetes health the nurse is required to perform complex interventions. The nurse needs to evaluate the person's needs and ensure the time required to provide the care is available. The nurse also needs to include the family and/or carer in the care process. At times the person may require additional assistance and the nurse will need to evaluate and interpret the person's blood and urine tests and provide nursing interventions to meet the person's needs.

Managing nursing workload and re-prioritising care activities for the person

Part of working as a nurse is the ability to manage and prioritise your workload. When caring for a person with diabetes it is usual to monitor their BGL before meals and administer insulin just before the meal arrives. If the person shows symptoms of hypoglycaemia it is vital that nursing actions are directed towards alleviating this condition as a matter of urgency. This can throw your work plan out the window. If a situation arises that increases your workload it is important to notify your supervising registered nurse to reallocate work tasks, or arrange for additional help with caring for your patient.

At times the person with diabetes may not be feeling well. Sick days can occur and the person needs to rest and recover. This might occur when a scheduled assessment is arranged so this information needs to be relayed to the registered nurse so that the appointments can be rescheduled.

Reflective practice 18.1

Time management

Using a time management planner, identify when time critical nursing actions are required. If a situation arose such as the diabetic patient developing hypoglycaemia, what other tasks are affected? How would you manage this situation?

Review the skill in Tollefson *Essential Clinical Skills* 2.1 Head-to-toe assessment

Complex care needs of a person with diabetes

The person with diabetes requires a care plan that is holistic. The care plan should specifically address those areas that are critical for this condition. A top-to-toe assessment should be carried out, or alternatively a systems approach to assessment can be used to assess the person. The top-to-toe assessment focuses on the information in **Table 18.6.**

TABLE 18.6 Top-to-toe assessment and diabetes

Assessment	Types of information	Problems
General survey	Does the person look well? Is their skin colour flushed or pale?	
Vital signs	Does the person have a temperature? Are pulses easy to palpate? What is their blood pressure?	Infection Circulation Cardiac problems
Height and weight measurement	Is their BMI within normal limits?	May indicate poor control of BGL if underweight May indicate poor dietary habits or alcohol intake
Head and neck assessment	Do they have a headache?	May indicate hypoglycaemic or hyperglycaemic state or neurological condition
Mental and neurological status and affect	Are they alert and orientated?	May indicate hypoglycaemic or hyperglycaemic state or neurological condition
Skin assessment	Are there any broken areas? Pressure areas? Wounds?	May indicate poor circulation or nerve impulses. Opportunity for infection
Thoracic assessment	Is their chest clear?	Infection Cardiac problems
Abdominal assessment	Any pain in the region? Is their urine normal? What is their BGL?	Poor control of diabetes Infection Ketones in urine may indicate insufficient insulin production
Musculoskeletal assessment	What is the strength like in their limbs?	Poor nerve supply Poor circulation

For the well diabetic patient, particular attention should always be paid to the feet, which are easily infected with fungal infections or ulcer formation that the person may be unaware of if neuropathy is in the early stages.

The person's insight and confidence in managing their disease is critical for the nurse to assess. This can point to the need for re-education, ongoing education or new education regarding best practice for the management of diabetes. New treatments and changes in lifestyle patterns can also highlight the need for education. The nurse through the therapeutic relationship may discover a gap or faulty knowledge in the patient's understanding of their disease. This is important to be addressed as part of the care planning process.

As discussed previously, once a thorough assessment is made the nurse then can identify actual or potential problems and implement strategies for care.

Activity 18.3

Understanding the disease

Diabetes is a complex disease process. The pathophysiology is technical. Imagine you are looking after a young person of 13 years. Try to translate your knowledge of the pathophysiology of diabetes into everyday language that this person will be able to comprehend.

Ongoing management of the person's condition

At all times when undertaking nursing interventions the patient needs to have the intervention fully explained and their consent obtained. The nurse needs to be aware of the responses of the patient, family or carers to the interventions put in place.

Radically changing the diet of a person may make the person unhappy and reluctant to eat. The person who usually prepares the meals may feel that they are being criticised. The person with diabetes may develop poor self confidence in their ability to manage their disease if criticism is directed at their method of management. Does this mean we cannot change anything for the person? No; but we need to be mindful of our approach to enable the person to adopt the changes. Using positive feedback for taking on a new habit or technique will help to reinforce the change in behaviour. It is important for the person to accept the need for change in order to effect a long-lasting change, otherwise after discharge old habits may reappear.

Reflective practice 18.2

Changing habits

Think about a time you wanted to adopt a new habit. Perhaps it was to take up exercising or eat healthier.

How difficult was it to achieve? How long did it take to make this new habit automatic where you did not have to consciously think about it, it just happened?

Administering prescribed emergency medication

Self-administration of insulin can be a daily activity for the person with diabetes and in some cases may take place more than once a day. You will need to assist the person to administer medication safely. For routine administration of medication via subcutaneous route, the insulin dose is usually administered via an insulin pen. The needle on these devices are very fine and the person can administer the insulin through their clothing if needed. As there are a lot of injections for the diabetic patient to contend with it is important to rotate the site of injections to prevent use of sites with poor absorption. The abdomen is the preferred site of injection using a calendar rotation to prevent problems with absorption.

In an emergency situation where the person is admitted and being treated for ketoacidosis (see **Table 18.4**), the method of administration is via the intravenous route. Insulin is normally administered in a continual dose via a medication pump. It is important that you understand how to use the pump, problem-solve issues where the pump is not administering the medication and be able to program and retrieve the administration history of the pump. Other medications in this scenario will be ordered on a needs basis by the intensivist who will be providing medical care to the person. The nurse needs to clarify orders that are given, administer as necessary doses or once-only doses in accordance with legislative and facility guidelines.

In the case of hypoglycaemia where the patient is unconscious, the nurse needs to administer medication, glucagon, via the subcutaneous site, intramuscular site or (if in a health-care facility) via the intravenous route. Refer to **Figure 18.2** for a guide on the equipment needed to administer subcutaneous injections.

Review the skill in Tollefson *Essential Clinical Skills* 5.3 Medication administration – injections & Part 6 Intravenous care

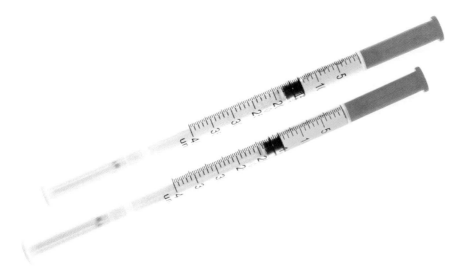

FIGURE 18.2 Equipment required to administer medication by subcutaneous injection

Alamy Stock Photo/LightField Studios Inc.

Activity 18.4

Diabetic medication

Check the resuscitation trolley in the workplace. Can you find glucagon? How is it presented – already to inject or needing to be made up with sterile water?

How long does it last in powder form and if in a pre-made preparation how do you prepare to administer it?

Research insulin. Where should it be stored? How is it presented? How long does it last for?

Evaluating and interpreting blood and urine test results related to diabetic conditions

Review the skill in Tollefson *Essential Clinical Skills* 3.8 Urinalysis and urine specimen collection

Monitoring the diabetic patient is one of the important nursing actions that is required. The patient will have doctor's orders for taking BGL measures. Depending on the condition of the patient, this could range from every 15 minutes (if having an episode of hypoglycaemia) to once daily. The doctor will leave a written plan with orders to notify if the BGL varies outside documented levels and an action plan to implement dependant on the BGL level of the patient.

With unstable diabetics it is important to also monitor their urine. If left untreated, a high BGL with ketones in the urine will indicate a serious medical condition of ketoacidosis occurring. Monitoring the urine in line with the BGL for the patient admitted with ketoacidosis will also assist in evaluating the patient's progress. As the BGL returns to normal, the level of ketones in the urine will also decrease.

Any time the BGL level is outside of normal limits or urine is showing ketones, the findings must be reported immediately to the registered nurse and doctor. The nurse caring for the patient will usually record their findings on special diabetic charts.

Activity 18.5

Urinalysis

Take a sample of urine from a diabetic patient to test. Usually the reagent strips are Multistix® that also predicate a number of other constituents that are not normally found in urine. What was the result of the urinalysis for the diabetic patient? Did any other abnormality show up? What do these results mean for the patient?

Alterations in the person's condition

When working as part of a team caring for people it is important to both document and verbally report on the person's condition to the registered nurse. This will enable the registered nurse to either report immediately to the doctor or alter the plan of nursing care to treat an actual problem or prevent a potential problem.

When a person is not medically stable, they are usually in a very anxious state. They will have fears about experiencing a hypoglycaemic event or be concerned about being out of control. Caring for this person requires not only physical nursing interventions but also psychological care.

CASE STUDY 18.2

Complex management

John, an elderly man of 68 years, had been admitted with an elevated BGL level. John was diagnosed as a type 2 diabetic over 10 years ago and had managed the condition well. Adrian was his nurse for the first three days of John's admission. On doing the nursing admission Adrian found that John had a number of significant problems that were impacting on his disease.

John lived in an upstairs apartment by himself as his wife had died 18 months ago. John had no children and no other family. His wife had a niece but she visited rarely as she lived quite a distance away. John lived independently but recently found it difficult to get downstairs and do the shopping for the week. He told Adrian that his neighbour often gave him meals, but as the neighbour was Indian, John found them to be too spicy for his taste. His physical assessment also showed a number of problems. John's vital signs were within normal limits but when Adrian assessed his skin he found that John had an ulcer the size of a 10-cent piece on his left lower leg. Adrian asked how long he had this and John replied that he only really noticed it a month ago. He told Adrian that initially it was only a speck but had got worse over the last two weeks. Adrian asked if John had sought treatment for this but John said that it did not bother him. John told Adrian that he thought he had burnt his leg slightly against the radiator. Adrian said

'that must have hurt'. 'No, not really, I did not even feel it', said John.

The next morning Adrian went to do the BGL for John. He found that John was pale, confused, trying to get out of bed and sweating. John's BGL was 2.8mmol/L. Adrian immediately reported the situation to the registered nurse in charge and gave John some oral glucose. Adrian stayed with John and repeated the BGL after 15 minutes. He was glad to see that it had responded and John was now more orientated. John's breakfast came and Adrian assisted John to get comfortable and was glad to see John eating. The doctor came and reviewed John and as John had recovered and was eating the doctor ordered John to have his normal insulin dose and medications. The registered nurse had instructed Adrian to monitor John closely over the morning and arranged for additional nursing support so Adrian was freed up to do this.

1. Describe the impact of the assessment for John, outlining what the findings may indicate for his condition.
2. Why should John have his normal medications?
3. What type of problem did John experience in the morning? With the problems that Adrian noted, why might this have occurred?
4. Was the treatment Adrian initiated correct for this condition?

18.4 Evaluating the care plan for a person with diabetes, and supporting self-management

The care plan for a person with diabetes can change constantly. The person's condition and uptake of knowledge is continually changing and the care plan needs to evolve to meet the person's changing needs.

Reviewing and modifying the care plan

The goal of the nursing care plan will be documented at the start of the nursing process. At times the care plan will contain smaller goals, indicating the person's progression to achievement and depending on how the person progresses the interventions may be modified to assist in achieving the goal. An example of this is where the person is receiving education regarding their condition. Initially it may be thought that the person required a specific type of education, such as the need to have a supply of glucose on hand if undertaking exercise. It may later become clear that the person needs education in meals and healthy food intake to plan for exercise, so the education plan may change.

No two people react the same way to illness. Some people will be angry that this has occurred to them while some are fearful. Emotions can play a large role in a person's ability to achieve goals. It is important to recognise these emotions and acknowledge a person's feelings.

At times you may feel that you are not assisting the person and this can cause you frustration, anger or sadness. It is important that you are able to debrief with another team member in an environment where you feel safe and supported.

Considering outcomes against evidence-based best practice

Evaluation is a critical component of the nursing care planning process. It is important to identify if an intervention is assisting the person achieve the outcomes or if it is ineffective or causing other problems.

The diabetic patient requires a lot of education and support. It is important to evaluate if they are receiving the right amount of education or if they are being overloaded with information and not able to process the required learning. Providing support is critical for the diabetic patient to take ownership of their condition and it is vital to provide enough support to enable this to occur but not too much support that results in the patient becoming dependent upon the support person.

As nurses we make clinical judgements about our actions based on evidence-based best practice. An example of this is to encourage the person to undertake self-checks of their BGL and adjust their insulin dose within the levels prescribed by the doctor, rather than the nurse administering the insulin. It is important to be aware of and respond to the person if they are having difficulty with this procedure, but rather than take over you need to encourage, supervise and guide the person to self-management.

Review the skill in Tollefson *Essential Clinical Skills* 2.4 Health teaching

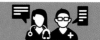
How do you teach?

When caring for people you become a role model and influence the learning behaviour of the person with each intervention that is undertaken. When you are learning a new skill, you watch your teacher, buddy or supervisor undertake this skill. You are participating in a learning activity.

Thinking about recent interventions you took, what learning did the person take away from the interventions you had with them?

The person's understanding of their diabetes condition, medications, therapeutic regimes and self-management

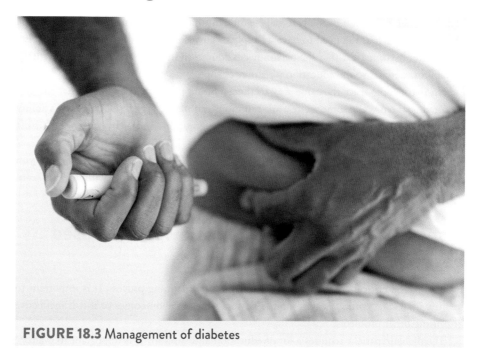

FIGURE 18.3 Management of diabetes

Source: Getty Images/IAN HOOTON.

How can the nurse evaluate the person's understanding of their condition and management practices (as shown in **Figure 18.3**). Monitoring the BGL measures, checking food diaries and asking questions are all useful. Listening to the person is also helpful because often they will talk about a behaviour or activity they believe is helpful.

The doctor also will monitor the person by taking fasting BGLs and a **HbA1c** blood test to assess the person's condition.

Assessing the person, as discussed, is also important as early signs of complications occurring may indicate poor control over their disease.

HbA1c
A blood test that gives an indication of how well a person's diabetes is being controlled by current lifestyle and treatment

Activity 18.6

Assessment

Review the patient's file. How do their blood test results now compare with those on their admission? Check out their vital signs and BGL measurements. Have they changed since admission?

Promoting the person's self-management of their condition

Diabetes is a complex condition that requires education and confidence to manage effectively. Education is not only necessary for the person who has the disease but also for the family or carer. The person needs to have confidence in their ability to manage their condition and ongoing support is required. When a person is first diagnosed with diabetes, education is targeted at giving the person knowledge and skills to control the condition. As the person ages, education is geared to assist them to manage the condition in line with the changes in their physical development and also lifestyle changes.

Review the skill in Tollefson *Essential Clinical Skills* 2.4 Health teaching

The family or carer needs education on the disease so that they can support the person achieve control and manage if the person requires assistance, such as if a person becomes unwell or has a hypoglycaemic event.

Education also is tailored for each individual and carer. The parent of a young teenager recently diagnosed with the condition may be given education about how to administer insulin while a young woman and her partner, who are expecting a child, will require quite different education.

Reflective practice 18.4

Education and diabetes

Compare the files and education given to two people diagnosed with diabetes.

1   What differences are there for each of these clients?
2   Why is the education different?

Specific health promotion initiatives to support self-management

Often patients, like ourselves, learn best from their peers. Providing the person with a support group can be beneficial as they can talk to others with the same conditions and know the other person can relate fully to their story.

Diabetes is a chronic disease that requires lifelong management. At times this can place a financial burden on families or individuals. It is important to link them to services that can supply aids or services that will assist them to manage their condition.

This is an important function of caring for the person with diabetes and needs to be fully documented in their file. This will also prevent other team members undertaking the same task.

CASE STUDY 18.3

The person with diabetes

Alison had completed the clinical component of her studies and was on her final placement in an acute medical/surgical unit. One of the people Alison was caring for was an elderly woman of 73 years, who had recently had a fall. One of the diagnosis that Mrs Breem had was type 2 diabetes. After the fall, Mrs Breem had a soft-tissue injury that prevented her from ambulating and her diabetes was out of control. Mrs Breem had currently been managing with oral hypoglycaemic medication and diet. The doctor now felt that Mrs Breem needed to commence a daily dose of insulin that needed to be administered subcutaneously.

Alison noted that over the first two days, Mrs Breem was able to ambulate short distances with assistance and by using a pick-up frame to the toilet. Alison noted that Mrs Breem also found that the level of pain experienced lessened over the two days. At the case conference, Alison reported the progress that Mrs Breem had made. The doctor also noted that Mrs Breem's BGL levels were more controlled. The team decided the Mrs Breem could go to rehabilitation and the diabetes education could take place in the rehabilitation facility.

One of the tasks that Alison completed each day was updating the care plan for her shift. Alison was pleased to note that over the two days that she provided care for Mrs Breem her mobility level had increased. Alison noted that Mrs Breem had initially been resting in bed but now could ambulate independently with her pick-up frame. Alison also changed the intervention from complete BGL QID to supervise Mrs Breem for her BGL measures.

Mrs Breem and her daughter asked Alison if Mrs Breem could still access the physiotherapy sessions when she had been discharged. Mrs Breem told Alison that she could feel the difference the exercise had made and that she was nervous about managing her diabetes and exercising independently. Alison told them that she would enquire and let them know. The diabetes educator told Alison that Mrs Breem would benefit from doing a structured gym program for older people with diabetes. The diabetes educator gave Alison some information on the latest research for exercise and diabetes control.

The diabetes educator invited Alison to sit in on the next education session where she would be evaluating

Mrs Breem's understanding of her condition and management techniques. At the session, Alison noted that while Mrs Breem was managing the injection she seemed uncertain about her medication regime. Mrs Breem told Alison and the diabetes educator that she had had the previous medications for years and with the changes could not remember when she should take what. The diabetes educator provided Mrs Breem with a written daily plan and suggested that the pharmacist provide the medications in a dose administration aid to assist her to remember when she needed to take them. The diabetes educator also told Mrs Breem and Alison that after discharge from rehabilitation the RDNS would visit to check that all was going well. Mrs Breem was happy with this plan.

Over the next two days Alison supervised Mrs Breem with using the dose administration aid. Mrs Breem progressed well and by the time of discharge needed little prompting, except late in the afternoon when she appeared to get tired. Mrs Breem's daughter was also involved in the medication sessions and told Alison that after discharge she would pop round to check on her mother before tea.

Alison provided Mrs Breem's daughter with some literature and brochures on diabetes. One of the brochures was for a support group for family members who cared for an older person with a chronic disease. Mrs Breem's daughter told Alison that she would give them a call and see if it was something that would assist her in caring for her mother.

After Mrs Breem's discharge her daughter called in and told Alison that she had contacted the support group. She thanked Alison for her care for her mother and her support for herself.

1. Why does the care plan need to be reviewed?
2. Give an example of best practice nursing intervention for a diabetic person.
3. Explain how community supports can assist both the person with the disease and their family/carer.
4. Why is it important to evaluate the person's understanding of their condition and management regime?
5. How does giving accurate information to the family or carer assist the person with their self-management?

SUMMARY

- There are many specialist services that are available to assist a person with diabetes that provide support and funding in the Australian health-care environment.
- It is essential when assessing the needs of a person with diabetes to assess their understanding of the condition, their current situation and their treatment regimes.
- At times the person with diabetes will present with emergency conditions that require immediate response and treatment. This will require the nurse to re-prioritise the care of the client.
- When evaluating the nursing process it is critical to evaluate the person's understanding of their diabetic condition, medications, therapeutic regimes and self-management.

SELF-TEST QUESTIONS

1   What diabetic care services in the Australian health-care environment are available to provide specialist support and funding for the person with diabetes?
2   How can the nurse ensure that the needs of the diabetic patient are being met?
3   What role does the family or carer play in assisting the person with diabetes manage their condition?
4   What are some of the tests that a person with diabetes will require?
5   How can the nurse assist the person to self-manage their condition?

BIBLIOGRAPHY

Australian Government Department of Health (2015). *Australian National Diabetes Strategy 2016–2020,* www.health.gov.au/internet/main/publishing.nsf/content/3AF935DA210DA043CA257EFB000D0C03/$File/Australian%20National%20Diabetes%20Strategy%202016-2020.pdf. Accessed 27 July 2017.

Clarke, L., Gray, S., White, L., Duncan, G. & Baumle, W. (2016). *Foundations of Nursing: Enrolled Division 2 Nurses* (ANZ Edition). Cengage Learning: South Melbourne.

Diabetes.co.uk (n.d.). *Hyperglycaemic Hyperosmolar Nonketotic Coma (HONK).* Retrieved from https://www.diabetes.co.uk/diabetes-complications/hyperglycaemic-hyperosmolar-nonketotic-coma.html. Accessed 27 July 2017.

Gray, S., Ferris, L., White, L., Duncan, G. & Baumle, W. (2018). *Fundamentals of Nursing* (2nd edition). Cengage Learning: South Melbourne.

JDRF (n.d.). *JDRF Resources Program.* Retrieved from https://www.jdrf.org.au/type-1-diabetes/community-resources-program. Accessed 24 July 2017.

National Diabetes Service Scheme (2015). *Support services.* Retrieved from https://www.ndss.com.au/support-services. Accessed 24 July 2017.

Primary Care Diabetes Society of Australia (PCDSA) (n.d.). *Who the PCDSA are.* Retrieved from https://pcdsa.com.au/. Accessed 24 July 2017.

Rizzo, D. (2015). *Fundamentals of Anatomy and Physiology* (4th edition). Delmar Cengage Learning: Boston, MA.

Royal District Nursing Service (2017), https://www.rdns.com.au. Accessed 24 July 2017.

Scott. A. & Fong. E. (2017). *Body Structures and Functions* (13th edition). Cengage Learning: South Melbourne.

Tollefson, J., Watson, G., Jelly, E. & Tambree, K. (2018). *Essential Clinical Skills: Enrolled Nurses,* 4th edition. Cengage: Melbourne.

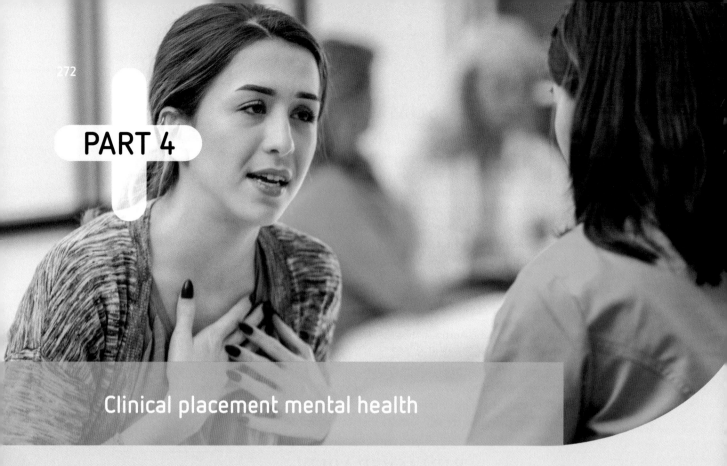

PART 4

Clinical placement mental health

Chapter 19: Care for a person with mental health conditions

The mental health experience

Mental health was an area that I really had no clue about. I mean, I had seen the effects of some mental health conditions, such as depression, in patients I had worked with in other placements, but just a mental health ward? Never. I was expecting patients to have varying levels of interaction, some might want to talk, others might have behaviours related to their illness that prevented them from communicating well or effectively. I was wrong on so many levels. Mental health nursing was an absolute eye opener. I was shocked at how many people are affected by it, and just how damaging it can be. Schizophrenia, for example, is life altering. I will never forget this one patient, who was only 23; he had never had any mental health or health issues at all. One day he was found wandering naked, muttering to people that were not there and convinced that there were people after him. It was utterly astonishing to see how debilitating the disease process could be. Other patients had chronic conditions where hospitalisation was required infrequently, or they required ECT (electroconvulsive therapy), which was also an eye opener for me. I honestly can say that when my placement was finished, I was upset that it was. I am in my final semester now and I am seriously considering working in mental health. Broken bones are visual, and can be fixed quickly; mental health conditions take so many different adjuncts and healing and recovery can be very slow. I would really suggest you go in with your eyes open and with a positive attitude, you really will get a great deal out of it.

For most of you this will be your second or third clinical placement. Mental health is a specialised area where you will be able to put into practice many of the skills that you have learnt at school to date, and rely heavily on communication and interpersonal skills to assist you with your patients.

What is mental health? Mental health encompasses many different forms of care from community-based care to in-hospital or acute care. Mental health care relies on communication between varying providers as many patients will have long-term mental illness that requires care in hospital and management in the community setting. Mental health nursing is provided in a variety of settings including hospitals, rehabilitation centres, medical centres, community-based mental health and community outreach programs.

What kind of patients are in mental health facilities?

Mental health affects one in five Australians aged 16–85. The most common forms of mental illness are depression, anxiety and substance abuse disorders. The onset of mental illness is generally around age 18, and alarmingly, 54% of people with a mental illness do not access any treatment (Black Dog Institute, 2017).

In this placement you will be based in a mental health-care facility – this can be an acute care facility such as a hospital, or a primary health-care facility such as community health facility. The patients you will come across will have a variety of mental health conditions and often patients can have dual diagnoses, meaning they have depression and substance abuse disorders, or have bipolar disorder and anxiety. No two mental health patients will be affected by mental illness the same way. This is the very nature of mental illness – while the symptoms can often be grouped together (for example, hallucinations, delusions and paranoia in schizophrenia) they are never the same for each individual.

Common experiences of student nurses in mental health

It can be confronting for students to see the many different presentations of mental illness. Often it can be difficult to see a person so debilitated by a condition that is not visible – mental illness is not comparable to any physical condition. Some patients will be unable to talk or communicate, others will be volatile, while others will be distressed and teary. Suicide is something that is discussed and questioned frequently and patients are assessed in terms of risk. There are many types of medications to administer and review, and the effects of these medications can have an impact on the patient's day-to-day functioning because they can make patients drowsy and dull their mental focus. Substance abuse and misuse of prescription medications is also something that you will most likely observe.

In acute care, mental health wards generally have common areas for patients to socialise and to convalesce. The big difference you will notice in mental health wards is the lack of clinical nursing equipment, and often observations are not recorded at all on patients while they are an inpatient. Patients are also offered day pass/leave, or will require leave to leave the hospital grounds for a cigarette.

There is a great deal of legislation relevant to mental health so ensure you ask about this while you are on placement and understand the ramifications of the relevant mental health Acts. The focus of this placement is to apply and consolidate the foundations skills of nursing care, including interpersonal skills, assessment skills and effective communication.

Objectives

The objectives for this placement need to be contextualised to the mental health-care setting. Here are some examples:

- application of nursing theory to a mental health context
- consumer and carer perspectives on mental health care

- impact of stigma, discrimination, culture and belief systems on a person with a mental health condition
- common mental health conditions and their treatment and management
- appropriate response to a person in distress or crisis
- principles of recovery in the mental health context
- principles of recovery-orientated practice
- mental health legislation.

Work allocation

How work will be undertaken in mental health varies according to each facility. Some facilities use a team approach where a group works together for their allocated patients. Other facilities may allocate you a designated patient load to care for under supervision or with a buddy. Medications may be administered by the student if the unit HLTENN007 has been completed and the student is supervised. For more complex management there will be a registered nurse who will undertake specialised activities. All enrolled nurses and support staff work under the supervision of a registered Division 1 nurse.

Enjoy your placement and ensure you make good use of the valuable time you have with this speciality in nursing practice.

Care for a person with mental health conditions

LEARNING OUTCOMES

After reading this chapter, you should have an understanding of:

19.1 State/territory mental health legislation requirements

19.2 Responding appropriately to signs of mental illness

19.3 Contributing to care planning and conducting initial clinical observations for a person with a mental health condition.

19.4 Contributing to the recovery of a person with a mental health condition

Placement within the mental health environment

I was next due to undertake my placement within a mental health facility. I was feeling very nervous of what types of clients I would be caring for and the treatments that they would require. In class we had learnt about different mental health illnesses, medications and treatments, but I was still apprehensive. I had seen a couple of movies regarding mental health and I was hoping that these would not be based on reality. I was scared about being in the same room with a person with a mental health illness. The sessions on how to look after yourself and avoid conflict in this environment were helpful but still did not fully allay my apprehension. It was not until I realised that everybody at some time in their life suffered from mental health issues, maybe not as serious as those that cause admission to facilities, that I was able to think about this area of nursing in a more realistic manner. I started to understand that I had been holding onto some negative stereotypes about mental illness that were based on fear and not on reality.

This chapter is cross referenced to Gray et al., *Foundations of Nursing 2e*, Chapter 24.

19.1 State/territory mental health legislation requirements

mental illness
When a client is unable to function effectively in society due to emotional stresses that impact on their behaviour and response to others

mental health problem
Where the person is unable to function to full capacity in society with others due to emotional stresses but is not totally isolated from reality

As a nurse you may be required to care for people with either a **mental illness** or a **mental health problem**. Mental health nursing is a specialised field that is based on a recovery model of care. The mental health nurse will be the liaison person between other health providers and include the support of the family or carer as part of their role. There is a major emphasis on the holistic approach to caring for the person with a mental health illness and the nurse is pivotal to providing information, education and support (ACMHN, n.d.).

In Australia there are efforts to ensure that each state and territory is embedding all of the United Nations' (UN) Principles for the Protection of Persons with Mental Illness and for the Improvement of Mental Health Care. Refer to **Table 19.1** for a list of some of the UN principles and an explanation.

TABLE 19.1 UN principles relating to mental health

Principle	Explanation
Promotion of mental health and prevention of mental disorders	Everybody should have access to the best possible measures to promote mental health wellbeing. This will include access to mental health promotion efforts and mental disorders prevention efforts. Suggested means to achieve this include promoting behaviours that enhance mental wellbeing and identifying and taking action to eliminate the causes of mental disorders.
Access to basic mental health care	All persons should have access to basic mental health care regardless of cost and location and it should be voluntary. The care provided should preserve the dignity of the patient, promote independence in the management of the mental health illness, provide care that minimises the impact of the mental health disorder and improves the quality of life and maintains mental health care outside of mental health facilities.
Mental health assessments in accordance with internationally accepted principles	Mental health assessments will include a full assessment and have a diagnosis, choice of treatment, determination of competence, determination if the person is at risk of harming themselves or others and only be undertaken when directly related to a mental health disorder.
Provision of the least restrictive type of mental health care	Health care should be the least restrictive. This is based on the disorder involved, treatment, level of autonomy, acceptance and cooperation and whether there is a risk of harm to self or others. Community-based treatment should be considered if appropriate. Treatments involving the use of physical and chemical restraints should only be used if attempts to discuss alternatives with the patient fail, they are approved by an approved health care provider and there is an immediate threat of harm to self or others. If restraints are used the client needs: • regular observation • reassessment of the need for restraint every 30 minutes • limited duration – four hours for physical restraint • be fully documented in the client's file.
Self-determination	Consent is required before any type of interference with a person can occur. Interference includes any form of therapy or restriction of liberty.
Right to be assisted in the exercise of self-determination	If a person is unable to understand fully their decisions they will be able to benefit from assistance of a knowledgeable person of their choice. This may occur for a general knowledge deficit, language difficulties and disabilities from other disorders.
Availability of review procedure	There should be a review process in place when decisions are made by an official or a representative of the person.

>>

Principle	Explanation
Automatic periodical review mechanism	If a decision is made that involves a long-lasting impact, an automatic periodical review should be undertaken.
Qualified decision maker	Decision makers, such as family or carer, an official or representative, should be qualified to do so. This means the person needs to be competent, knowledgeable, independent and impartial. It is best if it is a decision made by an official and that more than one person, drawn from different disciplines, makes or contributes to the decision.
Respect the rule of the law	Decisions should be made according to the law of the country at the current time.

Source: Adapted from World Health Organisation (1996). *Mental Health Care Law: Ten Basic Principles.*
Retrieved from http://www.who.int/mental_health/media/en/75.pdf. Accessed 4 March 2017.

Key features of mental health legislation

As a nurse working within the mental health area it is important for you to identify and correctly interpret the key features of mental health legislation to operate in both a legal and ethical manner that is consistent with the policies and procedure of the organisation as well as the state or territory in which you are undertaking your nursing practice.

From the principles outlined in **Table 19.1**, nurses need to respect the client and demonstrate this through maintaining the dignity of the person, allowing the person freedom of choice, obtaining consent before undertaking procedures and acting as advocates for clients.

The other important area that nursing needs to address is that of providing support and care in a holistic manner for each client. In the mental health facility this may involve the use of restraint if required and ensuring the safety of the person while being restrained.

Activity 19.1

Mental health legislation and restraint

Locate the policy and procedure manual in the clinical health facility and find the policies relating to admission and restraint.

Do they comply with the UN principles listed above?

For specific information relating to the state or territory in which you are undertaking nursing, access the following mental health Acts:

- *Victoria Mental Health Act 2014*
- *Mental Health Act 2007 NSW*
- *Mental Health Act 2009 South Australia*
- *Mental Health Act 2000 Queensland*
- *Mental Health Act 2014 Western Australia*
- *Mental Health Act 2015 ACT*
- *Mental Health and Related Services Act 2002.*

The values and philosophies that apply to mental health care

As discussed in the previous section, Australia is working to ensure that the UN principles are applied to people with mental health issues. As a nurse you can play a vital part in ensuring that the nursing care upholds these values, one of which is the principle of the least restrictive care.

For nurses following a recovery model of care, this means that nursing care is aimed at engaging the individual in an active life, personal autonomy, social identity, hope, understanding of abilities and disabilities and a positive sense of self. These principles of recovery for individuals with a mental health illness are outlined in **Table 19.2**.

TABLE 19.2 Principles of recovery orientated mental health practice

Principles	Explanation
Uniqueness of the individual	• Having opportunities for choices and living a meaningful, satisfying and purposeful life, and being a valued member of the community. • Recovery is unique for each person and is holistic in nature. • Person-centred care.
Real choices	• Assists the person to make their own choices for their life. • Builds on their strengths and to take responsibility for their life. • Balances duty of care and support with allowing the person to take risks.
Attitudes and rights	• Communication is two-way and person-centred. • Promotes and protects the individual's rights. • Assists to maintain activities that are meaningful to the individual. • Fosters hope for the individual's future.
Dignity and respect	• Is courteous, respectful and honest. • Sensitivity and respect for the person and their values, beliefs and culture. • Challenges discrimination and stigma.
Partnership and communication	• Works in partnership with the person and support them. • Values the sharing of communication. • Works in positive and realistic ways with people and carers to help them achieve their goals.
Evaluating recovery	• Continuous evaluation of recovery-based practice at several levels. • The individual and their carers can monitor their progress. • All care and interventions given are evaluated as part of a continuous quality improvement system. • Mental health system takes part in government reporting activities to measure key indicator achievement for individuals.

Source: Adapted from Australian Government Department of Health (2010). *National Standards for Mental Health Services 2010: Principles of recovery oriented mental health practice.* Retrieved from https://www.health.gov.au/internet/main/publishing.nsf/Content/CFA833CB8C1AA178CA257BF0001E7520/$File/servpri.pdf. Accessed 3 March 2017.

Review the skill in Tollefson *Essential Clinical Skills* 9.2 Establishing a 'therapeutic relationship' in the mental health setting

FS

Verbal skills, listening skills

The rights of the person

The nurse can support the rights of the individual by acting as an advocate if required and maintaining a person's dignity and respect, as discussed in Chapter 4.

In some cases it is difficult to complete the nursing care for activities of daily living (ADLs) due to the individual's mental health issues. Common problems that can arise concern hygiene and feeding. If the individual refuses to eat or shower you should contact your supervisor but also ensure that no other factors are causing this situation such as the individual not wanting to eat certain foods due to their cultural identity.

Activity 19.2

Food preferences as a result of cultural identity

For each person that you are caring for identify any cultural barriers to ADLs.

1 Is there any food that the person does not include in their diet due to cultural reasons?
2 Is there a specific pattern of behaviour that a person from that culture should display?

Legal issues in nursing

The recovery-orientated model of nursing care is what mental health nursing aims to follow, but what happens if the person is likely to harm themselves or someone else? Nurses have a duty of care for their client and others. It may be necessary for the individual to be restrained till this danger has passed. Sometimes it can be alleviated with medication or in extreme cases through physical restraint, which includes isolation of the person or restricting the movements of the individual.

The nurse's responsibility is to fully document and report the behaviour that the person is displaying. If restraint is required you should ensure that a rigorous checking system is maintained and documented. Ongoing observation of the person will ensure that when the episode of likely harm has abated the restraint can then be removed after gaining approval of the medical officer. It is important that good communication between the person, carer, doctor and nurse is maintained in this instance. All facilities will have policies and procedures that address these specialised areas of intervention.

Documentation and privacy are also legal areas that you must ensure you adhere to. All case files should be kept securely, and conversations about individuals outside the facility or not in the course of work should be avoided.

As discussed previously, consent should be obtained for all interventions including those of daily activities. It is important that you fully document and report any refusal of care to ensure that the individual does not suffer from neglect.

When caring for individuals that are experiencing a mental health illness it is important that you respect their privacy and dignity. This also means that you treat the person as a unique individual free of any **stigma** or **discrimination**. By using a person-centred model of care it is hoped to avoid these negative attitudes.

stigma
A mark of disgrace associated with a particular quality in which a person is exposed to discriminatory practices by other people based on fear and ignorance

discrimination
Unjust or prejudicial treatment of different categories of people, especially on the grounds of race, age or gender, where the physical, psychosocial, cultural and spiritual environment threatens individual/group safety and security (De Laune, 2016)

Review the skill in Tollefson *Essential Clinical Skills* 9.4 Assist with the management of a patient in seclusion

---

Reflective practice 19.1

Thinking about mental health clients

When thinking about an individual with a mental health issue, try to identify what is based on fact and what is being influenced by stereotypes. This is the basis of person-centred care and applies to every nursing environment. Choose a client that you have been caring for and review their client file.

1 How do you view this client?
2 What issues or behaviours does this client have?
3 Are they all due to a mental health issue or are some due to other factors?
   Try to identify the other factors that may be driving the behaviour or the symptoms that the client has.

19.2 Responding appropriately to signs of mental illness

Reading

Always try to be prepared for different behaviours that clients with a mental health illness may display. Before interacting with a client, spend time researching what type of mental health illness they have and what their pattern of behaviour has been. It can be quite confronting to encounter behaviours that are violent or against standards of accepted behaviour.

If a client exhibits behaviour that is abnormal in a situational context it is important to stay calm, always maintain personal safety and do not agitate the client by trying to reorientate them to reality at this point. Reorientation needs to be carefully monitored and implemented to avoid agitation and aggressive responses by a client.

Conditions and behaviours

As a nurse it is important to understand the underlying pathophysiology or cause of the mental health condition. Once a diagnosis has been made the causes and/or triggers of behaviours the person exhibits will be more clearly identified. Refer to **Table 19.3** for a broad outline of some of the major mental health illnesses.

TABLE 19.3 Mental health illnesses

Mental health illness	Explanation
Mood disorders	Unpredictable moods, depression or just feeling sad all the time.
Personality disorders	Conditions that are characterised by a pattern of long-term antisocial behaviour. Causes interpersonal connectivity problems and a different view of the world. Odd or eccentric disorders: • paranoid personality disorders • schizoid personality disorders • schizotypal personality disorder. Disorders that are dramatic, emotional or erratic: • antisocial/psychopathic personality disorders • borderline disorders • histrionic personality disorder • narcissistic personality disorder. Anxious or fearful disorders: • avoidant personality disorder • dependent personality disorder • obsessive-compulsive personality disorder.
Anxiety disorders	Everyone can suffer from anxiety but some people are unable to overcome anxiety and it interferes with their life and activities and leads to depression: • generalised anxiety disorders • social phobias • specific phobias such as agoraphobia • panic disorders • obsessive compulsive disorder • post-traumatic stress.
Psychosis	A serious mental health illness where the person has thoughts and emotions that indicate they have lost touch with reality.
Organic disorders	A disorder that is caused by a physiological or structural change in the brain.
Depression	A feeling of sadness, moodiness or feeling low that is intense and long lasting. Does not always have a reason for occurring.
Bipolar disorder	Bipolar disorder, may be called manic-depressive illness, is a disorder that causes unusual shifts in mood energy, activity levels and the ability to carry out ADLs.
Eating disorders	There are many different types of eating disorders that can affect both males and females. There is no one cause but a variety of factors that can lead to the disorder: • anorexia • binge eating • body image • bulimia nervosa • other specified feeding and eating disorders (OSFED).
Dementia	A progressive disorder that affects the working of the brain, in particular: • memory • thinking • reasoning. It is a collection of symptoms.
Delirium	A state of mental confusion that can occur from surgery, illness or medication.

Signs and symptoms

By having a good knowledge of mental health illness it will be possible to identify the signs and symptoms the person is displaying that are due to the illness. It can sometimes be difficult to understand a person's behaviour without the required background knowledge. At times the person will appear completely normal and may refuse care in a manner that appears the same as any other person, so knowing what to look for will assist you in determining if their behaviour is due to the illness or to another factor.

Biopsychosocial effects

When caring for a person with a mental health illness it is important to employ a holistic approach. This will identify all aspects of the person that are affected by the mental health illness. Biopsychosocial health is the state of physical, mental, emotional, social and spiritual wellbeing.

As outlined above, mental health illness can affect the way the person interacts with others, how they view the world and the behaviours they display. This can have impacts on their relationships, work, social, emotional and spiritual wellbeing. The nurse, through assessment, observation and therapeutic communication can identify if other areas of the person's life are disrupted by the mental health illness.

TIP 19.1

Knowing the signs and symptoms of mental health illness

When being assigned clients to care for it is important to review the mental health illness that they have been diagnosed with. Research on the Internet, read mental health textbooks and discuss these with the supervisor. This will make it easier to identify behaviours that the person exhibits that are due to the mental health illness.

IT skills

CASE STUDY 19.1

The effects of mental health illness on other components of the individual's life

Susan Parks was a 48-year-old woman who was admitted as an inpatient for a mental health illness. On admission Susan was noticed to be well groomed and quietly spoken. Susan's vital signs were within normal limits except for a low BMI. Her height was 170 cm and she weighed 43 kilos. On assessment and through communication with her husband, Susan was found to have been suffering from a mental health disorder for the last 10 years. This illness had gradually progressed and Susan was now paranoid about germs and dirt, to the

extent that her husband and two daughters, aged six and eight years, were unable to enter the home but instead lived in the garage that they had converted. At meal times it was noted that Susan would walk in a clockwise direction three times around the table before sitting. It was also noted that Susan would refuse any food that was unpackaged and spent a long time inspecting the packaging.

1   What type of symptoms was Susan displaying?
2   What impact was her mental health issue having on other aspects of her life?
3   Identify what type of mental health illness Susan was experiencing.

Stereotyping and stigma

It is important to recognise the effects that stigma and discrimination can have on an individual. The person may internalise the negative stereotypes and this may delay their recovery. It is important for the nurse to challenge discrimination and dispel myths about mental illness. You have a critical role in educating others, family and carers about the mental health illness. This will require honesty in communication both with the client and with others, and it is important to gain the consent of the person before these discussions take place.

The nurse also can promote mental health for all people through promoting healthy attitudes and coping mechanisms. This focus on wellness for mental health may be required for the person and their family, who may be grieving for the person.

Using negotiation skills

It is important that the nurse interacts with the person with a mental health illness in an ethical manner. This includes therapeutic communication and being honest. At all times you must seek consent before any intervention with the person. One way you can achieve a positive outcome with the person is to empower the person to 'own' their illness and take an active role in their recovery process.

It may not be possible for you to convince a person to undertake a specific nursing intervention when they are experiencing the florid symptomology of some mental health illnesses. In some instances trying to negotiate with the client may trigger other challenging behaviours.

In other individuals techniques that assist the person with recovery are reality testing, ventilation, motivation, modelling, symptom monitoring, problem solving, empathic understanding and reciprocal relating, as outlined in **Table 19.4**.

TABLE 19.4 Methods of interaction with clients suffering from a mental health illness

Method	Description
Reality testing	Assisting the person with determining if their perception is fact or fiction
Ventilation	How the person expresses their emotions and feelings
Motivation	Their desire to change their current situation
Modelling	Providing an example to follow
Symptom monitoring	Awareness of the person's current behaviours, emotions and thoughts
Problem solving	Being able to identify solutions to current issues or to achieve goals
Empathic understanding	Being able to understand another's view and experience
Reciprocal relating	Taking part in an exchange of views with another

19.3 Contributing to care planning and conducting initial clinical observations for a person with a mental health condition

At all times when a person enters a health-care facility for assistance with a mental illness or a physical condition it is important that a baseline measurement is taken. This allows the health-care team to determine if the person has progressed in a positive manner. This baseline measurement includes physical, emotional and social behavioural measurements.

Risk assessment

When a person is admitted to a mental health facility a risk assessment for suicide or self-harm is undertaken. As a student you need to perform this assessment under the supervision of a registered mental health nurse who is specially trained in risk assessment. A mental health illness can predispose a person to a number of triggers for suicide. These include but are not restricted to:

- stress
- a sense of failure
- unemployment
- discrimination
- loneliness

- isolation
- depression.

The risk assessment should also identify other symptoms the person is having and will elicit information that will assist in the care planning for the individual. A way of determining whether the client is depressed, suffering from delirium or dementia is included in **Table 19.5**.

TABLE 19.5 Comparison of depression, delirium and dementia

	Depression	**Delirium**	**Dementia**
Onset	Abrupt or gradual over weeks or months	Sudden, within hours or days	Slow and insidious, over several years
Aetiology	Multifactorial (genetic, physiological, psychological)	Related to general medical conditions or psychosocial changes	Genetic, specific medical conditions (e.g. HIV, Parkinson's disease)
Duration	Acute: from two weeks to six months Chronic: many years	A couple of days to a few weeks	Until death (months to years)
Progression	Self-limited or chronic without treatment	Fast and fluctuating, but temporary if underlying condition is treated	Slow, stable, with a continuous and permanent decline in abilities and cognition
Symptoms	Do not fluctuate	Fluctuate rapidly	Tend not to fluctuate
Cognitive changes			
Consciousness	Clear	Clouded	Clear
Orientation	Unaffected	Disorientated	Alters in accordance with severity of dementia
Speech	'I don't know' is a common response	Incoherent or unable to respond	May use confabulation, repetitive, aphasia in later stages
Thought content	Negative	Confused	Disorganised, sometimes delusional
Perception	May be distorted	Misinterpretations common	Occasionally distorted
Attention span	May experience some difficulty	Reduced	Fluctuates
Affect	Flat	Labile	Labile and apathetic
Memory	Generally unaffected	Impaired	Impaired
Insight	May be some impairment	May have some if lucid	Only in early stages
Judgement	Poor	Poor	Poor
Psychomotor activity	Agitation or retardation	Abnormally increased or reduced	Often normal
Behaviour	Fatigued, apathetic, occasionally agitated	Varies from agitation to unresponsiveness	May or may not have behavioural symptoms
Sleep	Early-morning wakening	Often disturbed	Often disturbed
ADL	Not inclined	Unable	Struggles

Source: Adapted from Neville, C. & Byrne, G. (2009). The older person experiencing mood symptoms. In G. Byrne & C. Neville (eds.), *Community Mental Health and Older People* (pp. 169–70), Elsevier: Sydney, NSW.

One of the major concerns nurses hold is whether a client is suicidal. The initial risk assessment should screen for this problem. See **Figure 19.1** for a checklist that nurses can use to assess the risk of suicide.

For further information on mental health and risk assessment, the following website contains information on assessment, diagnosis, treatment and sites to access for assistance: Sane Australia, https://www.sane.org/mental-health-and-illness.

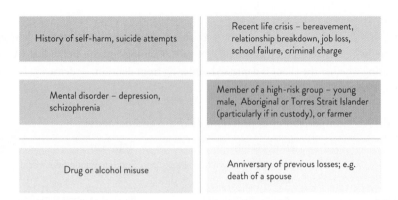

History of self-harm, suicide attempts	Recent life crisis – bereavement, relationship breakdown, job loss, school failure, criminal charge
Mental disorder – depression, schizophrenia	Member of a high-risk group – young male, Aboriginal or Torres Strait Islander (particularly if in custody), or farmer
Drug or alcohol misuse	Anniversary of previous losses; e.g. death of a spouse

FIGURE 19.1 Risk factors for suicide

Sources: Lifeline (2017). *Preventing suicide*. Retrieved from https://www.lifeline.org.au/get-help/topics/preventing-suicide?gclid=CjwKCAiAxJPVBRB4EiwAsCA4aYNBhO3q7gW4vuTGmgWb0GlUq5Eb_XbTFPn2HXrgmGlPbtrU12ALixoCr8AQAvD_BwE. Accessed 15 March 2017; Australian Psychological Society (2017). *Believe in change*. Retrieved from https://www.psychology.org.au/inpsych/2016/feb/dudgeon/. Accessed 15 March 2017.

TIP 19.3

Undertaking a risk assessment

When taking part in a risk assessment it is important to review the documentation prior to undertaking the assessment. Make sure that you have all the documentation and checklists before commencing the assessment.

Reading

The interdisciplinary health-care team

The enrolled nurse is part of the interdisciplinary health-care team and integral to the planning of care for the person (see **Figure 19.2**). The nurse is able to identify the individual's care needs. In order to do this the nurse must:

- design a care plan using the nursing process that will assist the person in a recovery model for the best outcomes

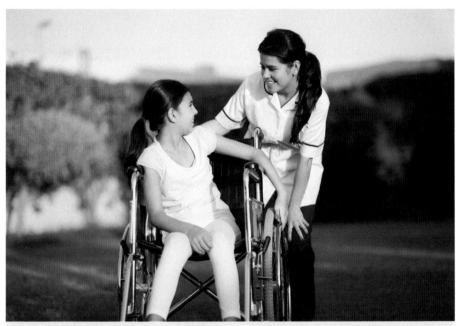

FIGURE 19.2 Caring for the individual

Getty Images/Katarina Premfors.

- monitor the person undergoing treatment and interventions
- establish and maintain the therapeutic relationship.

As discussed, the person with a mental health illness has a complex set of needs that requires a team approach. Beside physical and mental issues that require specialist assistance, the problems facing a person with a mental health illness may include unemployment, housing and social connections. By addressing all aspects of the person's life, a holistic care plan can be formulated.

Along with risk assessment for suicide, the enrolled nurse will also undertake assessments to identify mental health issues. This is usually done with a mental state assessment. This will gather information enabling the health-care team to make a judgement regarding the person's mental state and what interventions are required.

Observing the person's behaviour and physical health

The nurse, along with other members of the allied health team, is expected to observe and document the person's behaviour and identify any areas of change to the person's physical and mental health.

One important way to do this is by following the facility's routine checks. These will involve the reassessment of the person for each of the body systems as well as specific charts for behaviours. Examples of specific charts may include but are not limited to:

- food and fluid intake charts
- sleep charts
- behaviour charts (wandering, disruptive behaviour, aggression)
- interaction charts and responses by the person and nurse.

Some of the behaviours that might be noted are listed in **Table 19.6**.

TABLE 19.6 Behaviours in mental health illnesses

Mental health illnesses	Behaviours
Delusions	Fixed false beliefs that do not alter with logic.
	Delusions of reference – other people and events contain messages specifically for them.
	Delusions of grandeur – that they have great importance or powers.
	Somatic delusions – believe something is happening to their body.
	Delusions of persecution – believe they are being followed, poisoned or spied on.
Hallucinations	Auditory – hears voices that may be kind, demanding, critical or frightening.
	Visual – sees things or people that are not there.
	Olfactory – smells things that others cannot.
	Gustatory – food may taste bad or contaminated.
	Tactile – experiences sensations differently to what they are.
Delusional disorder	Strong belief in something that others do not believe to be true.
Schizophrenia	Hallucinations, delusions and thought disorder.
Bipolar affective disorder	The person experiences up and down moods.
Depression	Sadness, lack of energy, amotivation, changes in sleep patterns, changes in appetite, hopelessness, less enjoyment in activities, feelings of worthlessness and guilt, and depressive delusions.

Review the skill in Tollefson *Essential Clinical Skills* 9.1 Mental state assessment

Writing

TIP 19.4
Documentation
Ensure that you have collected all of the required charts at the start of each shift. Make certain that you understand how to complete the charting requirements according to the policies and procedures of the facility. It is important to update charts on a continual basis to ensure accuracy.

Review the skill in Tollefson *Essential Clinical Skills* 7.1 Documentation & 7.3 Clinical handover – change of shift

Writing

Review the skill in
Tollefson *Essential
Clinical Skills* 7.5
Health teaching

Verbal skills,
writing

Health promotion and educational strategies

If you notice that an individual is experiencing a change in their physical health status, it is important that this is documented and reported appropriately. It is important to provide the individual with the necessary knowledge and education to assist them to make informed choices.

In mental health, the person is entitled to the same access to health promotion and education as any other individual. In some instances, providing this education may alleviate anxiety that the person may experience due to the changes in their physical health.

Interdisciplinary team meetings and service providers

In the mental health environment it is usual that an interdisciplinary team meeting is held to review the ongoing treatment and care for a person with a mental health illness. The nurse may identify any areas of concern that they have regarding the individual's ability in ADLs and share information that the person or carer has communicated to them. Other members of the team will also reassess the care the person has received and evaluate the outcome. At this time new objectives may be set by the team and responsibilities may be delegated to a specific member of the team.

When the person is nearing discharge the team may identify further community supports, such as Meals on Wheels, home help and district nursing, that the enrolled nurse will need to liaise with to ensure a smooth transition from inpatient care to the community. The facility will have transfer documentation that the enrolled nurse will need to locate and complete.

Recovery principles with support from interdisciplinary team

In the Australian health-care system the team will consist of a variety of specialised personnel. It is important to have all members of the team involved in the care planning for a client with a mental health illness to maximise outcomes. In the mental health arena the health-care team will consist of a psychiatrist, psychiatric nursing staff, registered nurses, psychologists and social workers.

By referring the client to the appropriate member of the health-care team, a more targeted approach can be instituted and better outcomes achieved for the client. It allows each member of the health-care team who specialises in a particular area to assist in the assessment and care planning approach in response to the needs of the client.

19.4 Contributing to the recovery of a person with a mental health condition

When working in the mental health arena the nurse will be able to assist with the assessment, implementation and evaluation of strategies and provide input to the health-care team. Often the needs of clients with a mental health problem will change as their condition improves. When first admitted the focus is on managing the mental health illness. As the client improves the focus may move to reintegration into society.

The nurse can use many techniques that have been approved by the health-care team for managing the mental health illness. These have been identified previously in **Table 19.4**.

Planning, prioritising and implementing nursing interventions

The underlying philosophy behind care planning is patient-centred care. This will also involve the family, carers and members of the interdisciplinary team to contribute to the care plan as well as the individual and nurse.

Once the individual has been assessed holistically the team can then identify priority areas for intervention. Initially the nursing care required for the individual may need to be re-evaluated to address any needs that may be noted. This may be identified through communication with the person and through observation. Some mental health illness will have a direct impact on the ADLs.

Specific interventions such as ECT therapy may be a priority to treat mental health illness and a re-evaluation of the person after the intervention needs to be undertaken.

Respect for the person's dignity and uniqueness

It is important to always work in a manner that includes respect for the person. One of the ways that nurses can do this is to include the client in the care planning process. At times it may not be possible for this to occur as the person may be unable to identify reality, but allowing the opportunity for this to occur is important when the person is able to make decisions.

In Victoria, for example, people must be told about their rights under the *Mental Health Act 2014* and the process of being assessed or treated, including the right to:

*   communicate
*   have their preferences considered
*   get support to make treatment decisions (Victoria Legal Aid, 2015).

At all times the person's consent needs to given before nursing interventions. This can be problematic in the mental health arena but should always be attempted with an explanation given to the client before the intervention takes place. The *Mental Health Act 2014* contains a number of principles that aim to uphold the rights, dignity and autonomy of the client.

Assisting the client, carer or family in appropriate therapeutic interventions

The person is central to the care planning processes and always should be included. As discussed previously the person may not be able to verbally provide input due to their altered mental state. The family or carer can provide additional information as to how the person normally functions and this can be included in the care planning process. It also is important to include cultural requirements in the care plan. How does the person like to be addressed? What food do they prefer? Even if the person cannot convey this information, they may make the association and this can assist in reality reorientation.

It is important to determine who has the right to consent for treatments in the mental health arena. Is it the person? Is it the family? Or has an independent guardian been appointed. There is more information on informed consent and mental health illness here: https://www.humanrights.gov.au/our-work/disability-rights/publications/mental-health-legislation-and-human-rights.

Medication

It is important to fully explain the use and administration methods of any medications that are to be used in the therapy. The person or other responsible person needs to be given knowledge of the effects and side effects of any medication that is ordered.

Review the skill in Tollefson *Essential Clinical Skills* 9.5 Electro-convulsive therapy (ECT) – patient care pre- and post-treatment

Review the skill in
Tollefson *Essential
Clinical Skills*
5.1 Medication
administration – oral,
sublingual, buccal,
topical and rectal
& 5.2 Medication
administration – eye
drops or ointment, and
eye toilet

Depending on the type of mental health illness the individual is suffering from a particular method of administration may be ordered. This can be helpful for people who are experiencing the onset of dementia and may forget to take medication at set times. It may be more beneficial if the medication is given parentally or in a longer acting formulation.

As the person's illness progresses repeated education regarding medication may be required. It is important to note any cultural and language issues and present information in a manner that the person can access more readily.

Community resources and opportunities

There are a number of support groups for both the person with mental health issues and their families that may be useful. Most health-care facilities will have printed leaflets that can be given to family and individuals.

Other community resources will be decided upon in the team meetings prior to discharge but it is also important to involve the family or the individual in the planning of these resources when they are discharged. This may highlight other areas that need addressing and can be referred to the appropriate resource in the community by a member of the allied health team. An example of this may be the need for a taxi voucher to attend the community service, in which case the social worker can assist the family or individual.

Activity 19.3

Community resources

The mental health facility will be located within a region with specific community resources located within that region. Try to identify as many of the community resources that the facility will use to assist the individual after discharge.

CASE STUDY 19.2

Discharge from a mental health facility

Michael was a 58-year-old male that had been admitted as an inpatient on a voluntary basis for treatment of his depression. Michael had undergone ECT therapy and a medication review with a new medication treatment being ordered for him. Michael was supported by his wife Elaine, to whom he had been married for 26 years.

Unfortunately due to his mental health illness Michael had lost his position as a bus driver. Michael has two children who are both now independent.
1   What information regarding the new medications that Michael was prescribed should be given to him?
2   What community services should be accessed for Michael and his wife?

Supporting and valuing the person with a mental health illness

Part of the process of recovery for a person with a mental health illness is the re-establishment of their autonomy. The person should be provided with opportunities to decide on treatments and outcomes that will meet their needs.

The recovery model of treatment and the strengths building model are based on providing opportunities for the individual to build upon their individual strengths. As discussed previously, the person with a mental health illness may be subject to stigmatisation and discrimination. It is important that the nurse is a role model who upholds the rights of the person with a mental health illness.

SUMMARY

- Nurses are required to work within legislative boundaries. These can vary from state to state.
- By recognising the signs and symptoms of mental health conditions and their effects on the physical and social behaviours of an individual, the nurse will be able to respond appropriately.
- In the mental health arena it is necessary to undertake a holistic assessment of the person and to use specialised mental health assessments to determine both the health of the person and identify any risks to the person with a mental health illness.
- Assisting with the recovery of a person with mental health illness includes respecting the person's dignity and uniqueness and employing strategies that assist the person to contribute to their own plan of care.

SELF-TEST QUESTIONS

1   What are the values and principles that underpin the nursing care of a person with a mental health illness?
2   What strategies can the nurse use to negotiate with a person with a mental health illness?
3   How can the nurse contribute to the promotion of mental health?
4   What are the recovery principles that are applied to mental health nursing?
5   How can the nurse support the person to build on their strengths and make decisions?

BIBLIOGRAPHY

Australian College of Mental Health Nurses (ACMHN) (n.d.). *What is mental health nursing?* Retrieved from http://www.acmhn.org/about-us/about-mh-nursing. Accessed 3 March 2017.

Australian Government Department of Health (2010). *National Standards for Mental Health Services 2010: Principles of recovery oriented mental health practice.* Retrieved from https://www.health.gov.au/internet/main/publishing.nsf/Content/CFA833CB8C1AA178CA257BF0001E7520/$File/servpri.pdf. Accessed 3 March 2017.

Australian Psychological Society (2017). *Believe in change.* Retrieved from https://www.psychology.org.au/inpsych/2016/feb/dudgeon/. Accessed 15 March 2017.

Black Dog Institute (2017). *Facts & figures about mental health.* Retrieved from https://www.blackdoginstitute.org.au/docs/default-source/factsheets/facts_figures.pdf?sfvrsn=8. Accessed 15 March 2017.

Gray, S., Ferris, L., White, L., Duncan, G. & Baumle, W. (2018). *Fundamentals of Nursing* (2nd edition). Cengage Learning: South Melbourne.

Lifeline (2017). *Preventing suicide.* Retrieved from https://www.lifeline.org.au/get-help/topics/preventing-suicide?gclid=CjwKCAiAxJPVBRB4EiwAsCA4aYNBhO3q7gW4vuTGmgWb0GlUq5Eb_XbTFPn2HXrgmGlPbtrU12ALixoCr8AQAvD_BwE. Accessed 15 March 2017.

Neville, C. & Bryne, G. (2009). The older person experiencing mood symptoms. In G. Byrne & C. Neville (eds.), *Community Mental Health and Older People* (pp. 169–70), Elsevier: Sydney, NSW.

Sane Australia (n.d.). *Mental Health & Illness.* Retrieved from https://www.sane.org/mental-health-and-illness.

Tollefson. J. (2012). *Essential Clinical Skills: Enrolled Nurses* (3rd edition). Cengage Learning: South Melbourne.

United Nations (1991). *Principles for the Protection of Persons with Mental Illness and for the Improvement of Mental Health Care.* Retrieved from http://www.un.org/documents/ga/res/46/a46r119.htm.

Victoria Legal Aid (2015). *Rights of people receiving compulsory treatment.* Retrieved from https://www.legalaid.vic.gov.au/find-legal-answers/mental-health-and-your-rights/rights-of-people-receiving-compulsory-treatment. Accessed 5 March 2017.

World Health Organisation (1996) *Mental Health Care Law: Ten Basic Principles.* Retrieved from http://www.who.int/mental_health/media/en/75.pdf. Accessed 4 March 2017.

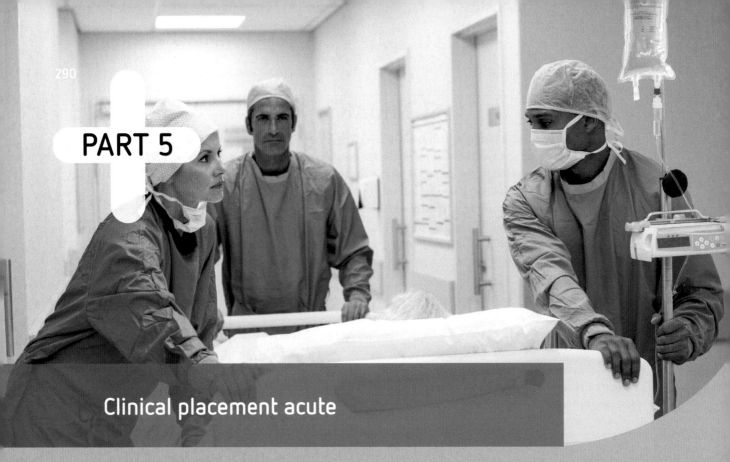

PART 5

Clinical placement acute

Chapter 20: Medicines and intravenous therapy
Chapter 21: Care for a person with acute health problems

The acute care experience

I was really excited to finally get my acute placement. I really wanted to see the patients who were in hospital for things like trauma, surgery, illness and not just aged care. What I soon realised, days into my placement, was that acute care deals with something that just happened, like trauma, on top of a host of other diseases and conditions. It is tricky and complicated! Some medications or treatments could not be started because of contraindications – like renal disease, or the fact that the patient was on blood thinning medications. My view of acute care was all bloody and gory, like on TV. It is not like that at all – and in fact, I think I like the reality better. I had to think of all the diseases and conditions the patient had and couple that with what the acute admission was for. It was so incredibly interesting to see how each of us are different in terms of healing, disease progression and injury. For example, you could break the leg of three patients, all the same age, but they would all take different amounts of time to heal – because they each have different disease processes, tolerance to pain, mobility concerns and different mindsets. Acute care nursing was so much more than I thought it would be. No patient was the same, and all patients were a mystery, with some having so many contributing factors it was like a puzzle trying to work out how to fix one aspect. Patients were varying in age, with the mean age (on the ward sign) as 64 years old. Which was another thing I did not realise – I assumed acute care would mean a younger patient population – not true! My acute experience really opened my eyes to how much you can do as an enrolled nurse, and how many different specialities there are available. It also made me revisit my anatomy and physiology for a quick revision of why the kidneys are so important for blood pressure!

For most of the students this will be your final placement. Acute care is a specialised area where you will be able to put into practice everything you have learnt so far! It is an area where you will need to be constantly assessing, evaluating and reviewing patient data.

What is acute care? Acute care encompasses a large patient population and involves care of patients who may have many co-morbidities or chronic conditions, or the hospitalisation may be a result of an injury or acute illness, or surgery. Patients who are in acute care settings are in a hospital environment, and acute care also covers pre- and post-procedure or operation nursing care. Acute care environments can also incorporate day surgery centres, or private procedure clinics. Acute care is not just surgery, it can be due to illness (such as pneumonia, cholelithiasis, or a urinary tract infection), trauma or injury. Acute care is also delivered through emergency departments.

What kind of patients are in acute care facilities?

Acute care is required by people of all ages. From neonates all the way up the ages! Acute care facilities will have specialised wards for paediatrics and for maternity patients, for example. There are also surgical wards which have a patient population of pre- and post-op patients, and then general medical wards where patients are admitted for acute intervention and management. In 2015–16 there were 10.6 million separations from hospitals (public and private) meaning that there were 10.6 million admissions/discharges! (AIHW, 2017).

In this placement you will be in a hospital environment – this can be a hospital ward (surgical, medical, maternity) or department, such as the emergency department. The patients you will come across will have a variety of illnesses or diseases that are termed 'co-morbidities'. You will need to perform a thorough health history on every admitted patient to determine past medical and surgical history, as well as medications, and assess activities of daily living. This is where you will be involved in planning nursing interventions and evaluating data from the patient.

Common experiences of student nurses in acute care

No two shifts are ever the same in nursing – and this adage will ring true in this placement. You will notice that patient turnover (admission and discharge) is frequent, with some patients discharged home the next day after some operations, or after initiation of intravenous antibiotics. Each patient will respond differently to interventions, and you will need to assess patients, for example, for pain, discomfort and mobility. You will be exposed to wound care, stoma care, medication management, and management of invasive devices such as indwelling catheters, intravenous cannulas and nasogastric tubes.

You will perform countless sets of observations in a single shift – acute care nursing requires frequent observation. Patients will have their observations recorded onto an Adult Deterioration Detection Score (ADDS) chart, which has designated prompts for ongoing patient assessment and intervention. While completing these charts can be overwhelming, get going and practise as soon enough it will be your sole responsibility for completing this documentation.

You might also witness a cardiac or respiratory arrest, or a medical emergency call. All of these are unfortunately common in the acute care arena, as patients can deteriorate or have further complications resulting in, for example, a myocardial infarction or a stroke. Death is something that does occur in the acute care setting, and you may very well witness your first patient death.

Objectives

The objectives that are to be set for this placement need to be contextualised to the acute care setting. Here are some examples of objectives:

- holistic approach to care in the acute care environment including nursing interventions and outcomes

- emergency management protocols for first-aid procedures and cardiac and respiratory arrest
- pre- and post-operative nursing management
- pain management strategies
- surgical nursing
- monitoring of patients with invasive devices such as PICC lines, nasogastric tubes
- frequent observations
- patient assessment including health history
- knowledge of acute health problems such as renal disorders, gastrointestinal disorders, pain, respiratory conditions, angina, sepsis, burns, cellulitis.

Work allocation

In acute care, often a patient workload is allocated to either a nurse, or to a team of nurses. Allocation is often specific to areas and facilities so make sure you are aware of what your role will be. Some facilities use team nursing, while others have a team leader and a designated nurse for four to six patients. Patient allocation in acute nursing also depends on the acuity of the patient. One post-operative patient may be very time-intensive requiring a great deal of nursing interventions and cares, while other patients may not have as many or as complex interventions. Patients' needs are reviewed when the allocation of nursing staff is made to ensure safe patient care can be delivered. Medications may be administered by the student if the unit HLTENN007 has been completed, and the student is supervised. For more complex management there will be a registered nurse who will undertake specialised activities. All enrolled nurses and support staff work under the supervision of a registered Division 1 nurse.

Enjoy your placement and ensure you make good use of the valuable time you have in this specialty area.

Medicines and intravenous therapy

CHAPTER
20

LEARNING OUTCOMES

After reading this chapter, you should have an understanding of:

20.1 Minimising potential risk to ensure safe administration of medications

20.2 Preparing for medication administration and infusion of IV fluids

20.3 Administering and storing medication

20.4 Monitoring and evaluating a person's response to administered medication, IV fluids and blood and blood products

20.5 Assessing the effectiveness of pain-relieving therapy

Administering medications

My whole training, I focused on this subject as being 'the subject' where I would become a 'real' nurse. I never realised how much danger lies in administering medication, and how it is about so much more than just popping a pill or drawing up an antibiotic. There is a great deal of responsibility and accountability in the administration of medications. Checking medications is a serious business – not just a quick glance, but a thorough check, because you could be preventing a medication error. In my short career I have already seen medication errors and the impact that they can have – not just on patients but on staff also. While I greatly enjoy the responsibility of medication administration, it is an area that I find myself constantly checking, re-checking and seeking further information on for safety. If I am not sure, I will always seek clarification.

20.1 Minimising potential risk to ensure safe administration of medications

Managing medication requires collaboration – from nurses, medical officers, nurse practitioners and pharmacists. Medications can be prescribed by dentists, medical officers and nurse practitioners. Registered nurses can prescribe certain medications for the enrolled nurse to administer, but this is reliant upon local policies and procedures (Clarke et al., 2016).

Drugs and poisons schedules and classifications

The role of Australian Governments in regulation of the pharmaceutical industry is to protect the health of the public by ensuring that medications are safe and effective. **Table 20.1** outlines the legislation governing Australia and New Zealand.

TABLE 20.1 Legislation governing drugs in Australia and New Zealand

Locality	Legislation
Commonwealth of Australia	*Therapeutic Goods Act 1989* *Therapeutic Goods Regulations 1990* *National Health Act 1953* *Narcotic Drugs Act 1967*
Australian Capital Territory (ACT)	*Drugs of Dependence Act 1989* *Drugs of Dependence Regulation 2009* *Medicines, Poisons and Therapeutic Goods Regulation 2008*
New South Wales (NSW)	*Poisons and Therapeutic Goods Act 1966* *Poisons and Therapeutic Goods Regulation 2008*
Northern Territory (NT)	*Medicines, Poisons and Therapeutic Goods Act 2012* *Medicines, Poisons and Therapeutic Goods Regulations 2012*
Queensland (QLD)	*Health Act 1937* *Health (Drugs and Poisons) Regulations 1996*
South Australia (SA)	*Controlled Substances Act 1984* *Controlled Substances (Controlled Drugs, Precursors and Plants) Regulations 2014*
Tasmania (Tas)	*Poisons Act 1971* *Poisons Regulations 2008*
Victoria (Vic)	*Drugs, Poisons and Controlled Substances Act 1981* *Drugs, Poisons and Controlled Substances Regulations 2006*
Western Australia (WA)	*Poisons Act 1964* *Poisons Regulations under the Act*
New Zealand	*Medicines Act 1981* *Medicines Amendment Act 2013* *Medicines Regulations 1984* *Misuse of Drugs Act 1975* *Misuse of Drugs Regulations 1977* *Dietary Supplement Regulations 1985*

Sources: Mckenna, L. & Lim, A.G. (2012). *Karch's Pharmacology for Nursing and Midwifery*, 1st Australian and New Zealand Edition. Lippincott Williams & Wilkins: Macquarie Park, NSW; Crisp, J., Taylor, C., Douglas, C., & Rebeiro, G. (2013). *Potter and Perry's Fundamentals of Nursing*, 4th Edition. Elsevier: Sydney, NSW.

Further to the legislation of drugs, there are also schedules of medications, of which there are nine. Records must be kept by all nursing staff and pharmacists for the dispensing and administration of controlled substances. This is referred to as a 'Controlled Drug Register'. **Table 20.2** outlines the standard for schedules of medicines and poisons.

TABLE 20.2 Standard for the schedules of medicines and poisons

Scheduled medications	Explanation of the scheduled medications
Unscheduled medicines	• These are medications sold in supermarkets. • There are guidelines surrounding therapeutic agent, dosage and total dose per packet. For example, paracetamol can be sold in supermarkets as unscheduled medicine, but only in small amounts per box. This is because paracetamol is considered safe and clients do not need to receive counselling before use. It is used for minor ailments and has a low potential for abuse. • Larger quantities of unscheduled medicines (e.g. 100 tablets per box) are categorised as schedule 2 and must be purchased from a pharmacy; for example, paracetamol is toxic in large doses.
Schedule 1	• This schedule is not currently in use.
Schedule 2 (S2)	• Drugs and poisons are pharmacy medicines that are considered to be relatively safe and used for minor ailments. • In small quantities (less than 24 tablets) these medications can also be purchased in a supermarket and other general stores. Examples include aspirin, paracetamol and ibuprofen.
Schedule 3 (S3)	• Pharmacy only medicines. They are substantially safe, but require pharmacist advice, management and, at times, monitoring. • Examples include cold and flu medicines that contain pseudoephedrine.
Schedule 4 (S4)	• Therapeutic agents available by prescription only from a medical, dental or veterinary professional with prescribing rights. • Examples include, but are not limited to, antibiotics, antihypertensives and diuretics.
Schedule 5 (S5)	• Drugs and poisons requiring caution when handling, storing or using. They have low toxicity and are moderately hazardous.
Schedule 6 (S6)	• Drugs and poisons with moderate to high toxicity, which may cause death or severe injury if swallowed, inhaled or if they come into contact with skin or eyes.
Schedule 7 (S7)	• Dangerous poisons that are extremely toxic and may cause death or severe injury at low exposure. Highly regulated and require special training. • These agents are not available for domestic use.
Schedule 8 (S8)	• Known as controlled drugs, these therapeutic agents have a high potential for abuse and addiction. They are highly regulated and possession without authority is illegal. • Examples include morphine, flunitrazepam and cocaine.
Schedule 9 (S9)	• Prohibited substances that, by law, can only be used for research purposes. • Examples include heroin, LSD and cannabis.

Source: Adapted from Therapeutic Goods Association (2014). Poisons Standard 2014. Retrieved from http://www.tga.gov.au/about/tga.htm#.VEm8qPmUd8E.

Purpose and function of prescribed medicine and intravenous (IV) therapy

Medication is prescribed to alleviate the signs and symptoms of illness or responses to events that impact on the health and wellbeing of a client. Medication can also be prescribed to prevent a complication from occurring, such as a deep vein thrombosis (DVT). In all cases the aim of medication administration is to attempt to assist the client maintain homeostasis.

Activity 20.1

Purpose and function of medication and IV therapy

Select one of the clients you are providing nursing care for. Make a list of the prescribed medications and IV therapy they are receiving.

1 For each medication and IV therapy list the reason why the person is receiving it.
2 Identify what potential or actual problem it has been prescribed for.

Pharmacology and substance incompatibilities when administering medication, blood and blood products

Pharmacology is the study of drugs and their interaction with the body. This is then further broken down into two different areas, *pharmacokinetics* and *pharmacodynamics*. *Pharmacokinetics* can be described as what the body does to the drug, while *pharmacodynamics* is described as what the drug does to the body (DeLaune et al., 2016).

A client's response to a medication can be affected for a variety of reasons. When caring for clients, remember that no two people are alike psychologically or physically. Response to medications can therefore vary and are dependent on factors such as those outlined in **Figure 20.1**.

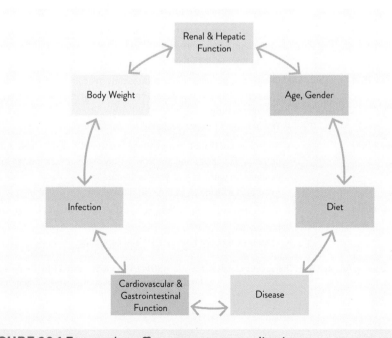

FIGURE 20.1 Factors that affect response to medications

Incompatibility is an undesirable chemical or physical reaction between a drug and a solution, or two or more drugs. Intravenous administration, as with all other routes of medication administration, has risks. An example of this would be the solution the medication is diluted in for administration and the drug itself. Certain medications (for example, phenytoin and diazepam) crystallise or precipitate IV fluids when mixed incorrectly or with incompatible fluids. Your hospital will have policies and procedures in place for you to dilute medications safely, and also you will have access to a pharmacist if in doubt (Broyles, 2017).

There are three groups of incompatibilities:

- Physical incompatibilities – these occur more frequently when there are multiple additives. Information on compatibility should be obtained if two drugs are going to be mixed in the same solution, or even if two drugs are administered concurrently through 'Y' connections. Examples are precipitation, haze, gas bubbles or cloudiness in the solution after dilution.
- Chemical incompatibility – these occur when two or more drugs are mixed together and lose their potency. Factors associated with chemical incompatibility include drug concentration, change in pH of the solution, volume of the solution to dilute the medications, length of time that the medications are in contact with one another and temperature and light.
- Therapeutic incompatibility – this is also referred to as physiological incompatibility. It occurs when prescribed drugs produce an undesirable effect in the patient. This includes overdose, incorrect dosage, contraindication for that specific patient, drug **synergy**, and drug **antagonism**.

Each ward should have a resource that contains comprehensive data allowing nurses to check substance compatibilities. Clinical areas should also have available a pharmacological compatibility chart of intravenous fluids and solution commonly used within the particular clinical area.

20.2 Preparing for medication administration and infusion of IV fluids

The aims of administering medication are to do it safely and efficiently and to observe the client for both desirable and undesirable effects. Prior to administering medications it is also important that the nurse is *accredited* to do so. For example, there are some medications which may not be administered by the enrolled nurse or even the registered nurse – such as intravenous chemotherapy or intravenous medications via central venous access – until they have been assessed as being competent/accredited to do so (see **Figure 20.2**).

Many health-care facilities will have their own accreditation process in place to promote both client and staff safety, however, it is important to also work within the nurse's scope of practice.

Explaining the processes of medication administration or IV fluid infusion

Patients rely heavily on health-care professionals to ensure that medications – of all routes – are administered safely and effectively. Patients also rely on health-care professionals to answer any questions they may have concerning the medication. With this in mind, it is essential that all nursing staff have excellent foundation knowledge in pharmacology. Simply giving a medication does not make you a great nurse – knowing what to look for, possible interactions or adverse reactions and long-term considerations make you a well-informed and *safe* nurse.

antagonist
Drug that blocks receptors, stopping what normally binds to the receptor and as a result inhibits normal response (Broyles et al., 2017)

synergy
Effect of the use of two or more agents that produces a pharmacological response greater than what would be expected by the individual effects of each agent (Broyles et al., 2017)

TIP 20.1

MIMS
Remember to utilise your MIMS or equivalent provided to ensure that you are aware of all ramifications of administering the medication. Ultimately it is your signature and your scope of practice for the responsibility of administering IV medications.

Explore the theory in *Foundations of Nursing* Chapter 22 Medication administration and IV therapy

TIP 20.2

Preparation of the client for medication administration
As with any nursing intervention it is necessary to obtain informed consent from the client before undertaking the intervention.

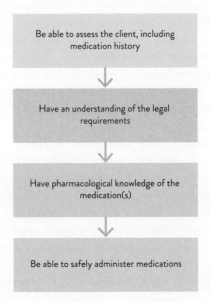

FIGURE 20.2 Steps to prepare and administer medication

Identifying correct administration route or site for each medication or IV fluid

To correctly identify the administration route for the medication or IV fluid the nurse needs to understand the terminology and abbreviations and symbols used in the Australian healthcare system.

Table 20.3 identifies common abbreviations and symbols used for medication administration.

TABLE 20.3 Routes of administration

Type of administration – enteral	Description
Oral (PO)	Medication is given by mouth and swallowed.
Sublingual (SL)	Medication is placed under the tongue to dissolve.
Buccal	Medication is placed against mucus membranes of the cheek to dissolve.
Type of administration – parenteral	**Description**
Intravenous (IV)	Medication is given through invasive intravenous cannula.
Subcutaneous injection (SC)	Medication is injected into subcutaneous tissue.
Intramuscular injection (IM)	Medication is injected into muscular tissue.
Epidural	Medication is injected into the epidural space (often through a catheter inserted by a medical officer).
Topical (top)	Medication is applied to the skin.
Inhalation (inh)	Medication is inhaled through the lungs.
Vaginal (PV)	Medication is inserted into the vagina.
Rectal (PR)	Medication is inserted into the rectum.
Intraocular (IOC)	Medication is administered into the conjunctiva of the eye.
Transdermal (Trans)	Medication is delivered across the skin.
Intranasal	Medication is instilled into the nose.

Source: White, L., Duncan, G., Baumle, W., Gray, S., & Ferris, L. (2018). Foundations of Nursing, Australian and New Zealand edition, 2nd Edition. Cengage: Melbourne.

Other nursing responsibilities include:
- privacy (if required such as when giving an injection)
- positioning (the position of the patient will vary according to the type of administration. e.g. lying on side for injection, sitting up for oral administration)
- education and consent.

TIP 20.4

Medications

When preparing medications for administration, ensure you complete medication administration one patient at a time. Errors are more likely to occur when multiple medication charts are being referred to for different patients; or if multiple pill cups are being carried or moved around the ward. Prioritise medications if required, and plan your time around administering medications at ordered times. More information can be found here: Standard 4: Medication safety, https://www.safetyandquality.gov.au/wp-content/uploads/2012/10/Standard4_Oct_2012_WEB.pdf.

Considering the medication's effect on the body

Some medications will have side effects or work quickly when administered. You need to be aware of these and plan nursing care accordingly. Examples of these effects are:
- Lasix – the diuretic may cause the client to pass urine frequently shortly after administration. This could cause the elderly client with mobility issues to fall if in a rush to get to the toilet or be incontinent of urine on the floor. Lasix can be ordered twice daily and you will notice it is given in the morning and at lunch time to avoid the diuresis effect occurring at night.
- Morphine – may cause the client to feel nausea and may require the administration of an antiemetic medication at the same time. It will also necessitate the nurse to have a vomit bag nearby and place the call bell within reach of the client.

Review the skill in Tollefson *Essential Clinical Skills* 5.1 Medication administration – oral, sublingual, buccal, topical and rectal

Activity 20.2

Effects of medication and nursing considerations and actions

For the following commonly used medications find out what nursing actions are required prior to administration and post administration:
- Actrapid insulin
- Warfarin
- Digoxin.

Calculating accurate dosages and IV infusion rates

For some, the concept of calculations may produce negative memories of school and mathematics, especially if maths was not your strongest subject.

However, in order to practise medication administration safely, you must develop the basic numeracy skills you will need to do the calculations. It is most important that you seek help if you need it and practise until you have those skills.

In science and medicine, the 'metric system' is a system of measurement that is based in general terms around a single unit known as a 'metre' – see **Table 20.4**. This system is used internationally and is the basis for the 'SI' units – also known as the 'International System of Units'.

TABLE 20.4 Metric system

	Unit	Abbreviation	Equivalents
Mass	gram (base unit)	g	1 g = 1000 mg = 1 000 000 mcg
	milligram	mg	0.001 g = 1 mg = 1000 mcg
	microgram	mcg or microg	0.000001 g = 0.001 mg = 1 mcg
	kilogram	kg	1 kg = 1000 g
Amount of substance (molecules/atoms)	Mole (base unit)	n or Mol	1 mol = 1000 mmol
	millimole	mM or mmol	0.001 mol = 1 mmol
Volume	litre (base unit)	L	1 L = 1000 mL
	millilitre	mL	0.001 L = 1 mL
Length	metre (base unit)	m	1 m = 100 cm = 1000 mm
	centimetre	cm	0.01 m = 1 cm = 10 mm
	millimetre	mm	0.001 m = 0.1 cm = 1 mm

Source: Brotto, V. & Rafferty, K. (2012). *Clinical Dosage Calculations for Australia & New Zealand.*
Cengage Learning: South Melbourne, Table 2.1, p. 42.

Medication calculations – conversions

The metric system enables us to either multiply or divide to obtain the dose equivalent. For example, to change grams to milligrams you multiply the number by 1000, for example, 4 g to mg = $4 \times 1000 = 4000$ mg.

To convert mg to g you divide the number by 1000, for example, 400 mg to g = 400 mg/1000 = 0.4 g.

TIP 20.5

10 rules to ensure accurately written and interpreted metric notation

Rule 1   The unit or abbreviation always follows the amount (e.g. 5 g not g 5).

Rule 2   Do not put a full stop after the unit abbreviation because it may be mistaken for the number 1 if poorly written (e.g. mg not mg.).

Rule 3   Do not add an 's' to make the unit plural because it may be misread for another unit (e.g. mL not mLs).

Rule 4   Separate the amount from the unit so the number and unit of measure do not run together because the unit can be mistaken as zero or zeros, risking a 10-fold or 100-fold overdose (e.g. 20 mg not 20mg).

Rule 5   Place thin spaces for amounts at or above 10 000 (e.g. 10 000 microg not 10000 microg).

Rule 6   Decimals are used to designate fractional amounts (e.g. 1.5 mL not 1½ mL).

Rule 7   Use a leading zero to emphasise the decimal point for fractional amounts less than 1. Without the zero the amount may be interpreted as a whole number, resulting in serious overdosing (e.g. 0.5 mg not .5 mg).

Rule 8   Omit unnecessary or trailing zeros that can be misread as part of the amount if the decimal point is not seen (e.g. 1.5 mg not 1.50 mg).

Rule 9   Do not use the abbreviation g for microgram because it might be mistaken for mg, which is 1000 times the intended amount (e.g. 150 microg not 150 g or 150 mcg).

Rule 10   Do not use the abbreviation cc for mL because the unit can be mistaken for zeros (e.g. 500 mL not 500 cc).
Always ask the prescriber to clarify if you are not sure of the abbreviation or notation used. Never guess!

Source: Brotto, V., & Rafferty, K. (2012). *Clinical Dosage Calculations for Australia & New Zealand.* Cengage Learning: South Melbourne, p. 44.

There are several different formulas to use when calculating drug doses, the most common is as follows:

$$\frac{\text{Does required} \times \text{Volume of stock}}{\text{Dose in stock}} = \text{Volume required}$$

Another simpler way to look at it is:

$$\frac{\text{What you want} \times \text{Quantity it comes in}}{\text{What you've got}}$$

Let's look at these examples to explain it further:

- Example tablets: 0.125 mg of digoxin is ordered orally (PO – per oral). The medication is available in tablets containing 0.25 mg.

$$\text{Dose required} = 0.125 \text{ mg}$$
$$\text{Stock strength} = 0.25 \text{ mg}$$
$$\frac{\text{Dose required}}{\text{Stock strength}} = \text{Amount to be administered}$$

$$\frac{0.125 \text{ mg}}{0.25 \text{ mg}} = \text{Tablets to be administered}$$

$$= \frac{1}{2} \text{ or } 0.5 \text{ tablet to be administered}$$

Legislative and organisational requirements

The most common routes for administration by injection are:

- subcutaneous
- intramuscular
- intravenous.

Review the skill in Tollefson *Essential Clinical Skills* 5.3 Medication administration – injections

---

CASE STUDY 20.1

Injections

Graham Taylor is a 54-year-old male who has been hospitalised with a pulmonary embolism. He is ordered 5000u of heparin, SC. You attend his bedside with the medication to administer it. He has significant bruising to his abdomen from 'all the other heparin injections'.

1 How would you select a suitable site for administering heparin for Graham?
2 Would you withhold the medication because the abdomen is so bruised?
3 How would you document this encounter?

Techniques and precautions specific to the person's situation

All medications must be administered in a safe manner and you must adhere to local policies and procedures, if relevant, when administering IV medications.

Within Australia the National Inpatient Medication Chart (NIMC) is used. Refer to **Figure 20.3** for the NIMC.

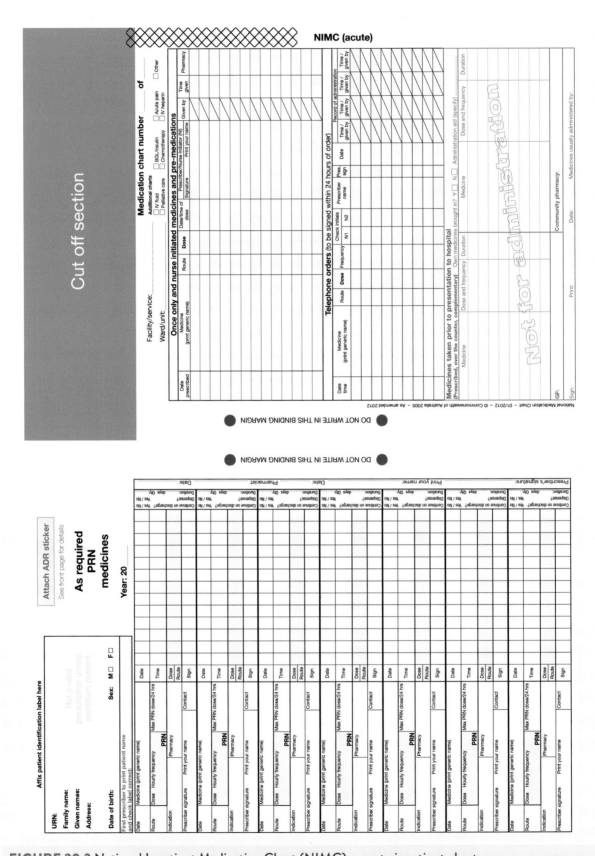

FIGURE 20.3 National Inpatient Medication Chart (NIMC) – acute inpatient chart

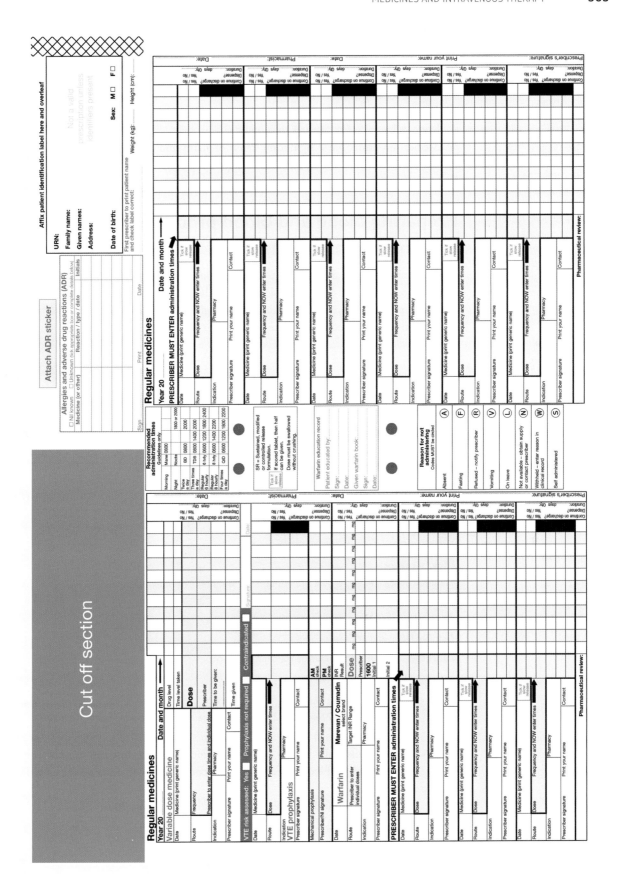

TIP 20.6

Equipment

While on placement, familiarise yourself with the types of infusion pumps and giving sets, and also needles for injections. Not every health-care facility carries the same brands and it is always interesting to see the differing types. Try to prepare as many medications as you can – particularly in cracking or snapping ampoules as practice truly makes perfect!

The NIMC was introduced by the Australian Commission on Safety and Quality in Health Care as an effective way to ensure consistency with prescribing and administering medications in Australia. There are two variations of the NIMC:

1   NIMC long stay version – for long-term stable clients in acute care settings (such as in a spinal rehabilitation unit)

2   Paediatric versions of the NIMC – short-term and long-term stay. The paediatric NIMCs have additional safety features to support safe prescription for children.

Medication errors are a significant cause of harm and disability in health care. The NIMC aims to reduce the number of errors through consistency throughout Australian health-care facilities.

Preparing blood and blood products for blood transfusions

A blood transfusion is administered to replace blood loss and can be an infusion of whole blood or components of blood. Whole blood products include red blood cells and plasma. Blood components or products include plasma, and albumin (Clarke et al., 2016).

Blood transfusions require frequent observations initially to ensure there is no transfusion reaction. Transfusion reactions can occur during the entire transfusion and are due to three reasons:

*   allergic reaction
*   haemolytic reaction
*   febrile reaction.

If a transfusion reaction occurs the actions as outlined in **Table 20.5** should be followed.

TABLE 20.5 Nursing actions for blood reactions

Immediate nursing action
Stop transfusion.
Keep vein open with 0.9% normal saline.
Notify the RN and treating doctor.
Other measures
Monitor client's vital signs every 15 minutes for four hours or until stable.
Monitor fluid balance (input and output).
Send IV tubing and bag of blood back to the blood bank.
Obtain a blood and urine specimen.
Label specimen 'Blood transfusion reaction'.
Process a transfusion reaction report.

Source: Clarke, L., Gray, S., White, L., Duncan, G. & Baumle, W. (2016). *Foundations of Nursing: Enrolled Division 2 Nurses* (ANZ Edition). Cengage Learning: South Melbourne, Table 22.7, p. 544.

Blood transfusions must be run on a single line – and the line can only be primed with 0.9% normal saline. Blood transfusions are incompatible with other intravenous fluids (Clarke et al., 2016).

Treatment of blood transfusion reactions are outlined in **Table 20.6**.

TABLE 20.6 Transfusion reactions, aetiologies, signs and symptom and treatments

Reaction	Aetiology	Sign and symptoms	Treatments
Acute haemolytic transfusion reaction (intravascular haemolysis)	Incompatible blood product transfused because of errors during processing the blood products and the type and cross-match, or the client identification process.	Fever, low back pain, pain at IV site, hypotension, tachycardia, abdominal pain, dyspnoea, nausea/vomiting, rash/hives, headache, anxiety, renal failure.	Stop the transfusion immediately. Keep the vein open with a 0.9% normal saline IV. Contact doctor stat. Support vital functions – may require haemodialysis. Complete lab tests necessary to determine if blood reaction occurred.
Non-haemolytic transfusion reaction	Reaction to donor leukocytes in the blood products.	Fever, anaemia, increased bilirubin levels.	Stop the transfusion. Give premedications to reduce reaction: • promethazine • hydrocortisone.
Allergic reactions	Recipient antibodies against donor antigens (foreign proteins).	Itching to rashes to anaphylaxis and shock.	Stop the transfusion. Treat with antihistamines. May resume slowly when symptoms resolved.
Transfusion-related acute lung injury (TRALI)	Anti-HLA antibodies and neutrophil antibodies.	Acute respiratory insufficiency, chills, fever, cyanosis, hypotension.	Stop the transfusion. Support respiratory function, IV steroids.
Bacterial contamination of blood product	Endotoxins from gram-negative and gram-positive bacteria.	Fever, shock, disseminated intravascular coagulation (DIC), renal failure.	High-dose antibiotics. Vital organ support, steroids.
Circulatory overload	Too rapid a flow rate for client's cardiovascular system/renal system.	Dyspnoea, cough, frothy sputum, tachycardia.	Support respiratory system. Administer diuretic between units. Slower infusion rates for clients with known cardiovascular compromise.
Citrate toxicity	Hypocalcaemia resulting from citrate binding with calcium in the recipient's bloodstream.	Tetany (cramps, muscle twitching, tingling lips, seizures).	Monitor for signs and symptoms. Monitor calcium level. Transfuse extra calcium, if warranted.

Source: Clarke, L., Gray, S., White, L., Duncan, G. & Baumle, W. (2016). *Foundations of Nursing: Enrolled Division 2 Nurses* (ANZ Edition). Cengage Learning: South Melbourne, Table 22.8, p. 545.

20.3 Administering and storing medication

Medication administration is a large component of your role as a nurse. As a student, on your placement you will be able to administer medications with your buddy nurse or clinical facilitator. You will notice on placement that the facility will either have a lockable 'pill trolley' or a designated medication room that will have swipe card access so as to maintain the safe storage of medications (see **Figure 20.4**).

It is important to store medication according to the manufacturer's instructions. Some medication needs to be stored in the refrigerator or at a set temperature, such as supplies of insulin or eye drops. Other medication needs to be stored out of direct sunlight such as anginine tablets.

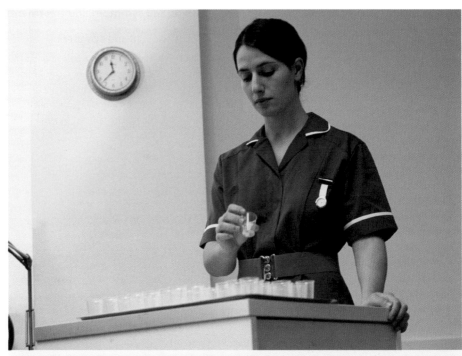

FIGURE 20.4 Using a medication trolley for the administration of medication

Applying the 'rights of medication administration'

Alongside the NIMC, for safe administration you will be required to adhere to the nine rights of medication administration. They are as follows:

1 Right client

The first step in medication administration is ensuring that the right person is given the right medication. A variety of checking procedures are carried out as listed below:

- Check the NIMC against the client's identity bracelet.
- Ask the client to verify their name, date of birth and any allergies they have.
- Check the adverse drug reactions on the front of the NIMC.

2 Right drug

To ensure that the right medication is delivered you must match the medication order on the medication chart with the name of the medication on the packet, bottle, ampoule or vial. In this step you should also be checking the *expiry dates of medications*. The expiry dates of medications can be found on the receptacle, container or packaging in which they are manufactured. This check is completed three times prior to administration:

- before removing the container from the drawer or shelf
- as the amount of medication is removed from the container
- before returning the container to storage.

3 Right dose

You must confirm you are administering the correct dose by checking the dose ordered on the medication sheet with the stock dose on the medication packaging. Again, this check is done three times before administration.

It is vital that you are confident about the unit measurements (grams, milligrams, micrograms) because you must have the same unit of stock and dosage ordered before applying your formula to calculate the correct dosage.

Pay careful attention to decimal points because an error could cause massive (and often lethal) overdosing. *Check, check and RECHECK your calculation.*

TIP 20.8
Calculating dosages
Work out your calculations on paper then recheck with a calculator. Ask the supervising registered nurse to check your calculation.

4 Right route

A drug may be presented in a variety of forms and administered via several different routes. Therefore, it is imperative that the correct route is followed as all drugs have a specific requirement for absorption. For example, anginine tablets are given sublingually and will not work if swallowed.

5 Right form

Medications are available in different forms such as syrups, suppositories and capsules. Always ensure the correct form is being used for your client.

6 Right time

To ensure that you understand the time written on the medication sheet you must be familiar with medical terminology associated with time, for example, TDS, BD, QID, daily. The NIMC also states that the prescriber must enter the administration time.

A frequent error in medication administration is when the nurse administers at the times listed without checking the frequency ordered; for example, if the drug is ordered TDS but times are charted as QID then the patient could receive an extra dose daily if this is not rectified.

7 Right documentation

The nurse must check the medication chart to ensure that the prescription is legal and clearly written. If anything is unclear, then they must check with the prescriber and have the documentation made clear. The nurse must also check to see if the medicine has already been given or if there is anything else wrong with the documentation before administering the medicine and signing the necessary documentation themselves.

8 Right response

The right response incorporates your assessment and you must monitor the patient for the desired outcome. Evaluating the effect of medication is vital for the patient's wellbeing.

9 Right to refuse

Clients have the right to refuse a medication, however, most are more likely to take the medication if they know why they are taking it. If a client refuses to take a medication the nurse charts this on the medication chart, informs the registered nurse or doctor and enters this into the client's file notes (Clarke et al., 2016).

Coupled with the nine rights is the responsibility of knowing what the drug does, what a normal dose is and how to administer it. These are all aspects of medication administration and you will need to ensure you understand these prior to administering the medication.

TIP 20.9

Safe storage of
medication
Always lock medication
away before leaving
the area. It is easy
for 10 minutes to go
by if an incident or
interruption occurs.
There can be serious
consequences if clients
or visitors access
dangerous medication.

Securing medications in a safe manner

When medications are being administered it is important to ensure the safety of the client and others. In acute wards some clients may be experiencing delirium or have dementia and may self-administer medications if the trolley is left unlocked. Visitors also need to be safeguarded so that children visiting relatives don't have access to dangerous medications.

For some clients, in areas where the medications are stored by the bedside, it is important for the above reasons to keep this drawer locked. The effect of some medications may cause confusion and the client may self-medicate or, if experiencing no relief and not being fully educated on the dangers of the medication, may also self-medicate in an attempt to hasten recovery.

Applying quality practices and undertaking risk assessment

Aside from the quality practices already discussed the Australian Commission on Safety and Quality in Health Care has a list of measures it advocates to reduce medication errors and harm from medicines. **Table 20.7** outlines these measures.

TABLE 20.7 Safe medication administration measures

Quality measure or action	Reason
Medication charts: https://www.safetyandquality.gov.au/our-work/medication-safety/medication-charts/	To standardise medication management and increase safety.
Medication reconciliation: https://www.safetyandquality.gov.au/our-work/medication-safety/medication-reconciliation/	To ensure the patient is given the medication that is prescribed.
Safer naming, labelling and packaging of medicines: https://www.safetyandquality.gov.au/our-work/medication-safety/safer-naming-labelling-and-packaging-of-medicines/	To ensure safe naming, labelling and packaging of medication.
High risk medicines: https://www.safetyandquality.gov.au/our-work/medication-safety/high-risk-medicines/	To prevent harm or death when using high risk medication.
Electronic medication management: https://www.safetyandquality.gov.au/our-work/medication-safety/electronic-medication-management/	To improve safety and quality of health care.
Quality use of medicines in hospitals: https://www.safetyandquality.gov.au/our-work/medication-safety/quality-use-of-medicines-in-hospitals/	To measure the safety and quality of medicines, identify improvement process and change health-care practices.
Medication safety in mental health: https://www.safetyandquality.gov.au/publications/medication-safety-in-mental-health/	To prevent serious side effects for people with a mental health illness who require long term medication therapy.
Medication safety tools and resources: https://www.safetyandquality.gov.au/our-work/medication-safety/medication-safety-tools-and-resources/	To ensure tools develop to increase medication safety.

Source: Australian Commission on Safety and Quality in Health Care (n.d.). Medication safety. Retrieved from https://www.safetyandquality.gov.au/our-work/medication-safety/. Accessed 9 January 2018.

Reporting refusal of medication or IV therapy or suspected incomplete medication ingestion

As it is important to gain consent before the administration of medication or IV therapy it can sometimes occur that the client refuses the intervention. This can be due to a variety of reasons. Some of these are:

• lack of knowledge
• false beliefs about the intervention
• religious or cultural beliefs
• mental health illness that causes faulty perception of intervention
• previous adverse side effects.

If the client refuses you cannot force them to undergo the intervention (see Chapter 4 on legal and ethical issues in nursing). You should report the refusal to the registered nurse and document according to the policies and procedures of the facility.

At other times it may occur that the person vomits after administration of medication or the intravenous cannula does not work and needs resiting. Both instances will result in the client not having the correct dose of medication administered. You must report these occurrences to the registered nurse and the doctor may order a new prescription or blood test to assist the client in having the correct dose.

Handling and storing of medications and blood products

As discussed previously medications may need to be stored in special conditions to ensure they are effective when administered. Some medications that are administered intravenously also have special storage or administration requirements. Some will need to be administered in a flask that is covered to prevent sunlight from inactivating the medication. Blood and blood products have special storage requirements. If left out of the refrigerator for a period of time blood will clump or coagulate. In some instances blood will need to be administered via a blood warmer to prevent complications for the client.

Activity 20.3

Blood and blood products

Locate the policies and procedures for blood and blood product administration.

1   When should blood or blood products be administered
2   Who can administer blood and blood products in the facility?
3   What checking requirements are needed before the administration of blood and blood products?
4   If an adverse reaction to the blood or blood product occurs what actions are required?

20.4 Monitoring and evaluating a person's response to administered medication, IV fluids, blood and blood products

Administering medications is just one of the many complex tasks a nurse needs to accomplish during the course of a shift. It requires knowledge of the actions, uses, and therapeutic and adverse reactions that occur with drug use. It is an integral part of many client's treatment and offers the nurse an opportunity to increase knowledge and skill and to observe the effects of various medications on disease processes as well as to educate clients in the effective use of their medications.

Documenting and monitoring the person's response

The concepts of safe and effective documentation are outlined in many previous chapters, such as Chapter 6. After you administer the medication, you need to document this. A component of administering medication is assessing and monitoring the client for their response to the medication. This can be a desired response, such as analgesia, or an adverse reaction, such as nausea and vomiting after administration of an opioid agent.

Acute and delayed adverse reactions

A drug allergy is an antigen-antibody immune reaction that occurs when a client has been exposed to a drug and has developed antibodies against the drug. The types of reactions can vary from mild, such as a rash, headache or nausea, to severe such as anaphylaxis, which is life threatening and requires immediate intervention. You will need to ask your client every time you administer a medication if they have allergies. Overlooking this and becoming familiar with a client can cause an error and potentially cause harm. It is always important to remain vigilant regarding allergies and ascertaining them.

CASE STUDY 20.2

Allergies and medication

Megan Ruiz is a 40-year-old female who has been admitted for community acquired pneumonia. Megan has been prescribed benzylpenicillin 2 g IV. She has no allergies documented on her NIMC. When you attend her bedside with another nurse to check and administer the medication Megan says she thinks she is allergic to penicillin, but is not sure what happens or if she has ever had it, as her mother is allergic to penicillin.

1 What would you do?
2 How would you document this?

Managing adverse drug reactions

Your management of an adverse drug reaction will depend upon the type of reaction, the severity of the reaction and whether the reaction is acute or delayed. If the adverse drug reaction is severe, additional medication or clinical procedures may be required; for example, if the reaction includes respiratory depression, you may need to initiate respiratory support. If the reaction is milder, such as a rash, then discontinuing or modifying the dose will be effective.

Your response to the adverse reaction will be relevant to the type of reaction. If the patient is experiencing anaphylaxis then a medical emergency call needs to be made and the support necessary for the patient must be provided – CPR, medications etc.

After any adverse drug reaction or event you need to document this in the client's notes and ensure the allergy is recorded so that the medication is not given again. **Figure 20.5** highlights the ADR table on the NIMC.

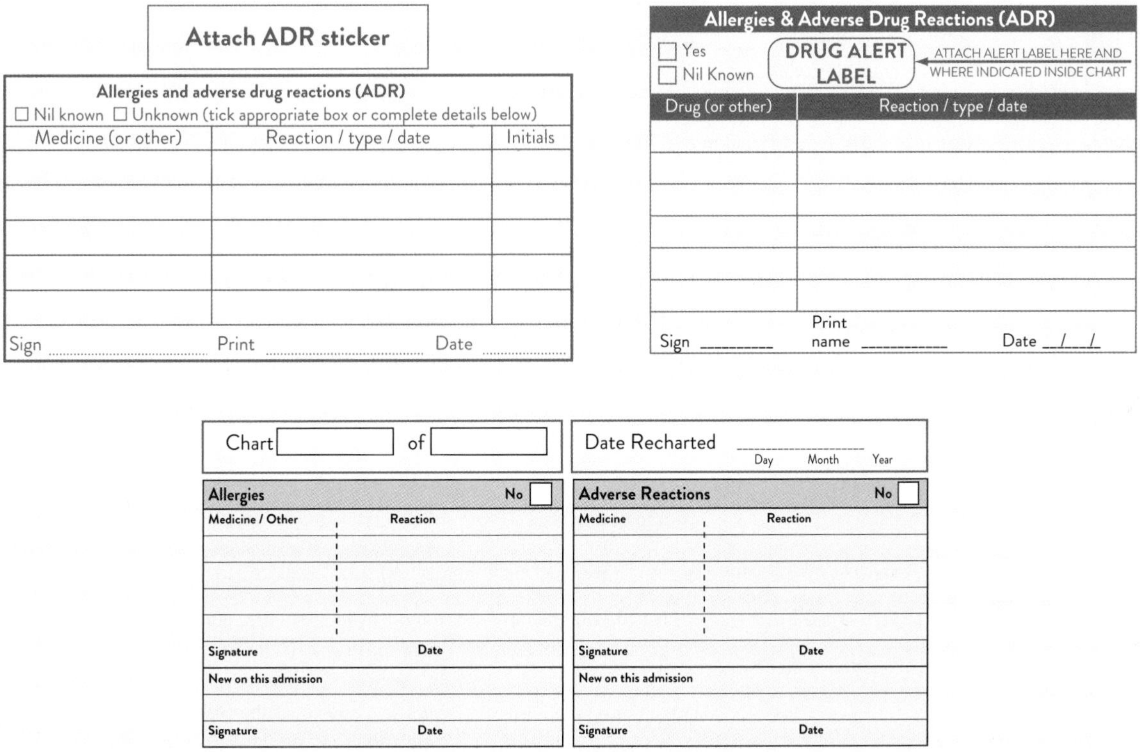

Attach ADR sticker

Allergies and adverse drug reactions (ADR)
☐ Nil known ☐ Unknown (tick appropriate box or complete details below)

Medicine (or other)	Reaction / type / date	Initials

Sign .... Print .... Date ....

Allergies & Adverse Drug Reactions (ADR)
☐ Yes   **DRUG ALERT LABEL** ATTACH ALERT LABEL HERE AND
☐ Nil Known   WHERE INDICATED INSIDE CHART

Drug (or other)	Reaction / type / date

Sign _____ Print name _____ Date __/__/__

Chart ☐ of ☐   Date Recharted ____ Day Month Year

Allergies   No ☐
Medicine / Other	Reaction
Signature ____ Date ____
New on this admission
Signature ____ Date ____

Adverse Reactions   No ☐
Medicine	Reaction
Signature ____ Date ____
New on this admission
Signature ____ Date ____

FIGURE 20.5 Adverse reactions and allergies chart on the NIMC

Source: Australian Commission on Safety and Quality in Health Care.

Fluid and electrolyte imbalances

Intravenous fluid is frequently used to maintain and restore fluid and electrolyte balance. When administering IVF there are three types of fluids:
- Hypotonic fluid – lowers osmotic pressure and makes fluid move into cells.
- Isotonic fluid – increases only extracellular fluid volume, does not change cell volume.
- Hypertonic fluid – increases osmotic pressure and draws fluid from the cells causing them to shrink.

Some examples of IVF can be seen in **Table 20.8**.

Measuring and recording all IVF and all output is often essential in ensuring that your patient is being monitored appropriately for a response to the IVF and medication administration.

Removing the IV cannula

IV cannulas are by far the most common access device you will monitor and administer medications via. They are short-term devices with most hospitals using a 72-hour rule for replacement. Evidence has shown that removing the cannula and resiting every 72 hours results in less incidence of phlebitis and associated infections.

TIP 20.10

Checking IV fluids
When checking IVF, discard the bag if it is wet when removed from the outer wrapper as this indicates the integrity of the bag is compromised. If the fluid is not clear, or there is sediment also discard the fluid. IVF should be clear and the bag should be intact.

TABLE 20.8 Common IV solutions

Tonicity	Solution	Contents (meq/l)	Clinical implications
Hypotonic	Sodium chloride 0.45%	77 Na$^+$, 77 Cl$^-$	Daily maintenance of body fluid and establishment of renal function.
Isotonic	Dextrose 2.5% in 0.45% saline	77 Na$^+$, 77 Cl$^-$	Promotes renal function and urine output.
	Dextrose 5% in 0.2% saline	77 Na$^+$, 77 Cl$^-$	Daily maintenance of body fluids when less Na$^+$ and Cl$^-$ are required.
	Dextrose 5% in water (D$_5$W)	38 Na$^+$, 38 Cl$^-$	Promotes rehydration and elimination; may cause urinary Na$^+$ loss; good vehicle for K$^+$.
	Ringer's lactate	130 Na$^+$, 4 K$^+$, Ca^{2+}, 109 Cl$^-$, 28 lactate	Resembles the normal composition of blood serum and plasma; K$^+$ level below body's daily requirement.
	Normal saline (NS), 0.9%	154 Na$^+$, 154 Cl$^-$	Restores sodium chloride deficit and extracellular fluid volume.
	Dextran 40 10% in NS (0.9%) or D$_5$W	zero Na Cl K Ca – just 50g of Dextrose	A colloidal solution used to increase plasma volume of clients in early shock; it should not be given to severely dehydrated clients and clients with renal disease, thrombocytopenia or active haemorrhaging.
	Dextran 70% in NS	Na 154 Cl: 154 no potassium or calcium	A long-lived (20 hours) plasma volume expander; used to treat shock or impending shock caused by haemorrhage, surgery or burns. It can prolong bleeding and coats the red blood cells (RBCs) (draw type and cross-match before administering).
Hypertonic	Dextrose 5% in 0.45% saline	77 Na$^+$, 77 Cl$^-$	Daily maintenance of body fluid and nutrition; treatment of fluid volume deficit (FVD).
	Dextrose 5% in saline 0.9%	154 Na$^+$, 154 Cl$^-$	Fluid replacement of sodium, chloride and calories (170).
	Dextrose 10% in saline 0.9%	154 Na$^+$, 154 Cl$^-$	Fluid replacement of sodium, chloride and calories (340).
	Dextrose 5% in lactated Ringer's	130 Na$^+$, 4 K$^+$, 3 Ca^{2+}, 109 Cl$^-$, 28 lactate	Resembles the normal composition of blood serum and plasma; K$^+$ level below body's daily requirement; caloric value 180.
	Hyperosmolar saline 3% and 5% NaCl	856 Na$^+$, 865 Cl$^-$	Treatment of hyponatremia; raises the Na osmolarity of the blood and reduces intracellular fluid excess.
	Ionosol B with dextrose 5%	57 Na$^+$, 25 K$^+$, 49 Cl$^-$, 25 lact., 5 Mg^{2+}, 7 PO^{4-}	Treatment of polyionic parenteral replacement caused by vomiting-induced alkalosis, diabetic acidosis, fluid loss from burns and postoperative FVD.

Source: Kee, J., Paulanka, B. & Polek, C. (2009). *Fluids and Electrolytes with Clinical Applications: A Programmed Approach* (7th edition). Delmar Cengage Learning: Clifton Park, NY.

A client receiving intravenous medication therapy requires especially close observation and the nurse needs to be aware of the signs and symptoms of any possible complications. Common complications are infiltration, phlebitis, thrombophlebitis and bleeding. Other complications include:

- circulatory overload
- hypersensitivity
- infiltration
- systemic infection
- venous spasm
- speed shock.

Pain, swelling, redness and ooze are all signs indicating that the cannula requires removal for patient safety and comfort. Best practice currently adheres to the Visual Infusion Phlebitis Score (VIPS) as shown in **Figure 20.6**. This is a scale where the cannula is reviewed and monitored and resited if any element of phlebitis is present.

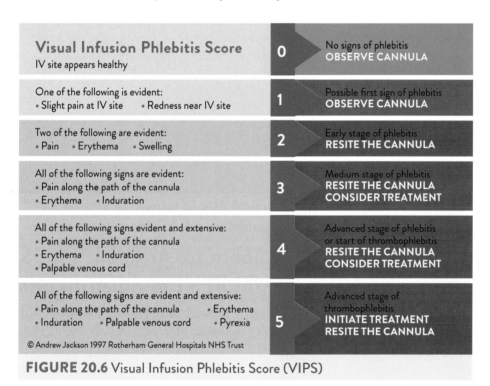

FIGURE 20.6 Visual Infusion Phlebitis Score (VIPS)

With permission from Andrew Jackson, IV Nurse Consultant, The Rotherham NHS Foundation Trust, UK. Copyright Andrew Jackson 1997.

The removal of the IV cannula (IVC) needs to follow the principles of infection control. If the IVC is being removed because the client is being discharged or if the IVC has become a source of infection, the removal is the same.

Reflective practice 20.1

Cannulas here there and everywhere

Over the course of my career, I have made it my 'thing' to ensure I assess all my patients and review cannulas every shift. This started five years ago because in one patient a cannula was left in for five days. No one noticed it, including myself, because she had another cannula we were using. The patient was a 78-year-old lady, who wore a cardigan all the time. She had a large bore IV cannula in her cubital fossa. It was inserted most likely by the ambulance and was not documented in any admission notes. This is by no means an excuse. Her fevers increased, her response to antibiotic therapy was poor, and we were all at a loss for the source of infection. The cannula, when found, was red, inflamed, tracking infection up her arm and clearly the source of her blood borne infection. Ever since this incident, I check all limbs on my patients for cannulas and if it is not labelled (for instance if they are a transfer) or I cannot tell when the cannula was put in, I will remove it. It also highlighted to me that all IVs are a potential source of infection and infection control in using/accessing the IV is paramount.

Whenever I have a student buddy with me, I will always go through a skin inspection with them to show them the importance of assessing skin integrity and IVC placement.

Justin, 38, Enrolled Nurse

1 Why do you think skin inspection is crucial in patient assessment?
2 What do you think could have occurred if the cannula was not found?
3 Where do you think IVC sites should be documented?

Review the skill in Tollefson *Essential Clinical Skills* 6.3 Peripheral intravenous cannula (PIVC) and therapy (PIVT) management

Educating the person, their family or carer on administration of medicines

No matter what the type of medication, or the route, it is essential for you to discuss the whole process with the client. How well the client understands the medication will be an important factor in their willingness to comply with a regimen.

The four most important components to ensure your client understands are:

1 action and purpose of the medication
2 importance of regular dosage
3 proper administration methods and techniques
4 possible side effects.

A good way to ascertain the client understands the medication or dose is to ask them to explain it to you.

20.5 Assessing the effectiveness of pain-relieving therapy

Pain is a phenomenon found in all nursing specialties. The experience of pain can have a significant impact upon the client and their health. Assessment of pain is essential to determine if analgesia can be administered in order to provide relief for your client (Clarke et al., 2016).

Identifying signs of pain or discomfort

Assessment of pain in your client is an essential nursing intervention. It should be noted that pain is a personal experience with many influencing factors such as age, previous experience with pain, and cultural norms. Pain assessment requires both subjective and objective data.

Subjective data can be obtained by asking the client to rate their pain on a scale of 1–10 with 10 being the worst pain imaginable. It is also useful to assess pain using the PQRST process. **Figure 20.7** outlines this assessment.

MEMORY TRICK

Pain assessment: PQRST

P = What Provokes the pain (aggravating factors) and palliative measures (alleviating factors)

Q = Quality of pain (gnawing, pounding, burning, stabbing, pinching, aching, throbbing and crushing)

R = Region (location) and radiation to other body sites

S = Severity (quantity of pain on 0–10 scale: 0 = no pain and 10 = worst pain experienced) and setting (what causes the pain)

T = Timing (onset, duration, frequency)

Adapted from Estes, 2010.

FIGURE 20.7 PQRST process for pain assessment

Source: Clarke, L., Gray, S., White, L., Duncan, G. & Baumle, W. (2016). *Foundations of Nursing: Enrolled Division 2 Nurses* (ANZ Edition). Cengage Learning: South Melbourne, p. 582.

Clarify the location and nature of pain

When assessing your client, there are some objective signs that indicate pain:

- increased heart rate
- increased blood pressure
- increased respiratory rate.

This information coupled with a client's subjective data can provide you with the information required to administer analgesia. It is important to ask the following questions:

- Where is the pain?
- When did it start?
- What type of pain is it? (dull, sharp, crushing)
- Does anything relieve the pain?
- How would you rate the severity of the pain? (use of pain scale)

Interpreting observations and evaluating the person's pain

The use of a documented chart for pain assessment is useful for:

- evaluating whether pain management strategies are working
- consistency of staff assessing client's level of pain.

Other documentation that assists in interpreting and evaluating the person's pain is the documentation of vital signs. By comparing the pain chart with the vital sign chart we should be able to see a correlation. For example, if blood pressure is elevated with the pain experience we should see a drop in the blood pressure when the pain is relieved.

Review the skill in
Tollefson *Essential
Clinical Skills* 7.1
Documentation

The documentation in the client's file should also reflect the situation and the outcome of interventions.

Prescribed medications and complementary strategies that may alleviate pain and discomfort

There are many forms of analgesia. Simple analgesia begins with medications such as paracetamol and ibuprofen. Other forms of analgesia include:

- morphine
- oxycontin
- fentanyl
- hydromorphone
- tramadol.

The type of analgesia used will depend on the condition that person has. For example a surgical patient may require administration of morphine for the first 24 hours post-operatively but then have the pain controlled by oral analgesia.

With pain relief nursing interventions can also involve:

- massage
- repositioning
- heat packs
- education – if a person is uncertain of why they are experiencing pain their response may be intensified due to fear and anxiety.

Assessing effectiveness of pain-relieving medication and non-medication therapies

When giving pain relieving medication and other therapies (see **Figure 20.8**) it is important to note what is working to relieve the pain for the person and what is not working. This may alert the doctor to change the pain relief medication or the frequency or method of administration. Examples of this are the breakthrough dosages that are ordered or the combination of both parental and oral medication to alleviate the pain. It will also be necessary to document in the care plan and client file notes what is working for the client so oncoming staff can undertake these interventions.

Recording observations of the effectiveness of pain management strategies

Working as part of the health-care team includes good communication skills. By documenting in the client's file and on their charts their episodes of pain and response to interventions the team can adjust the care plan to achieve the best outcome for the client. Your evaluations of the effectiveness of the pain management strategies are also important to give a clear picture of the response to the interventions. It is important to record data that is objective or subjective comments from the client and not your own opinion. An example of this is 'after administration of analgesia the client reported a lessening of the level of pain and was able to ambulate to the bathroom with supervision'.

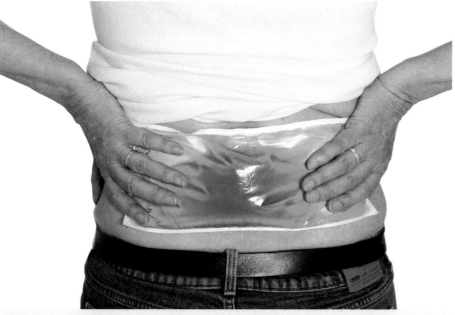

FIGURE 20.8 Non-pharmacological pain relief therapy

Science Photo Library/Lea Paterson.

CASE STUDY 20.3

Pain assessment

Harmony Williams is a 28-year-old female who has presented to hospital for abdominal pain. She is sitting upright in bed and when you walk in to assess her pain she is texting on her phone. During the conversation Harmony continues to text and interact on her phone. Her blood pressure, pulse and respirations are within normal limits. When you ask her to rate her pain out of 10, she states it is 10/10.

1   How would you document this pain assessment?
2   What type of analgesia would you consider offering Harmony if her ordered medication was paracetamol and Oxycontin?
3   Do you think her pain score is accurate?

SUMMARY

- In order to minimise risk with medication administration it essential to know the purpose and functions of prescribed medications and intravenous therapy.
- Medications and blood and blood products may have substances that the patient is incompatible with.
- To prepare for safe administration of medication and intravenous fluids the nurse must prepare the client, consider the effects of the medications, calculate the correct dosage and prepare the medication according to legislative and regulatory requirements.
- Medications and intravenous fluids may need special storage and administration requirements.
- Refusal of medication needs to be reported and documented according to the facility's policies and procedures.
- When administering medication and intravenous fluids the nurse must monitor the effects on the client and assess the effectiveness of the treatment.
- Pain relief may be given in the form of medication and alternative treatments. The nurse needs to monitor the effectiveness of the interventions and document the patient's response to them.

SELF-TEST QUESTIONS

1 What strategies are you aware of that are used to minimise the potential risks of medication administration?
2 Can you list the steps required for the preparation of medication administration and infusion of IV fluids?
3 What responsibilities does the nurse have in the administration and storage of medication?
4 How can the nurse monitor and evaluate a person's response to medications, IV fluids and blood and blood products?
5 Outline the actions the nurse needs to take to assess the effectiveness of pain-relieving therapy.

BIBLIOGRAPHY

Australian Commission on Safety and Quality in Health Care (n.d.). *Medication safety.* Retrieved from https://www.safetyandquality.gov.au/our-work/medication-safety/. Accessed 9 January 2018.

Australian Commission on Safety and Quality in Health Care (2011). *Recommendations for terminology, abbreviations and symbols used in the prescribing and administration of medicines.* Retrieved from http://www.safetyandquality.gov.au/wp-content/uploads/2012/01/32060v2.pdf. Accessed 14 March 2017.

Australian Commision on Safety and Quality in Health Care (2012). *Standard 4: Medication safety.* Retrieved from https://www.safetyandquality.gov.au/wp-content/uploads/2012/10/Standard4_Oct_2012_WEB.pdf.

Australian Commission on Safety and Quality in Health Care (2014). *National Inpatient Medication Chart user guide.* Retrieved from http://www.safetyandquality.gov.au/wp-content/uploads/2014/07/NIMC-User-Guide.pdf.

Australian Institute of Health & Wellness (2017). *Admitted patient care 2015-16: Australian hospital statistics.* Retrieved from https://www.aihw.gov.au/reports/hospitals/admitted-patient-care-ahs-2015-16/contents/table-of-contents. Accessed 14 March 2017.

Brotto, V. & Rafferty, K. (2012). *Clinical Dosage Calculations for Australia & New Zealand.* Cengage Learning: South Melbourne.

Broyles, B.E., Reiss, B.S., Evans, M.E., McKenzie, G., Pleunik, S. & Page, R. (2017). *Pharmacology in Nursing* (2nd edition) Cengage Learning: South Melbourne.

Bullock, S., Manias, E. & Galbraith, A. (2010). *Fundamentals of Pharmacology* (5th edition). Retrieved from http://wps.pearsoned.com.au/au_hss_bullock_fundpharma_5/56/14448/3698900.cw/index.html. Accessed 12 March 2017.

Clarke, L., Gray, S., White, L., Duncan, G. & Baumle, W. (2016). *Foundations of Nursing: Enrolled Division 2 Nurses* (ANZ Edition). Cengage Learning: South Melbourne.

Crisp, J., Taylor, C., Douglas, C., & Rebeiro, G. (2013). *Potter and Perry's Fundamentals of Nursing,* 4th Edition. Elsevier: Sydney, NSW.

DeLaune, S.C., Ladner, P.K., McTier, L., Tollefson, J. & Lawrence, J. (2016). *Australian and New Zealand Fundamentals of Nursing* (revised edition), Cengage Learning: South Melbourne.

Harris, P., Nagy, S., & Vardaxis, N. (eds) (2010). *Mosby's Dictionary of Medicine, Nursing and Health Professions* (2nd edition). Elsevier: Sydney.

Kee, J., Paulanka, B. & Polek, C. (2009). *Fluids and Electrolytes with Clinical Applications: A Programmed Approach* (7th edition). Delmar Cengage Learning: Clifton Park, NY.

McCallum, L. & Higgins, D. (2012). 'Care of peripheral venous cannula sites', *Nursing Times,* 108(34/35).

Mckenna, L. & Lim, A.G. (2012). *Karch's Pharmacology for Nursing and Midwifery,* 1st Australian and New Zealand Edition. Lippincott Williams & Wilkins: Macquarie Park, NSW.

MIMS Australia (2013). Retrieved from http://www.mims.com.au/. Accessed March 12, 2017.

PainEdu.org (2013). *The pathophysiology of pain.* Retrieved from https://www.painedu.com/tools/pathophysiology_pain.asp. Accessed 12 March 2017.

RMIT University (2011). *Nursing calculations.* Retrieved from https://emedia.rmit.edu.au/learninglab/content/nursing-calculations. Accessed 12 March 2017.

Tollefson, J., Watson, G., Jelly, E. & Tambree, K. (2016). *Essential Clinical Skills: Enrolled Division 2 Nurses* (3rd edition). Cengage Learning: South Melbourne.

Care for a person with acute health problems

LEARNING OUTCOMES

After reading this chapter, you should have an understanding of:

21.1 Identifying the impact of acute health problems on a person, family or carer

21.2 Planning care for a person with acute health problems

21.3 Performing nursing interventions to support health care of a person with acute health problems

21.4 Contributing to pre- and post-operative nursing care of a person with acute health problems

21.5 Contributing to an emergency response in the acute care environment

Undertaking acute placement

This was my final placement before qualifying as an enrolled nurse. I was determined to show how competent I was and was looking forward to delivering acute nursing care to people.

I had already completed aged care and rehabilitation placements and had gained a lot of experience in administering medications, so I felt confident of being able to do so in this acute area.

The first day on placement was a real eye opener. The hospital was enormous with many departments and a large team of staff. I was assigned to the surgical area and from the time I stepped onto the floor till I completed the shift I ran. Patients needed to be made ready for theatre and then before you knew it they were coming back and required post-operative care. I had never seen so many intravenous drips and the number of intravenous medications were huge. The clinical supervisor instructed me to take my time and complete the checking procedure correctly. I was glad that she was there as so many medications sounded the same and it took me a while before I was able to really recognise the treatments without having to look them up.

Surgical dressing wounds were also a steep learning curve. There were many different types of dressings, some with vac dressings that had been applied in theatre and some that were surgical sites with only a transparent cover on top. My buddy showed me where to look in the post-operative orders for the nursing care that was required and this made my life a little easier as I was worried that I would not know what to do. At the end of the placement I felt that this was an area that I would really enjoy working in.

21.1 Impact of acute health problems on the person, family or carer

Acute health covers accidents and injuries, so you will learn quickly about the different types of fractures and traumatic injuries and their treatment and management. Eventually it will not surprise you that yet another person has come into hospital because of a misadventure or senseless accident!

One of the biggest challenges you will face will be remembering the clinical terms for the vast array of pathophysiological states and injuries associated with acute health. You will notice 'hyper' and 'hypo' are used for many terms, so if you can remember the meaning for both it will enable you to start picking apart the terms to gain understanding.

There will be many acute conditions to which you will gain exposure and experience across not only your clinical placement but also your nursing career. One of the skills required when working in acute care is the ability to identify acute problems that require urgent medical and nursing interventions. It is often a very stressful environment with patients requiring urgent attention and often anxious family members in attendance.

Reflective practice 21.1

Emergency department presentations

Emergency departments typically have a large number of patients presenting on a daily basis. In Australia during 2015–16 there were 7.5 million presentations to public hospital emergency departments nationally (AIHW, 2016). There are many reasons for this number of presentations, including after-hours need for medical assistance and free access to medical services, for example, X-ray, pathology and physiotherapy. The top three presentations to emergency departments for 2015–16 were:

1 abdominal and pelvic pain
2 pain in throat and chest
3 injury of unspecified body region.

Almost every patient that presents to emergency is presenting with an acute illness or injury (AIHW, 2016).

Preliminary health assessment and the health-care team

Acute care nurses should assess the client for urgent and emergency conditions, using both physiologically and technologically derived data, to evaluate for physiological instability and potential life-threatening conditions. It is always important to address the basic life functions – airway, breathing and circulation – on presentation of a client to an acute health-care facility.

Once this has been completed you will then undertake a preliminary assessment of the client, as discussed in Chapter 5. A more focused assessment is then undertaken concerning the reason for the patient's arrival at the hospital. At times the problem is evident, such as a broken leg where you can see the actual bone coming out of the skin, but at other times it is more difficult, such as in the case of abdominal pain that can have many causes.

The myriad of conditions and injuries that are acutely caused is too exhaustive to list, but common acute conditions are the result of accident or injury or an infective process (such as appendicitis) systemically. There are systemic responses to acute injury, such as hypovolaemic shock, that occur due to volume depletion, which can have many causes – bleeding, both internal and external, fluid loss through diarrhoea and vomiting, and multiple injuries. Other common acute conditions are fractures, respiratory distress and chest pain.

As in all areas of health-care the staff work together as a team to address the person's problems. General assessment is usually undertaken by the doctor and the nurse on presentation of the client. When the client is more stable other team members will undertake a more specific assessment such as assessing mobilisation by the physio or assessing swallowing by the speech therapist.

The most important clinical skills in acute care that you will use will be your observational skills – patient assessment is paramount as no two injuries are the same! You could have two patients with exactly the same mechanism of injury who will respond to it completely differently. They will have different levels of pain (as pain is personal), different amounts of bleeding and inflammation, and different recovery time. Even when comparing an operation – for example, laparoscopic appendectomy – each patient will have varying levels of post-operative pain, varying levels of nausea and vomiting post-anaesthesia and varying differences in mobility post-operatively.

Review the skill in Tollefson *Essential Clinical Skills* 3.1 Professional workplace skills – including time management, rounding and personal stress management; 2.3 Temperature, pulse and respiration (TPR) measurement; 2.4 Blood pressure measurement; 3.3 Assisting the patient to ambulate; 3.4 Assisting the patient with eating and drinking; 3.8 Urinalysis and urine specimen collection

Activity 21.1

Bleeding

I will never forget my placement in Emergency. I was so incredibly surprised about just how much injuries can bleed. Some lacerations to fingers bled so much that I was worried that the patient would not stay conscious. It really assisted with quantifying blood loss and seeing the immediate effects of blood loss on a patient. One man came in and was perfectly calm. He said to the triage nurse that he had cut himself. My preceptor and I were then asked to take his dressing down and review it – we took off the dressing and there was blood spurting out! He had nicked his artery with a saw – and all the signs of blood loss were present – he was pale, sweaty and hypotensive! There was blood everywhere. And the smell! Blood has a very specific smell. I highly recommend placement in emergency to see so many little accidents and injuries to make you appreciate how much can go wrong, but also how to assess bleeding, and basic patient assessment.

Emma, 26, EN

1   What physiological changes occur in blood loss, in particular to the cardiovascular system?
2   What would you do if a patient presented with to you with a wound that was spurting blood?

Physical and psychological impacts of acute problems on the client and the family or carer

The nature of acute injury and illness is diverse. Almost all acute illnesses and/or injuries are unexpected. This generally means that the client and their family will not be prepared for the impact of the acute health condition. Your role will include discussing the processes and planned care with the client alongside the medical and allied health-care team. Families and the client alike will most likely have many questions, and this is where you will need to consider the impact the injury or illness can have on the client, and plan your care around this. An acute health problem can see a client go from being independent with self-care to one requiring full assistance with activities of daily living.

Reflective practice 21.2

Acute nursing

Some of the most challenging shifts in my nursing career have been due to the nature of the injury or illness. Families and the patient don't have time to prepare, everything is all new, all frightening and there are always so many questions. Someone having an accident on the way home from work is potentially devastating to a family. There are many emotions, and it is always not just about the patient. The family will call, they will attend, and they will have so many questions. I always think that if it were me in that situation I would want someone to answer all of my questions, so I really try to be empathetic and as patient as possible, because every single one of us reacts differently to stress.

Megan, 40, EN

1   What are two non-verbal communicating factors you could employ when liaising with family?
2   What would you do if you were asked a question concerning your patient that you did not know the answer for?

Pathophysiology

There are many common acute care conditions, these include:

- fractures
- myocardial infarction
- cerebrovascular accident (stroke)
- laceration
- allergic reaction
- pneumonia
- pneumothorax
- migraine.

You will need to rely upon your foundation anatomy and physiology and the application of this to your client's condition. Some conditions will be unusual or 'weird' – you will need to source information regarding treatment methods or the pathophysiological process of the condition. Some overdoses or ingestions of medicines or poisons can occur rarely or infrequently, so staff may not be aware of the impact and will need to source information.

CASE STUDY 21.1

The interrelatedness of body systems

Margaret Jason is a 39-year-old who has presented post a motor vehicle accident. She has been in hospital for two days. The injuries sustained are:

- fractured clavicle
- lacerated liver
- fractured #4 rib.

1   With these injuries, what are some pathophysiological processes in place that could affect Margaret's recovery?
2   What nursing considerations would you have for Margaret?

21.2 Planning care for a person with acute health problems

All patients with acute health conditions will commence their hospital journey through the emergency department. All patients go through the emergency department and are managed for either admission or discharge. This may be the first presentation of the client to the facility or a repeat presentation. In all cases a new plan of care is formulated to address the needs of the client on the current presentation.

Health-care team and care planning

Upon admission to either emergency or to the ward you will need to perform and document a complete system-focused or symptom-specific physical assessment. A client, for instance, may be presenting for a laparoscopic open cholecystectomy. The nurse needs to assess the health status not only related to the operative region, but also to the whole body. For example, this client may have an associated respiratory condition that will increase the risk in the operative and post-operative phase.

Although other medical problems are not often the priority of the admission, it is important to understand how they will impact on the present treatments. The current acute episode could also exacerbate other underlying medical conditions. These assessments then can be used to plan the care required for the client.

All members of the health-care team are involved in the creation of the care plan for the client. Some of the team will have specialised knowledge and skills that can be utilised to address the needs of the client. Communication of the assessments may be verbal such as in meetings or written in the client file.

When assessing the status of an acute care client, all body systems must be assessed.

Activity 21.2

The health-care team

For the area that you are working in, identify the different health-care members involved in providing support to clients.

1   What are their specialised skills?

Gather information, document and report changes to health-care team members

Explore the theory in *Foundations of Nursing* Chapter 23: Assessment

It is the nurse's role to constantly evaluate the client's progress in achieving the goals of the planned care. You will use subjective and objective data to evaluate the client's condition and needs and clearly document this in the care plan or the client file.

In some instances, the client's condition may deteriorate and you need to communicate this information clearly and quickly to the different members of the health-care team. In an emergency situation you may need to call a Code Blue in response to the client's condition. In other less critical situations, you may need to communicate to a member of the health-care team via telephone, such as when the client is experiencing pain despite receiving the pain relief ordered.

TIP 21.1

Communicating changes in the client's condition

When communicating with other members of the health-care team for a specific reason, the nurse needs to have assessed the client and recorded the vital signs and focused assessments (such as pain or wound bleeding). Always have all the client's records and assessment charts at hand before ringing another member of the health-care team.

A client may be too tired or ill due to disease processes to advocate for themselves and will need another person to take on this role. Client advocacy refers to speaking on behalf of a client in order to protect their rights and help them obtain needed information and services.

CASE STUDY 21.2

Advocacy

Brendan Tysoe is a 19-year-old male who has been brought to hospital via ambulance following a motor vehicle accident. Brendan has sustained a lacerated liver and requires a blood transfusion. He has consented to the blood transfusion. When you are checking the blood products with another nurse Brendan's mother arrives and in a raised voice says 'Get that blood away from my son! He cannot receive blood products. What are you doing?'

Brendan has consented to the blood products and has not identified any religious beliefs on the patient administration information.

1   How could you advocate for Brendan in this situation?
2   What questions would you need to ask both Brendan and his mother?
3   In what instances would blood products be withheld?

21.3 Performing nursing interventions to support health care

Often in the acute area the client will require specialised nursing interventions to address their health needs. An example of this is the client who has chest tubes and underwater seal drainage in situ to reinflate the lung. Training is given to staff to manage specific acute nursing interventions. See **Table 21.1** for an overview of specific nursing interventions in the acute nursing arena.

Activity 21.3

Blood transfusions

Locate the policies and procedures manual for administering blood transfusions to a client.
1   Is there any specialised equipment required?
2   When can blood transfusions be administered?
3   Where is the blood obtained from?
4   What do you need to monitor when administering a blood product to a client?
5   What should you do if you notice an adverse reaction to a blood transfusion?

Compromised airway

Airway obstruction or a compromised airway can be partial or complete and constitutes a medical emergency. An airway can be threatened for many reasons, including a decreased level of consciousness related to medication administration or a head injury. Any threatened airway warrants a medical emergency call. Remember that the airway compromise may not be related directly to the acute health condition with which the patient presented. Refer to **Table 21.1** for further information on nursing interventions required for respiratory care.

TABLE 21.1 Acute nursing interventions

Intervention	Reasons why the intervention is undertaken	Tollefson Clinical Skill
Isolation nursing	For immunosuppressed clients For staff protection from infectious diseases	*8.1 Oxygen therapy (includes peak flow meter)*
Gowning and gloving	For infection-control management for clients who are compromised such as the client with a CVC/Picc line When undertaking invasive procedures such as catheterisation	*4.9 Gowning and gloving (open and closed)*
Catheterisation	To drain the bladder for clients who cannot mobilise To obtain accurate fluid output measures When the bladder is unable to be emptied normally	*8.6 Catheterisation (urinary)*
Chest tubes and underwater seal drainage	For clients who have a collapsed lung due to disease or a build-up of fluid in the pleural space	*4.11 Chest drains and underwater seal drainage (UWSD) management*
Nasogastric tube insertion	For clients when the gut is not functioning to drain off secretions When clients have a bowel obstruction For short-term feeding	*8.11 Nasogastric tube insertion* *8.12 Enteral feeding (nasogastric and gastrostomy tube)*
Pre-operative care	To prepare a client for a surgical procedure	*8.2 Pre-operative care*
Post-operative care	To provide nursing care for a client who has undergone a surgical procedure	*8.4 Post-operative care*
Tracheostomy care	A stoma that is made to enable the client to take in air through an opening in the trachea	*8.9 Tracheostomy care*
Pulse oximetry	Monitoring of a client's oxygen level to ensure adequate oxygenation of circulating blood	*2.5 Pulse oximetry*

Prioritising and modifying nursing interventions to reflect changes in the person's condition

All acute care interventions are relative to the needs of the patient and the severity of their injuries. For example, a client admitted via the emergency department after a road trauma will have had basic priorities to sustain life addressed, but the admitting nurse will also be considering other needs such as support and family. As the client moves from the emergency department to a non-acute ward, other needs of the client are prioritised.

Observe and identify the need for psychological support and care

As previously discussed, maintaining clients' independence is important as dependency disempowers clients. Clients or their family members can gain self-satisfaction by achieving even the smallest of tasks when they are recovering from acute illness and dependency.

Holistic care ensures that these needs are all incorporated into the nursing care as they all interrelate and impact upon health outcomes. A client who isn't having their emotional or psychosocial needs met is at risk of not being able to meet the physical demands of the nursing interventions. For example, the client may be anxious and scared of what is happening to them. This increases stress, which increases the client's blood pressure and can increase pain. The client is less likely to tolerate nursing interventions in this emotional state.

In the acute nursing arena clients are facing acute changes in their normal functioning. This change from being independent to relying on others to meet needs can cause anxiety and depression. For some clients having a barrage of medical equipment can also cause stress. The nurse needs to provide clear explanations of treatments and observe the client for signs of stress and anxiety.

21.4 Pre- and post-operative nursing care

After the assessment and planning phases, what happens next? In many facilities, an efficient admission with a well-designed checklist can confirm that the patient is appropriately prepared for theatre and assist with early detection of any issues.

A thorough health assessment of the client helps to identify and correct problems prior to surgery, and establishes a baseline for post-operative comparison. When performing the assessment you will need to not just focus on the problem area indicated by the client's history but also the body system that is being operated on.

Activity 21.4

Preparing clients for surgery

Locate the folder or file on how to prepare a client for a specific surgical intervention.

1   What pre-operative care do they require?
2   Where do you obtain the specialised equipment such as specific body washes and theatre clothing for clients?
3   What type of labelling is required to be placed on the patient prior to going to theatre?

Review the skill in
Tollefson *Essential
Clinical Skills*
8.2 Pre-operative care

Your role may include the preparation of the client for diagnostic tests pre-operatively, such as laboratory tests.

Laboratory tests may include:

* full blood count
* urea and electrolytes
* prothrombin time
* activated partial thromboplastin time
* urinalysis.

Activity 21.5

Blood tests

Locate the blood tubes for taking blood. Can you identify which tube is used for each of the blood tests listed above? How much blood do you need to obtain for each of the tests? Where do you take the blood tubes when you have obtained the blood samples?

1   What specific documentation is required to complete for blood testing?

Considerations prior to the operating room are as follows:

- nutritional deficiencies
- steroid use
- radiation or chemotherapy
- drug or alcohol abuse
- metabolic diseases such as diabetes
- smoking.

These are important as medications used can be altered in their distribution, for example, if the patient abuses alcohol or drugs. It is essential to obtain a holistic history of your client prior to the surgical procedure, unless of course the surgery is life sustaining!

When collating data, the client's allergy status should be noted. If the client does have an allergy, ensure that it is documented on the National Inpatient Medication Chart (NIMC) and in any other component of the chart such as the allergy register.

Reflective practice 21.3

Theatre preparation

The first few times I looked after a pre-operative patient I could not believe all the checklists and paperwork involved. There were three pages of checklists that needed to be completed by three different nurses. It was then I realised the seriousness of an operation. Not just the actual operation, but also the correct limb, correct patient, there are so many variables. Then there are the potential complications intra-operatively and post-operatively. Surgery is a BIG deal!

Caitlyn Jane, 22, EN

1 What are the National Safety and Quality Health Service (NSQHS) standards relevant to this situation?
2 Your patient asks you 'why are you asking me my name and all that bizzo again?' How would you explain the reasoning?

Post-operative care for your client is going to require ongoing education and support and collaboration with allied health professionals, such as a physiotherapist for post-operative exercises and activities. Examples include deep breathing exercises, coughing instructions (splinting an abdominal wound, for example), TED stockings and mobilisation.

It is also a good idea to discuss post-operative matters with your client, such as:

- multiple intravenous lines
- drainage tubes
- dressings
- monitoring devices.

Promoting post-operative comfort using pain management strategies

Pain management is the primary concern for many clients having surgery. Pre-operative instruction should include information about the pain management method that they will utilise post-operatively.

Finally, the client should understand long-term goals such as when he or she will be able to eat solid food, go home, drive a car and return to work.

Refer to **Table 21.1** for more information on pre- and post-operative care.

21.5 Emergency response in the acute care environment

Emergency situations happen every day in hospitals. With the introduction of observation charts that focus on the detection of the deteriorating patient, the emergent situation is more likely to be pre-arrest rather than a full cardiac arrest. Anaphylaxis is also a very real situation in the acute care environment.

Emergency equipment is commonly kept together on an emergency trolley in most health-care facilities. It is essential that nursing staff are familiar with this equipment, can access it quickly in an emergency, and can assist in its use. It is a nursing responsibility to ensure that the trolley has all items on it, and is checked as per the unit/hospital protocol. While the layout of the emergency trolleys can vary between facilities, the equipment used is essentially the same. Many health services have standardised emergency trolleys, which assist in staff being able to locate items quickly.

Emergency trolleys contain adjuncts for advanced life support so there is equipment to provide an artificial airway, medication to initiate cardiac response, and other equipment to initiate or administer treatment. Then there is the defibrillator. Getting familiar with the emergency trolley is a good thing – no matter how overwhelming it can be; you never know when an emergency may occur.

Activity 21.6

The resuscitation trolley

Locate the resuscitation trolley. Volunteer to check the trolley. You may need permission to do so and may also require a registered nurse to assist in this action.

1. How often is the trolley checked?
2. Can you identify all the equipment on the trolley?
3. Locate the medication protocols for resuscitation. What is the protocol for a person who has a cardiac arrest?

Medical Emergency Team

Medical Emergency Teams (METs) are pre-planned groups of health-care practitioners who respond to acute deteriorations in hospitalised clients. They are usually identical to hospital 'code' teams, with the exception that they respond prior to clients developing cardiac arrest.

Since the inception of METs the incidence of cardiac arrests on the wards has been significantly reduced. This does not mean that they don't happen and every nurse should be prepared for the possibility. The decrease in cardiac arrests also correlates to the use of the Adult Deterioration Detection System (ADDS) chart, where patients are monitored using a deterioration score.

Any member of a hospital clinical staff (including nurses, physiotherapists, social workers, speech therapists, residents and members of senior medical staff) can activate the MET. The members of the MET usually include the duty intensive care doctor, a designated intensive care nurse and the receiving medical doctor.

Activity 21.7

Emergency response

Locate the emergency response policies and procedures in the clinical area to which you are assigned.

1. When do you need to call a medical emergency?
2. Who forms part of the emergency response team for the area?

Identifying emergency situations and responding to first-aid requests

It is important to constantly monitor clients while in the acute nursing arena as a person's condition can change rapidly. Knowing the normal parameters for vital signs is essential to recognise abnormal functioning. Not everything is a medical emergency and a good knowledge of first aid may prevent a situation from escalating to a medical emergency. An example of this is a person who chokes while eating and where being able to administer appropriate first-aid actions may relieve the situation. The nurse can then report the incident and more specialised assessment of the client's swallowing reflexes can be undertaken by the speech therapist.

Cardiopulmonary resuscitation

Basic life support (BLS) is the act of maintaining airway patency and supporting breathing and circulation. The aim of BLS is to temporarily maintain circulation sufficiently to preserve brain function until specialised treatment can commence. Sudden cardiac arrest is a leading cause of death and survival rates are optimised when BLS is commenced immediately.

The steps required for successful resuscitation are as follows:

1   early recognition and call for help
2   early CPR
3   early defibrillation
4   early advanced life support (ALS).

BLS should be commenced if the patient displays no signs of life – is unconscious, unresponsive and not breathing effectively or normally.

The ratio of compressions to ventilation is 30:2. This ratio is recommended for all age groups, regardless of the number of rescuers. Compressions should be delivered at a rate of 100/minute, and aim to achieve the full compression depth of 4–5 cm for an adult or 1/3 of the chest depth. The guidelines recommend rescuers alternate in performing compressions every two minutes, where feasible, to reduce fatigue and ensure effective compression rate and depth.

SUMMARY

- The nurse needs to work as part of the health-care team and provide information to the team to enable nursing care plans that meet the client's needs.
- The family of the client also requires support and information and the nurse is ideally situated in the team to provide this support.
- Effective assessment skills are required to enable identification of actual and potential health problems of the client with an acute illness or procedure.
- Nursing interventions are specialised for many areas of acute nursing. The nurse may require additional training and skill development to undertake these interventions.
- Pre- and post-operative care are specialised nursing interventions to assist in caring for a person undergoing a surgical procedure.
- An emergency situation can develop quickly in the acute area and the nurse has a responsibility to ensure all equipment is kept ready to use. The nurse also needs to maintain knowledge and skills in response to emergency situations.

SELF-TEST QUESTIONS

1   How can you identify the impact of acute health problems on a person, family or carer?
2   What is your role in planning care for a person with an acute health problem?
3   What training and support will you require to undertake specialised nursing interventions for the client in the acute nursing arena?
4   What is your role in the pre- and post-operative care of clients?
5   How can you contribute to emergencies in the acute care environment?

BIBLIOGRAPHY

Australian Institute of Health and Welfare (AIHW) (2016). *Emergency department care 2015–16: Australian hospital statistics.* Retrieved from http://www.aihw.gov.au/publication-detail/?id=60129557372. Accessed 11 March 2017.

Brown, D. & Edwards, H. (eds) (2012). *Lewis's Medical Surgical Nursing: Assessment and Management of Clinical Problems* (3rd edition). Mosby Elsevier: Sydney.

Clarke, L., Gray, S., White, L., Duncan, G. & Baumle, W. (2016). *Foundations of Nursing: Enrolled Division 2 Nurses* (ANZ Edition). Cengage Learning: South Melbourne.

Tollefson, J., Watson, G., Jelly, E. & Tambree, K. (2016). *Essential Clinical Skills: Enrolled Division 2 Nurses* (3rd edition). Cengage Learning: South Melbourne.

PART 6

Clinical placement community

Chapter 22: Nursing practice in the primary health-care setting

Chapter 23: Aboriginal and/or Torres Strait Islander health care

Chapter 24: Maternal and infant health care

The community experience

Community nursing – I tried to think about all of the theory we had covered and what exactly would be involved in this placement. I thought about possible nursing roles in the community and what my role could be on placement. I really did not have a clear idea of what I would be doing. Let me tell you – no two days were the same and no two patients where the same. My patients ranged in age from 3 to 101, and the care they needed was all different. Some of the patients during my placement got progressively better and their need for interventions was reduced.

Working in the community setting entailed driving to client's homes, entering their homes and looking at how to perform dressings and other nursing interventions in a home environment. It could be tricky at times working out the safest way and the most hygienic way to perform nursing interventions. It was certainly a case of thinking outside of the box! I also got the chance to really look at effective communication, documentation and what it means to be a nurse. Remove the ward or the hospital and the role of a community nurse is all of what is required in hospital and then some. Hanging IV antibiotics and using a coat hanger (metal!) to raise the line. Thinking about how to dress a wound when the client is on the couch, thinking about safety, your back and your personal safety are all constant thoughts and processes. I found that this placement was a mixed bag and I really got to put so much of my learning into action. I could see the effects of diseases or a multi trauma like a car accident and the ongoing care or recovery processes required. This placement really enabled me to consolidate my learning and prepare me for my role as an enrolled nurse.

The community placement will generally be towards the end of your diploma. It will enable you to consolidate your learning from many subjects, such as acute care, anatomy and physiology, complex and chronic health conditions, and communication.

What is community nursing? Community nursing is a component of primary health care. Community health services provide universal access to a large range of services and also include focused services based on federal government initiatives. Primary health is a method for integrating services between hospitals and community and ensuring ongoing care and management exists (Department of Health, 2018).

What kind of patients are in the community setting?

Community care is for a broad range of nursing interventions. Patients can be managed in the community setting for a range of chronic and complex conditions, palliative care, wound care, intravenous antimicrobial therapy, medication management (such as diabetes, anti-thrombotic medications or high-risk medications) or assistance with activities of daily living (ADLs) post-surgery. Community nursing has no age limits – your patients can range from young children right through to elderly patients living in their homes.

In this placement you will be working in people's homes or at a community health centre, or both. Community nursing is delivered depending on what is required – patients are often assessed prior to discharge from hospital and their care handed over to the community health team. You will soon notice that there is a great deal of communication between health-care providers. The patients you will come across will vary in age, life experiences and socioeconomic circumstances. You will be entering people's homes, and will need to be mindful of respect for property while managing your levels of safety and hygiene.

Common experiences of student nurses in the community setting

Community nursing is more than driving around to clients' homes. Community nursing requires a great deal of communication and patient management between health-care professionals. You may be involved in case management where you are discussing planned interventions and ongoing management with the medical team, allied health team and any other health professionals involved in the care of the client. Community nursing will also involve 'hospital-in-the-home'-type patients to assist in reducing the length of hospital stays for eligible patients. Some patients may require community nursing for long periods while others may only require intervention for weeks or months.

Objectives

The objectives for this placement need to be contextualised to the community setting, for example:
* health challenges facing Australian communities
* workplace health and safety concerns in the home environment
* infection control concerns and methods to manage in the home environment
* critical thinking and problem-solving strategies
* emergency and first-aid management of conditions and injuries
* age-specific health issues for infants, children, adolescents, adults and the elderly
* community and in-hospital resources and services available for clients.

Allocation

In community nursing, often allocation is based on the daily schedule and what is required in terms of client needs. The morning shift nurse may cover one geographical area, and the other nurse may cover a different area. There are often both morning and afternoon shifts in community care. The workload allocation takes into consideration the travelling time and the care required at each client's home. As a student you may administer medications if the unit HLTENN007 has been completed and you are supervised. For more complex management there will be a registered nurse who will undertake specialised activities, such as administration of high-risk medications in the home environment. All enrolled nurses and support staff work under the supervision of a registered Division 1 nurse.

Enjoy your placement and ensure you make good use of the valuable time you have in this specialty area.

Nursing practice in the primary health-care setting

LEARNING OUTCOMES

After reading this chapter, you should have an understanding of:

22.1 Working as part of an interdisciplinary health-care team in a primary health-care environment

22.2 Recognising the impact of a health problem on a person in the primary health-care environment

22.3 Providing health education and health promotion for illness prevention

22.4 Performing nursing interventions that support a person's health-care needs

22.5 Evaluating outcomes of planned primary health care and promote suitable resources

Community placement

I was excited to be attending my community nursing placement. I really felt that this was an area in which I could make a difference to the health and wellbeing of people before they became ill. I was placed in a mother–baby unit and I found the experience very rewarding helping mothers and fathers to manage their child's behaviour. A number of the families had presented with referrals due to a lack of knowledge regarding diet and nutrition. I found that I could apply my knowledge from a number of subjects that would help me in this area. It was good being able to interact with dieticians and other health professionals and I found my knowledge increased as a result of working with these individuals.

22.1 The interdisciplinary health-care team in a primary health-care environment

Primary health care (PHC) is a person's first contact with the health-care system. It aims to maintain health and wellbeing and prevent illness and disease.

In Australia, primary health care provides personal care for the individual while also taking the opportunity to provide health promotion, to provide education on the prevention of illness and to assist communities to maintain health and wellbeing.

This is reflected in the definition of primary health care developed by the Australian Primary Health Care Research Institute (APHCRI):

> Primary health care is socially appropriate, universally accessible, scientifically sound first-level care provided by health services and systems with a suitably trained workforce comprised of multi-disciplinary teams supported by integrated referral systems in a way that: gives priority to those most in need and addresses health inequalities; maximises community and individual self-reliance, participation and control; and involves collaboration and partnership with other sectors to promote public health. Comprehensive primary health care includes health promotion, illness prevention, treatment and care of the sick, community development, and advocacy and rehabilitation.

It can also be helpful to review the World Health Organization (WHO) definition of primary health care, which can be accessed here: http://www.who.int/publications/almaata_declaration_en.pdf.

Primary health-care principles and philosophical framework

Primary health care has a person-centred approach and strives to be a service that is accessible to all individuals in the community. It seeks to empower the individual and community through increased knowledge, and provides opportunities for individuals to access specialist health services according to the needs of the individual and the community.

The primary health-care facilities will be unique to that community as they try to meet its specific needs. The type of services offered by the health-care facilities will be based on social, economic, cultural and political determinants that underpin the community in which it is located and health promotion activities will be tailored to the community.

Service model and the roles of the interdisciplinary health-care team

In order to be successful health-care education, interventions and planning need to meet the needs of the individual and the community. There are a variety of health-care professionals who work together in a team approach in order to achieve the objectives of primary health care.

---

primary health care (PHC)

A person's point of entry into the health-care system, which includes personal care with health promotion, prevention of illness and community development (DeLaune et al., 2016)

Activity 22.1

Primary health care and the team

Identify the members of the health-care team who are involved with the clients to whom you provide care. For each health-care member outline their role within primary health care and why they have been assigned to the client.

Your role in community health-care service

As a nursing student on a clinical placement within the community health sector it is important that you follow the organisation's policies and procedures. It will be helpful to do research on the clients who attend the centre and the reasons why they are accessing primary health-care services. You can gain this information from attending centre meetings with all the members of the health-care team. Policies and procedures within the organisation outline how specific problems that clients present with should be addressed. This information may also be contained within job descriptions, in pamphlets that are available for distribution and in the admission documentation outlining the appropriate referrals to members of the team dependent on the specification of the problem.

It is important that you operate within the role of the enrolled nurse. Information about role limitations is outlined in the Nursing and Midwifery Board of Australia's decision-making framework (2016) and in its *Enrolled Nurse Standards for Practice* (2016): http://www.nursingmidwiferyboard.gov.au/Codes-Guidelines-Statements/Professional-standards/enrolled-nurse-standards-for-practice.aspx.

Effective decision making in primary health care

Effective assessment is essential to defining the problems the person is presenting with to the primary health-care facility. Once the problems are identified they will then be assessed according to priority of need. This will occur as a team approach to identifying solutions and level of priority. The member of the health-care team who specialises in this area will become responsible for initiating the priority intervention.

One theory that supports this practice is Maslow's hierarchy of needs where it is proposed that until the basic needs for survival are met other higher needs cannot be addressed. See **Figure 22.1**.

Reflective practice 22.1

Prioritising needs of individuals

Select one of the individuals that you are providing nursing care for.
1 What were their needs on admission to the health-care service?
2 Have those needs changed over the time they have been involved with the health-care service?
3 Are there any needs that have to still be addressed? Why have these been less of a priority?

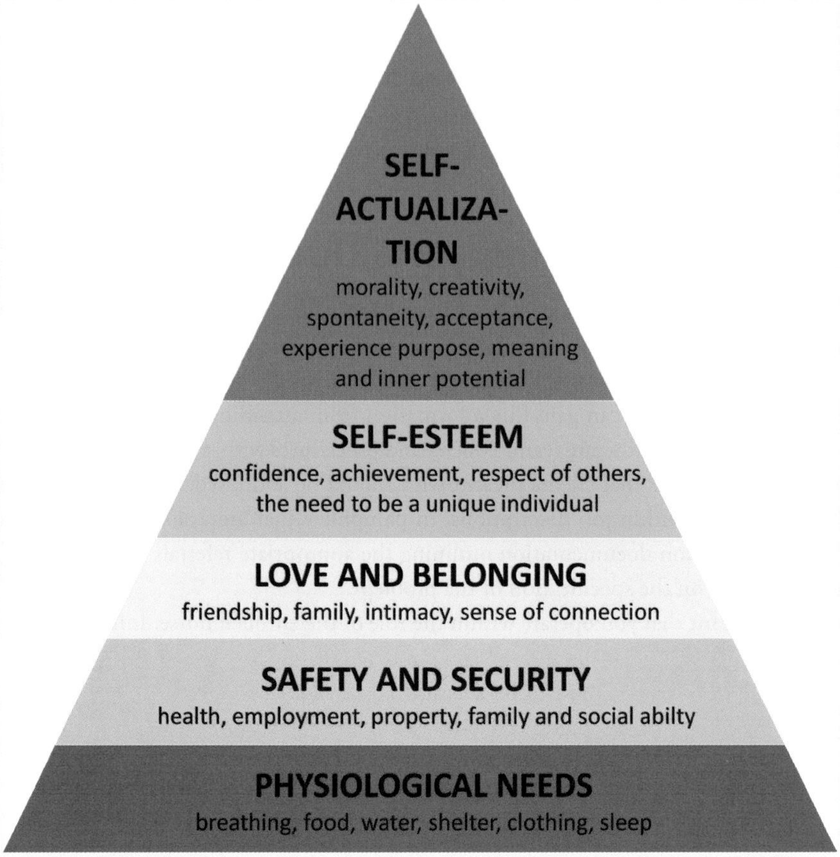

FIGURE 22.1 Maslow's hierarchy of needs

Alamy Stock Photo/Elena Elenaphotos21.

22.2 Impact of health problems on a person in the primary health-care environment

Before commencing nursing interventions the client needs to be assessed and actual problems and potential problems identified. This will ensure the client is referred to the correct health services for their identified problems.

Health issues affecting the Australian community

In Australia the health-care system is under more demand than ever before. One of the major contributory factors is the ageing population and a consequent rise in chronic health conditions. In 2016, the Australian Government identified nine areas that primary health care should focus on (http://www.health.gov.au/internet/publications/publishing.nsf/Content/health-oatsih-pubs-linkphc~health-oatsih-pubs-linkphc-systems~health-oatsih-pubs-linkphc-systems3). These include:

1 cancer control
2 cardiovascular health

3   injury prevention and control
4   mental health
5   diabetes mellitus
6   asthma
7   arthritis and musculoskeletal conditions
8   obesity
9   dementia.

While on clinical placement it is helpful to keep these in mind. Some of the most common factors that you will come across on clinical placement are discussed below.

Environmental and lifestyle factors

Environmental and lifestyle factors have an effect on the origin and development of cancer and the nine identified primary focus areas previously mentioned. Studies have identified three main risk factors that primary health care can address in the form of education and primary prevention (http://www.health.gov.au/internet/publications/publishing.nsf/Content/health-oatsih-pubs-linkphc~health-oatsih-pubs-linkphc-systems~health-oatsih-pubs-linkphc-systems3). These are:

* diet
* exposure to sunlight
* smoking.

Special populations

While care for every person is a basis of primary health care, there are some populations that require special consideration, including:

* Aboriginal and/or Torres Strait Islander people
* migrants
* socioeconomically disadvantaged groups, such as homeless people
* aged care residents.

It has been found that access to health education and screening programs are either not easily accessible by these groups or are not being accessed (Australian Nursing Federation, 2009).

Cancer control

The government found that the number of individuals diagnosed with cancer is rising due to the ageing population, population growth and better detection of cancer. With cancer control the main areas that the government identified were:

* lung cancer
* skin cancer
* cervical cancer
* breast cancer
* colorectal cancer
* prostate cancer.

Table 22.1 lists the types of cancer that the federal government has identified as being of most concern.

TABLE 22.1 Types of cancer the government has identified as being of most concern

Type of cancer	Government actions
Lung cancer	Second most common cancer in Australia Affects more males than females Prevention is able to reduce incidence of cancer by: • Promoting cessation of smoking and decreasing rates of people taking up smoking • Restriction of tobacco sales and consumption
Skin cancer	Australia has the highest rate of skin cancer in the world with non-melanocytic skin cancer being the most common Directives by government have focused on: • Raising awareness of the dangers of exposure to sunlight • Opportunistic detection by general practitioners and targeting specific high-risk groups
Cervical cancer	The eighth most common cancer among Australian women Pap smear screening has led to mortality rates falling Culturally appropriate strategies have been implemented to encourage Aboriginal and/or Torres Strait Islander women and older women to take part in this screening program
Breast cancer	The most common cancer affecting women Early detection and treatment is key to preventing mortality and BreastScreen Australia is a national initiative
Colorectal cancer	Second most common cancer affecting males and females Early diagnosis allows for effective treatment Faecal occult blood testing screening for adults over the age of 50 has commenced as a national screening tool
Prostate cancer	Other than skin cancer prostate cancer is the most common cancer affecting Australian men Currently no benefits have been seen with screening procedures

Source: Australian Institute of Health and Welfare (2017), https://www.aihw.gov.au/reports-statistics/health-conditions-disability-deaths/arthritis-musculoskeletal-conditions/overview. © Australian Institute of Health and Welfare 2018. Creative Commons BY 3.0 AU. www.creativecommons.org/licenses/by/3.0/au/.

Cardiovascular health

Heart, stroke and cardiovascular disease are the largest causes of death in Australia. Coronary heart disease is the major cause of death for people less than 70 years and stroke is the major long-term disability seen in Australian communities (https://www.aihw.gov.au/reports-statistics/health-conditions-disability-deaths/chronic-disease/overview).

Risk factors for poor cardiovascular health have been identified as:

• smoking
• low physical activity
• obesity
• poor nutrition (https://www.heartfoundation.org.au/images/uploads/publications/RES-115-Aust_heart_disease_statstics_2015_WEB.PDF).

Special populations such as Indigenous people, people living in rural and remote areas and socioeconomically disadvantaged people are at greatest risk. The government has identified three approaches to address these populations:

• improve living and working conditions
• reduce poverty and unemployment
• influence people's health-related attitudes and behaviours (https://www.aihw.gov.au/reports-statistics/health-conditions-disability-deaths/chronic-disease/overview).

Mental health

A variety of services are available for people with a mental health illness. This is provided by a range of health-care professionals in different health-care environments incorporating both inpatient and community facilities.

Approximately more than a third of people who accessed services did so for mental health issues in a 12-month period (Australian Institute of Health and Welfare, 2016).

Musculoskeletal conditions

Chronic musculoskeletal conditions affect a number of people in the community. Musculoskeletal conditions affect all areas of the body's musculoskeletal system, including bones, tendons, muscles and cartilage and more than 30% of the population that accessed health-care services in 2017 sought care for a musculoskeletal condition (AIHW, 2018). When the initial acute period is finished the person often requires ongoing care for chronic symptoms. The most common musculoskeletal conditions among the Australian population and their definitions are listed in **Table 22.2**.

TABLE 22.2 Common musculoskeletal conditions

Type	Definition
Back pain and problems	Many different causes. Usually arises from muscle strain or displacement of an intervertebral disc. May be due to disease or injury.
Osteoarthritis	Degenerative joint condition that affects the weight-bearing joints of the body. Pain starts as a reaction to activity and progresses to be constant.
Rheumatoid arthritis	Auto-immune disease causing inflammation of the joints and can lead to joint deformity.
Osteoporosis	Progressive loss of bone density and decrease in the strength of the skeleton.
Juvenile arthritis	Occurs in children under 16 years of age.
Gout	Inflammatory arthritis due to excess uric acid in blood leading to uric acid crystals in joints.

Injury

Suicide and transport accidents are a major cause of death in Australia, while falls are the main cause of hospitalisation due to injury (AIHW & Australian Department of Health and Family Services, 1998b). **Table 22.3** indicates the type of injury related to age.

TABLE 22.3 Type of injury related to age

Age	Type of injury
Early childhood	Drowning and near-drowning
Young adulthood	Self-harm and road accidents
Elderly	Falls and scalds

Source: AIHW & Department of Health and Family Services (1998b). *NHPA report on injury prevention and control 1997*. Cat. no. PHE 3. AIHW: Canberra, ACT.

Diabetes

It has been found that beside genetic factors, lifestyle-related risk factors such as obesity and levels of activity have an effect on the development and progression of diabetes. Type 1 diabetes cannot be prevented but type 2 can, and sufferers can improve their health status through diet and exercise (AIHW & Australian Department of Health and Aged Care, 1999b).

Obesity

Levels of obesity are rising in Australia with 63% of adults being overweight or obese, while 25% of children are overweight or obese. This has been shown to be a major risk factor for the development and progression of many diseases (https://www.aihw.gov.au/reports-statistics/behaviours-risk-factors/overweight-obesity/overview).

BMI or Body Mass Index gives a person an indication of whether their weight is in a healthy weight range. **Table 22.4** shows the weight categories based on height of the individual. It is important to note that different population groups may not fit into these categories and waist circumference measurement is now also taken.

TABLE 22.4 BMI classifications

BMI (kg/m²)	Classification
Less than 18.5	Underweight
18.5 to less than 25	Normal weight range
25 to less than 30	Overweight
30 or more	Obese

Source: National Health and Medical Research Council (2013). *Clinical practice guidelines for the management of overweight and obesity in adults, adolescents and children in Australia.* NHMRC: Melbourne.

Waist circumference measurement is used as an indicator of health risks associated with excess fat around the waist. **Table 22.5** outlines waist circumference measurements that indicate an increased health risk.

TABLE 22.5 Waist circumference and increased risk

Gender	Increased risk	Substantially increased risk
Men	94 cm	102 cm
Women	80 cm	88 cm

Source: National Health and Medical Research Council (2013). *Clinical practice guidelines for the management of overweight and obesity in adults, adolescents and children in Australia.* NHMRC: Melbourne.

Review the skill in Tollefson *Essential Clinical Skills* 2.1 Head-to-toe assessment

Reading, writing, numeracy

Clinical manifestations of health conditions

As part of the admission process the nurse will undertake a variety of clinical assessments that will identify symptoms of health conditions affecting the health status of the client. In Table 22.6 are some of the common signs and symptoms that may be present in clients presenting with the six of the nine priority areas identified by the Australian government as discussed in the previous section. It is important to always undertake assessment and baseline vital signs on all clients that present to the facility. **Table 22.6** outlines some of the diseases of the Australian population and signs and symptoms associated with that condition.

TABLE 22.6 Diseases, signs and symptoms

Condition		Signs and symptoms/clinical manifestations	Tollefson Clinical Skill
Cancer	Lung cancer	Persistent cough Changes in coughing and breathing Pain in the chest area Wheezing Changes in voice Drop in weight Bone pain Headache	 2.9 Pain assessment

>>

Condition		Signs and symptoms/clinical manifestations	Tollefson Clinical Skill
	Skin cancer	Changes in skin that are: • Raised, pearly, waxy or shiny • Firm and taut • Oddly coloured such as yellow, violet or blue • Crusty, scaly or bleeding	Step-by-step self examination, http://www.skincancer.org/skin-cancer-information/early-Detection/step-by-step self-examination
	Cervical cancer	No symptoms	
	Breast cancer	Lump in breast Change in size and shape of the breast Change to the nipple such as crusting, ulceration, redness or dimpling Pain	Breast self-exam, http://www.breastcancer.org/symptoms/testing/types/self_exam/bse_steps
	Colorectal cancer	Bleeding from the rectum or blood in the bowel motion A change in bowel habits Unexplained tiredness Abdominal pain	 3.7 Assisting the patient with elimination – urinary and bowel elimination 3.9 Faeces assessment and specimen collection
	Prostate cancer	Painful or difficult urination Frequent urination at night Loss of bladder control Reduced urinary flow Blood in urine	 3.7 Assisting the patient with elimination - urinary and bowel elimination
Cardiovascular health	Heart	Chest pain Shortness of breath Palpitations A fast heartbeat Weakness or dizziness Nausea Sweating	 2.3 Temperature, pulse and respiration (TPR) measurement 2.10 12-lead ECG recording
	Stroke	FAST assessment • Face – droopiness of mouth • Arms – limited movement • Speech – slurred speech • Time – critical (Stroke Foundation, 2017)	 2.7 Neurological observation
	Vascular Disease (legs)	Leg pain Cramps Varicose veins	 2.8 Neurovascular observation
Mental health	Depression	*Mood:* Sadness, anxiety, guilt, lack of enjoyment, hopelessness *Physical:* Tiredness, eating changes, sleeping changes, stomach problems, headaches chest pain *Mind:* Poor concentration, indecisiveness, forgetfulness, slow thinking, difficulty in problem solving, difficulty in planning	 9.1 Mental state assessment 9.2 Establishing a 'therapeutic relationship' in the mental health setting

>>

Condition		Signs and symptoms/clinical manifestations	Tollefson Clinical Skill
Musculoskeletal conditions	Back pain	Sciatica – pain that radiates down the back of the legs Lower back strain	 2.9 Pain assessment 3.3 Assisting the patient to ambulate
	Osteoarthritis	Limited motion or stiffness that goes away after movement Clicking or cracking sound when bending joints Mild swelling around a joint Pain that worsens after activity or at end of the day	
	Rheumatoid Arthritis	Fatigue Joint pain and tenderness Joint swelling Joint redness and warmth Loss of joint range of motion Joint deformity Anaemia Fever	
	Osteoporosis	Weakening of bones Bone pain Loss of height	
	Gout	Swelling, pain, tophi, kidney stones, itchy skin, red and hot joints, fever, joint fluid	
Injury	Drowning Road accidents Falls	Symptoms may vary from mild symptoms to severe brain injury affecting all areas of the body. Falls may restrict mobility due to damage or anxiety	 2.7 Neurological observation
Obesity	Obesity and overweight	Increased BMI or waist circumference	 2.6 Blood glucose measurement

Source: White, L., Duncan, G., Baumle, W., Gray, S. & Ferris, L. (2018). *Foundations of Nursing*, (ANZ edition). Cengage: Melbourne.

Activity 22.2

Identifying symptoms

Select one of the individuals for whom you are providing nursing care. Review your assessment on admission and ongoing care plan.

1   What symptoms did the person present with?
2   Have these symptoms changed?
3   What health condition do they relate to?

Technology

Priorities and potential areas of risk

One of the most important methods to determine priorities and potential areas of risk for implementation is a thorough assessment and collation of the client's data. These will then be compiled into the client's file and analysed by members of the health-care team.

Source-orientated records where each health-care professional makes separate entries is the traditional mode of patient recording. In primary health care a problem-orientated medical record, where the data is organised under the problems and all members of the health team contribute to this data, may be used. Another form of documentation called *case management* may also be used.

It is important that the confidentiality of the client's personal data is maintained. This will necessitate the client's file being kept secure and all discussion of the client information by the team to be undertaken within a private area.

A risk assessment of the problems that have been identified will be undertaken with members of the health-care team to determine priority interventions.

Writing

Sharing information

Information may be shared via a variety of means: verbal reports, case file notes and documentations, care plans and case conferences.

The case conference is based on a person-centred approach and each member of the health-care team who is involved in providing assistance to the person contributes to the information sharing. This model allows for other members of the health-care team to contribute or identify additional areas of concern that may impact on the client's progress.

Review the skill in Tollefson *Essential Clinical Skills* Part 7 Documentation

---

Activity 22.3

Care plans

For your client and with the supervision of the registered nurse complete the required documentation to ensure the care plan is updated.

1 What were their specific primary health-care needs?
2 What symptoms did they have?
3 What interventions did you decide on to meet the individual's needs?

Physical, psychological and social impacts on activities of daily living

One of the most important aspects of nursing care is to assess the impacts of health problems on the activities of daily living (ADLs) of an individual (see **Figure 22.2**). The nurse is the best person to assess these activities. A holistic assessment of the individual by the nurse will identify areas of need. In primary health care this may occur within the health-care facility or on a visit to the person's home. Documentation of how the person undertakes ADLs needs to be completed. Some of the many different forms of documentation include client file notes, fluid balance charts, and food and fluid intake charts.

Identification of the client's problem may be through observation of the person undertaking the activity or through therapeutic conversations with the client and their family/carer. It is important when discussing areas of concern with individuals other than the client that consent to do so is obtained.

Review the skill in Tollefson *Essential Clinical Skills* 3.3 Assisting the patient to ambulate, 3.4 Assisting the patient with eating and drinking, 3.5 Assisting the patient to maintain personal hygiene and grooming needs – sponge (bed bath) with oral hygiene, hair wash in bed, eye and nasal car & 3.7 Assisting the patient with elimination

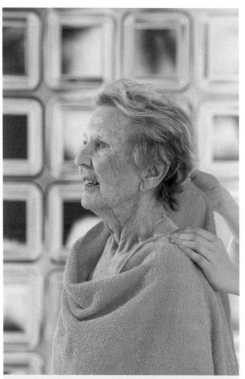

FIGURE 22.2 How nurses assist a person with activities of daily living

Alamy Stock Photo/BSIP SA.

Documentation

Actual or potential environmental health issues

After a thorough assessment of the problems that the person has presented with, it will be necessary for the nurse, in collaboration with other members of the health-care team, to identify factors that arise through environmental health issues. These may be identified through observation or communication on admission and general assessment.

After the problems have been prioritised by the health-care team, the member who specialises in the area may undertake a more thorough assessment of the problem. Underlying causes that have contributed to the problem will be attempted to be identified, for example, poor nutrition and diet. Compiling a food diary may be undertaken and reviewed by a dietician and a resulting education session may be scheduled for a client with a lack of knowledge in this area.

22.3 Providing health education and health promotion for illness prevention

It is important that the nurse is able to identify any factors that may stop or prevent an individual from accessing, understanding, evaluating and communicating information that will maintain and improve the individual's health.

Assessment of the person's communication and knowledge of the health problems they are presenting with is essential to identifying any barriers. Physical observation of the person's sensory abilities is essential and you need to address questions such as: Does the person require any aids for communication and are they working?

Using questioning techniques to assess knowledge and explore areas that have contributed to illness (as shown in **Figure 22.3**) is another strategy the nurse can use to identify barriers. Perhaps the client is from a non-English-speaking background and requires interpreter services to understand complex communication.

Oral communication

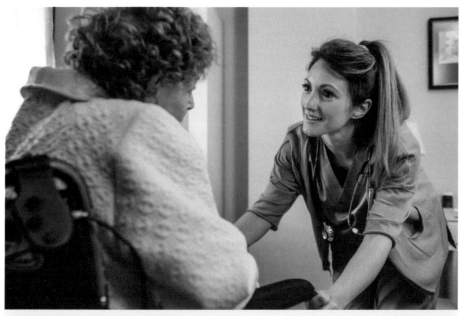

FIGURE 22.3 Barriers to communication

Getty Images/doble-d.

Strategies to support the person

The World Health Organization (2017a) defines health education as being:

> ... any combination of learning experiences designed to help individuals and communities improve their health, by increasing their knowledge or influencing their attitudes.

As previously discussed, the nurse may employ a variety of strategies to enable effective health education for a client. These may include, but are not limited to:

- providing information in the client's preferred language (interpreter services and written communication)
- ensuring communication aids are present and working
- undertaking education in appropriate time frames
- using terminology that the individual can engage with and avoiding jargon
- using educational aids to enhance the health education
- employing effective questioning techniques to assess learning.

Health promotion programs

The World Health Organization (2017b) defines health promotion as:

> ... the process of enabling people to increase control over, and to improve, their health. It moves beyond a focus on individual behaviour towards a wide range of social and environmental interventions.

There are three key elements of health promotion, as shown in **Figure 22.4**.

TIP 22.1

Barriers
Ensure that clients who need to wear glasses have these and that hearing aids are working when communicating with clients. It may be helpful to have a quiet area if complex communication is being undertaken. Provide written material to support verbal communication.

Review the skill in Tollefson *Essential Clinical Skills* 7.5 Health teaching

- Good governance – this is done at a political level and includes levying products that are harmful to health such as tobacco and alcohol. It also relates to sanitation, buildings, pollution and laws to increase desired behaviours such as wearing seatbelts.

⬇

- Health literacy – giving people the information to make healthy choices.

⬇

- Healthy cities – healthy living conditions to promote health.

FIGURE 22.4 Three key elements of health promotion

TIP 22.2

Effecting change

As a nurse you cannot make a client change. It is important to give the client all of the information regarding the issue. The nurse must maintain a non-judgemental attitude to encourage ongoing communication with the client.

As a nurse the contribution that you can make in the area of health promotion is to provide the person with information and also act as a role model. Modelling can assist in demonstrating desired behaviour/s to a client, allowing them to learn from and imitate the desired behaviour.

Reflective practice 22.2

Health promotion

Identify two health promotion campaigns that have caused a change in your behaviour. Reflect on the knowledge that you gained from these campaigns and how they altered your subsequent behaviour.

1   What were some of the successful strategies that you used to effect a change in your behaviour?

22.4 Performing nursing interventions that support a person's health-care needs

A client's care plan needs to be individualised. Everyone is unique and the care plan for an individual is unique. Unless factors of culture, age, religion, gender, as well as physical, psychological and social issues are considered the care plan will not fully address the needs of the person.

CASE STUDY 22.1

Person-centred care

Anthony was a 35-year-old man who was referred to the local community health centre from his local GP. Anthony suffered from confusion due to long-term alcoholism. Anthony currently lives in a caravan at the local caravan park. He does not have any next of kin. It was found that Anthony was often targeted by youths who would 'wind him up' and end up physically ill-treating him. When speaking with Anthony he referred to these youths as 'his mates'. Anthony was of Italian background and always documented his religion as Roman Catholic. The GP letter highlighted a number of concerns:

- inappropriate housing conditions
- continuing alcohol abuse
- smoking
- poor nutrition and diet
- poor dental health
- poor hygiene.

1 What would the priorities be for Anthony?
2 What nursing interventions would you employ for Anthony?
3 What education would be appropriate for Anthony?

Nursing practice to support dignity and privacy

It is important to treat each person as an individual and to respect the individual as a person. One of the ways that the nurse can demonstrate this is by employing a non-judgemental manner and a person-centred approach to care.

It is important to always gain the person's consent before undertaking any intervention and to provide an area of privacy.

Families and carers

Families and carers of the person also need to be given information and education on how they can assist the person to achieve their desired goals. This can vary according to the needs of the person. An example is the individual who wants to implement a healthy eating plan. If the spouse or the carer does the shopping and cooking they will be vital to assist the person to achieve their goal.

When giving information and education to families or carers, they too need to be assessed as to culture, religion and any other factors that may affect their ability to take on the desired behaviours. Written information should also be given to support their education.

TIP 22.3
Privacy and dignity

- Always close curtains and doors before undertaking a nursing intervention that will involve undressing a patient.
- Always knock on the person's door before entering their room.
- Always introduce yourself before commencing an intervention.
- Always keep patient files secure.
- Always undertake personal communication in a quiet area.
- Always address the person by their preferred name. It is best to be formal and take your cue from the person.

Oral

CASE STUDY 22.2

Dietary change in behaviour

Mr and Mrs Rosello were referred to the community health centre for education regarding health eating plans. Mr Rosello was presently categorised as obese with a BMI at 38. Despite numerous attempts to lose weight, Mr Rosello's weight had steadily increased over the last 10 years. Mr Rosello was 68, recently retired and had been diagnosed with type 2 diabetes. On discussing their

current diet it was found that they enjoyed pasta-based meals with snacks consisting of pastries and cheese.

1 What stage of change is Mr Rosello currently at?
2 What factors may have contributed to Mr Rosello's weight gain?
3 What information should be given to Mr and Mrs Rosello?
4 How can the nurse remain non-judgemental when discussing their food choices?

Adjusting nursing interventions

The process of meeting a person's needs to achieve their ADLs will be constantly changing. Orem's self-care theory, as shown in **Figure 22.5**, proposed that any change in the individual's capacity or actions will have a direct action on their care needs and the nursing interventions that are required (Wayne, 2012). This is encapsulated in the nursing process, especially during evaluation, and highlights the fact that the provision of nursing care is dynamic and constantly changes.

Documentation

Orem's Self-Care Theory
Conceptual framework

Self-Care

Conditioning Factors

Self-Care Agency

Self-Care Demands

Conditioning Factors

Deficit

Nursing Agency

FIGURE 22.5 Therapeutic self-care demand

Source: Wayne, G. (2012). *Orem's self-care theory*. Retrieved from https://nurseslabs.com/dorothea-orems-self-care-theory/#therapeutic-self-care-demand.

CASE STUDY 22.3

Mrs Grey

Mrs Grey was a 78-year-old lady who lived at home with her married daughter and family. Mrs Grey was referred to the hospital by her local GP who found that Mrs Grey was requiring increasing assistance to meet her ADLs, especially with showering, which had led to a series of falls. The nurse observed Mrs Grey showering and found that Mrs Grey was unsteady and had limited reach, in particular when trying to wash her back and feet.

The nurse assigned to Mrs Grey documented and discussed these issues with the allied health team. A referral to a physiotherapist and occupational therapist

was made. The care plan noted that currently Mrs Grey required assistance with personal hygiene.

After a physiotherapy session focusing on balance and the supply of aids from the occupational therapist the nurse found that Mrs Grey was now independent and only required supervision. The nurse then adjusted Mrs Grey's care plan to reflect this change.

1   Describe the changes required by Mrs Grey using the nursing process.

2   What impact did the physiotherapist and occupational therapist make to the nursing care interventions?

Prioritising nursing interventions according to the person's needs

Individuals need to be ready to change their behaviours. Nurses can provide positive feedback, assist with overcoming the barriers the person faces and focus on the positive benefits of the individual's changed pattern of behaviour. As discussed in Chapter 16 in relation to chronic diseases, one of the areas that the nurse must be knowledgeable in for effective health education and health promotion is the stages of change a person goes through when changing their behaviour. The stages of change are:

* pre-contemplation
* contemplation
* preparation
* action
* maintenance
* relapse
* termination.

The stage of change the person is at will directly affect the nursing interventions that the person will require. As the person moves through each stage the nursing interventions need to be modified. Recap your understanding of each stage by reviewing **Table 16.2** in Chapter 16.

Reading

Activity 22.4

Aids

For the individuals you are caring for, identify any aids that may assist them to maintain their independence with ADLs. Describe what function the aid performs for the person.

Emergency treatment

At all times the nurse must be prepared to administer first aid in the workplace if required. First aid or emergency treatment may be required if a person has an adverse reaction to an intervention. An example of this is an adverse drug reaction such as hypertensive medication and fainting.

The nurse should ensure that their first-aid knowledge is current and they know the facility's policy and procedures for managing such situations.

22.5 Evaluating outcomes of planned primary health care and suitable resources

At all times while the person is receiving care it is necessary to evaluate their progress towards planned goals. Achieving these goals may indicate a need to formulate a new action plan or indicate that the person is ready to move into the discharge planning stage. At other times there may not be significant goal achievement and by evaluating the progress further interventions may be required.

TIP 22.4

First aid and emergency treatment

It is important that you know what the process is for alerting other staff to an emergency in your area. Do you know the number to access the switchboard to notify other team members?

Always do the assessment of:

A Airway: Is the airway clear?

B Breathing: Is the person breathing?

C Can you feel a pulse?

D Defibrillator: Do you need to obtain the defibrillator?

Evaluating care and how to access resources

It is important to continually document and report the person's progress towards primary health goals to all members of the allied health-care team. The nurse can achieve this by:

- accurately charting vital signs and measurements
- updating the care plan
- completing progress notes in the person's file
- taking part in the health-care team's case meetings.

Community supports

When working with the person and family the nurse will be able to identify barriers to the person maintaining independence or changing behaviour. You will need to ensure that health education is supported by written literature for the person to take with them. During interactions you may be able to identify community supports that are required to support the person or the family. Other members of the allied health team may also suggest community supports that will be helpful for the individual.

It is important that all services are contacted and details are given both verbally and in writing to the person. Examples of some of the community supports are:

- Meals on Wheels
- home help
- support groups
- transport agencies if needed.

At times it may be appropriate to enlist the aid of other members of the allied health team to achieve these outcomes.

TIP 22.5

Documentation

Check the policies and procedures manual or ask the supervisor when documentation needs to be undertaken. In some cases it is needed to be completed every shift, while at other times it is documentation by exception.

Documentation, verbal or oral

Activity 22.5

Community supports

Identify the community supports in the local area.

1 What supports will the person you are caring for require?
2 What other members of the health-care team will need to assist with referral of the person to the support centre?
3 What documentation will be required to be sent to the support service?
4 What documentation will be given to the person?

SUMMARY

- The enrolled nurse is part of the health-care team. By working as a cohesive group a plan can be put into place that meets the needs of the client.
- When a client accesses the health-care service a holistic assessment is undertaken. The needs of the client and their family/carer are identified. This ensures that physical, psychological, social and environmental issues are identified and addressed.
- Health education and health promotion are delivered in a manner that accommodates the person's needs and respects their dignity.
- Nursing interventions are tailored to individual needs and take into account factors of culture, religion, age, and gender as well as physical, psychological and social needs.
- Evaluation is a critical step in ensuring the interventions are assisting the person meet their planned goals.

SELF-TEST QUESTIONS

1   What is the role of the enrolled nurse as part of the health-care team?
2   How can the enrolled nurse ensure that nursing interventions meet the needs of the individual?
3   What actions can the enrolled nurse take to ensure health promotion and health education is appropriate for individual clients?
4   When providing or formulating nursing interventions, what factors does the enrolled nurse need to take into account to ensure the person's dignity and privacy are maintained?
5   Why is it necessary to review nursing interventions on a regular basis?

BIBLIOGRAPHY

Australian Government Department of Health (2018). *National Primary Health Care Strategic Framework*. Retrieved from http://www.health.gov.au/internet/main/publishing.nsf/Content/nphc-strategic-framework. Accessed September 2017.

Australian Institute of Health and Welfare (AIHW) (2016). *Mental health services: In brief*. Retrieved from https://www.aihw.gov.au/getmedia/681f0689-8360-4116-b1cc-9d2276b65703/20299.pdf.aspx?inline=true. Accessed 16 July 2017.

Australian Institute of Health and Welfare (AIHW) (2018). *Arthritis and musculoskeletal conditions*. Retrieved from https://www.aihw.gov.au/reports-statistics/health-conditions-disability-deaths/arthritis-musculoskeletal-conditions/overview. Accessed 5 January 2018.

Australian Institute of Health and Welfare & Australian Government Department of Health and Aged Care (1999a). *NHPA report on cardiovascular health: A report on heart, stroke and vascular disease, summary*. Cat. no. PHE 12. Canberra, ACT: AIHW. Retrieved from http://www.aihw.gov.au. Accessed 31 October 2017.

Australian Institute of Health and Welfare & Australian Government Department of Health and Aged Care (1999b). *NHPA report on diabetes mellitus 1998, summary*. Cat. no. AIHW 4463. Canberra, ACT: AIHW. Retrieved from http://www.aihw.gov.au/publication-detail/?id=6442467059. Accessed 6 March 2017.

Australian Institute of Health and Welfare & Australian Government Department of Health and Aged Care (1999c). *NHPA report on mental health: A report focusing on depression 1998, summary*. Cat. no. PHE 14. Canberra: AIHW, http://www.aihw.gov.au/publication-detail/?id=6442467058. Accessed 6 March 2017.

Australian Institute of Health and Welfare & Australian Government Department of Health and Family Services (1998a). *NHPA report on cancer control 1997*. Cat. no. PHE 4. Canberra, ACT: AIHW. Retrieved from http://www.aihw.gov.au/publication-detail/?id=6442466961. Accessed 6 March 2017.

Australian Institute of Health and Welfare & Australian Government Department of Health and Family Services (1998b). *NHPA report on injury prevention and control 1997*. Cat. no. PHE 3. Canberra, ACT: AIHW. Retrieved from http://www.aihw.gov.au/publication-detail/?id=6442466968. Accessed 6 March 2017.

Australian Nursing Federation (2009). *Primary health care in Australia: A nursing and midwifery consensus view*. Retrieved https://anmf.org.au/documents/reports/PHC_Australia.pdf. Accessed 20 December 2017.

Australian Primary Health Care Research Institute (APHCRI) cited in Australian Department of Health and Ageing (2009). *Primary health care reform in Australia: Report to Support Australia's First National Primary Health Care Strategy*. Department of Health & Ageing: Woden, ACT. Retrieved from http://trove.nla.gov.au/work/29254941?selectedversion=NBD44711214. Accessed 10 December 2017.

DeLaune, S.C., Ladner, P.K., McTier, L., Tollefson, J. & Lawrence, J. (2016). *Australian and New Zealand Fundamentals of Nursing* (revised edition), Cengage Learning: South Melbourne.

National Health and Medical Research Council (2013). *Clinical practice guidelines for the management of overweight and obesity in adults, adolescents and children in Australia*. NHMRC: Melbourne.

Nursing and Midwifery Board of Australia (2016). *Enrolled Nurse Standards for Practice*. Retrieved from http://www.nursingmidwiferyboard.gov.au/Codes-Guidelines-Statements/Professional-standards/enrolled-nurse-standards-for-practice.aspx.

Nursing and Midwifery Board of Australia (2016). *Frameworks*. Retrieved from http://www.nursingmidwiferyboard.gov.au/Codes-Guidelines-Statements/Frameworks.aspx.

Stroke Foundation (2017). *About stroke*, https://strokefoundation.org.au/About-Stroke. Accessed 7 March 2017.

Tollefson, J., Watson, G., Jelly, E. & Tambree, K. (2016). *Essential Clinical Skills: Enrolled Division 2 Nurses* (3rd edition). Cengage Learning: Melbourne.

Wayne, G. (2012). *Orem's self-care theory*. Retrieved from https://nurseslabs.com/dorotheaorems-self-care-theory/#therapeutic-self-care-demand.

World Health Organization (1978). *Declaration of Alma Ata, International conference on PHC, Alma-Ata, USSR, 6–12 September*. Retrieved from http://www.who.int/publications/almaata_declaration_en.pdf. Accessed 13 March 2017.

World Health Organization (2000). *Obesity: Preventing and managing the global epidemic. Report of a WHO consultation*. WHO technical report series 894. WHO: Geneva.

World Health Organization (2017a). *Health education*. Retrieved from www.who.int/topics/health_education/en/. Accessed 13 March 2017.

World Health Organization (2017b). *Health promotion*. Retrieved from www.who.int/topics/health_promotion/en/. Accessed 13 March 2017.

Aboriginal and/or Torres Strait Islander health care

LEARNING OUTCOMES

After reading this chapter, you should have an understanding of:

23.1 Identifying cultural safety issues in the workplace

23.2 Modelling cultural safety in your own work

23.3 Developing strategies for improved cultural safety

23.4 Evaluating cultural safety strategies

Learning about Aboriginal and/or Torres Strait Islander cultures

I found the unit on Aboriginal and/or Torres Strait Islander cultures fascinating. I had not had any previous interaction with this group of people and except for stories that had been broadcast on news programs I really knew very little about the people or their cultures.

I found it very confronting to learn about the impact of European culture on the Aboriginal and/or Torres Strait Islander people and I very nearly cried when we learnt about the Stolen Generations. I could not believe that we had done this to a group of people who were part of Australia.

On a more positive note it was very informative learning about their traditional bush medicine and health practices. They were very different from any I had previously known and I wondered how they had been able to come to some of the remedies and cures that we learnt about.

As a nurse I found that the stories about health care in present-day society very interesting. I was surprised that Aboriginal and/or Torres Strait Islander people were not always accepting of mainstream health care (Australian Indigenous HealthInfoNet, 2017).

23.1 Identifying cultural safety issues in the workplace

Being culturally aware of all people with a different cultural upbringing from our own is an important aspect in the provision of health care. With respect to Aboriginal and/or Torres Strait Islander people, health-care provision is complex due to many historical events, but predominantly due to cultural differences. In providing care for Aboriginal and/or Torres Strait islander patients, as with all patients, we should ensure cultural sensitivity and respect.

When cultures differ, it is very easy for misunderstandings to occur because each culture brings with it differing experiences that will have an impact on the person's understanding of what is being communicated. When working with a client in health care, it is important that the client understands exactly what they are being asked to do or the treatment may be ineffective. Effective communication is an essential component of health-care provision.

Australia today is made up of many groups of people who have their own languages, religions, race and nationality (see **Figure 23.1**). Different groups within Australian society are defined by their ethnicity. This means they are identified as belonging to another racial group within the wider Australian population. As with all cultural differences, there are *stereotypes* – many people overseas see Australians as simply 'sports-mad beer drinkers'.

In Australia, it has been highlighted for some time that there is a 'chasm' in the provision of health-care information for Aboriginal and/or Torres Strait Islander people. This impacts greatly upon services provided, on nursing care and on cultural respect, cultural competence and the appropriateness of care and interventions (Bainbridge et al., 2015).

Some resources to prepare you for placement can be found here: http://www.lowitja.org.au/sites/default/files/docs/Beyond-Bandaids-CH8.pdf; http://www.healthinfonet.ecu.edu.au/cultural-ways-home/resources/practice-resources/guidelines.

Communication strategies to ensure effective communication with Aboriginal and/or Torres Strait Islander people are broad and generalised. Each Australian is different, and if you stopped and thought about communication with all of your clients you would realise that your methods change depending on the client.

Health to Aboriginal and/or Torres Strait Islander people is more than merely the absence of disease. It encompasses the social, emotional and cultural wellbeing of the community as a whole. This notion can be difficult for Western health professionals to understand along with the concepts of bush medicine treatments (Lowell et al., 2005).

Critical issues that influence relationships and communication

Aboriginal and/or Torres Strait Islander history is evident for more than 100 000 years in Australia. Based on strong ties to the land, Aboriginal and/or Torres Strait Islander people focused their health care on treatment of illness and injury with traditional or bush medicine. The illness and disease introduced with the arrival of the First Fleet in Australia in 1788 had a lasting impact upon the health of Aboriginal and/or Torres Strait Islander people.

Nurses needs to bear in mind that there has been gross inequity and inequality within recent history in Australia – the 'Closing the Gap' scheme and the apology to the Stolen Generations have attempted to address the impact on Aboriginal and/or Torres Strait Islander people.

Reading the history of the Aboriginal and Torres Strait Islander people post-colonisation can be a traumatic experience. Over the decades, many issues have arisen which have widened the gap between Aboriginal and/or Torres Strait Islander and non-Aboriginal and Torres Strait Islander people. In 1997 publication of *Bringing them Home – Report of the National Inquiry into the Separation of Aboriginal and Torres Strait Islander Children from their Families*, brought a broader awareness of the 'Stolen Generations'.

TIP 23.1

Communication

There are many cultural differences specific to Aboriginal and Torres Strait Islander people. Try not to assume that the patient or their family share your understanding of Western cultural concepts. An example of this would be the underlying effects of cardiovascular disease and the actual effects on the heart itself and the medication used to treat cardiovascular disease. This does not indicate that there is a lack of insight or awareness; it is a completely different perspective. Medication and the use of it regularly is a Western concept. So try to remember that information and beliefs that you may take as a baseline view are not always going to be shared, and the medication used to treat cardiovascular disease can also vary across cultures (Lowell et al., 2005).

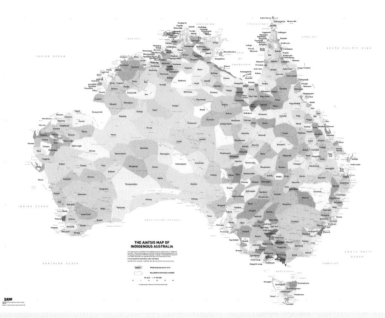

FIGURE 23.1 Map of Aboriginal and Torres Strait Islander Australia

This map attempts to represent the language, social or nation groups of Aboriginal Australia. It shows only the general locations of larger groupings of people which may include clans, dialects or individual languages in a group. It used published resources from 1988–1994 and is not intended to be exact, nor the boundaries fixed. It is not suitable for native title or other land claims. David R Horton (creator), © Aboriginal Studies Press, AIATSIS, 1996. No reproduction without permission. To purchase a print version visit: www.aiatsis.ashop.com.au/.

The *Bringing them Home* report also identified instances of official misrepresentation and deception, such as when caring and able parents were incorrectly described by Aboriginal Protection Officers as not being able to properly provide for their children, or when parents were told by government officials that their children had died, even though this was not the case. One firsthand account referring to events in 1935 stated:

> We was at the post office with my Mum and Auntie [and cousin]. They put us in the police ute and said they were taking us to Broome. They put the mums in there as well. But when we'd gone [about ten miles (16 km)] they stopped, and threw the mothers out of the car. We jumped on our mothers' backs, crying, trying not to be left behind. But the policemen pulled us off and threw us back in the car. They pushed the mothers away and drove off, while our mothers were chasing the car, running and crying after us. We were screaming in the back of that car. When we got to Broome they put me and my cousin in the Broome lock-up. We were only ten years old. We were in the lock-up for two days waiting for the boat to Perth.

The report discovered that removed children were, in most cases, placed into institutional facilities operated by religious or charitable organisations, although a significant number, particularly females, were 'fostered' out. Children taken to such places were frequently punished if caught speaking Aboriginal and/or Torres Strait Islander languages, and the specific intention was to prevent them being socialised in Aboriginal and/or Torres Strait Islander cultures with the boys raised as agricultural labourers and the girls as domestic servants.

Documentary evidence of a range of rationales for such action exists in newspaper reports and reports to and appearances before parliamentary committees. Motivations evident include child protection, beliefs that given their catastrophic population decline that Aboriginal and/or Torres Strait Islander people would 'die out', and a desire to maintain Caucasian racial purity (Australian Human Rights Commission, 1997; Berndt & Berndt, 1998).

There are many critical issues that have affected Aboriginal and/or Torres Strait Islander people and they have had a great impact upon trust, health care and self-determination. Deaths in custody, Maralinga and native title are just a few examples.

Reflective practice 23.1

Identifying bias

Choose a client that is from a different cultural background to yourself.

1   What aspects of care need to be considered for that client?

2   Do you think that different approaches to caring for such clients should be considered or should health care be standardised for all?

Cultural safety guidelines

The following link is to a document issued by the Royal Australian College of General Practitioners (RACGP), and is an introduction to cultural protocols and perspectives for health-care providers: http://www.racgp.org.au/download/Documents/AHU/2012culturalprotocols.pdf.

Activity 23.1

Cultural safety

Australia is a multicultural society and health care needs to be accessible to all people in society. Locate the policy and procedures that relate to cultural safety in your workplace.

1   What strategies are proposed to make the workplace safe for all people who access the workplace?

23.2 Modelling cultural safety in your own work

Cultural safety is not specific to the care of Aboriginal and/or Torres Strait Islander people. You will remember the term *cultural safety* from Chapter 9. It was coined by Irihapeti Merenia Ramsden, who trained as a registered general and obstetric nurse at Wellington Hospital in New Zealand. Her research outlined the concept of cultural safety and this term has since been adopted worldwide (Clarke et al., 2016).

Put very simply, cultural safety addresses the following components:

- All patients are treated with dignity
- All patients are individuals – not all non-Aboriginal and Torres Strait Islander people are the same
- Recognising that there is more than one way to complete a task
- All patients are respected and treated with respect for culture, experience and knowledge
- Respect for patient's identity (Williams, 1999).

Cultural safety incorporates an environment that is socially, spiritually and emotionally safe, and physically safe for all patients – free from assault, challenge or denial of their identity. This means that in order to provide a culturally safe environment, we need to consider holistic care, and importantly, if a patient has identified as Aboriginal and/or Torres Strait Islander people that this is not challenged, denied or questioned. Cultural safety is also about respect, dignity, trust and working together to create meaning from the interactions. Any behaviour that 'diminishes, demeans or disempowers the cultural identity and wellbeing of an individual or group' is unsafe cultural practice (Williams, 1999, p. 15).

Figure 23.2 outlines the process involved in achieving cultural safety in your nursing practice.

Cultural awareness is a beginning step towards understanding that there is a difference.

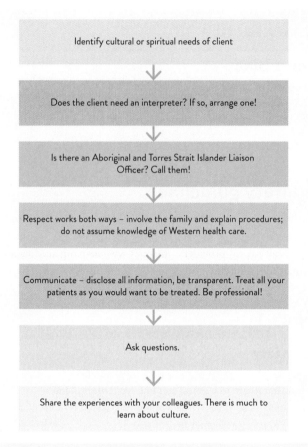

FIGURE 23.2 The process of achieving cultural safety

Communication techniques

RACGP (2012) outlines that there are many ways to support Aboriginal and/or Torres Strait Islander people to take greater control over their health care. These include:

- create opportunities for Aboriginal and/or Torres Strait Islander patients/interpreters and health-care workers to work together to develop a shared understanding based on their perspectives and practices
- respond to the needs and priorities of the patient
- increase the patient's control over the interactions – allow patients to set the topic, determine the language and the time and place if possible

Finally, the RACGP places emphasis on listening with our ears as well as our eyes – that is, taking note of body language and non-verbal cues. Silence is not always an indicator of the patient not understanding. The patient may be reflecting, waiting on an elder or simply just thinking (RACGP, 2012).

23.3 Developing strategies for improved cultural safety

Like any culture, Aboriginal and/or Torres Strait Islander people have specific terms or 'jargon' that may evoke a different meaning for health-care providers. You will notice that in varying states in Australia there are slang words specific to that area – imagine the variances in Aboriginal and/or Torres Strait Islander jargon! Some examples you may come across are:

- 'Elder' does not always mean men or women over 60 years of age. A relatively young (30–40-year-old) male or female may be given the status of an elder because of their highly respected position in their community. Aboriginal elders often possess specific skills, attributes and knowledge, which further endorses their title.
- 'Women's business' – information pertaining to women's business should remain that way! It is culturally significant for Aboriginal and/or Torres Strait Islander people that women only know about 'women's business'.
- 'Men's business' – again, information pertaining to men's business should be kept as that if at all possible. It is highly significant.
- 'Death and Sorry Business' – is a continuous cycle which impacts greatly on families and communities. The mourning process may take up to several days or a number of weeks, depending on the community. It is not appropriate for health-care service providers to enter communities at this time. In order not to offend, any printed material with Aboriginal and/or Torres Strait Islander people on it must bear the warning that deceased persons may be pictured. Death is dealt with differently in every Aboriginal and/or Torres Strait Islander community. To find out what mourning process is undertaken, refer to the Aboriginal liaison officer for information, as it will be different in almost every community (RACGP, 2012).

Strategising and managing care with Aboriginal and/or Torres Strait Islander health workers or liaison officers is a key to success. Such workers can best interpret the true understanding of cultural differences. What is available where you are completing placement? (RACGP, 2012). Here is an example of the services provided from the Aboriginal Liaison Unit within the Women's and Children's Hospital South Australia: http://www.wch.sa.gov.au/services/az/other/allied/aboriginal/documents/alu_services_factsheet.pdf.

An Aboriginal and/or Torres Strait Islander health worker will be invaluable to you and will assist you in communicating effectively with Aboriginal and/or Torres Strait Islander clients – there should be one available in every facility or at least covering several smaller hospitals.

Another significant and unique trait is the close relationship and kinship ties that all Aboriginal and/or Torres Strait Islander groups have. For example, uncles/aunties are also seen as parents, cousins are seen as brothers/sisters, and grandparents are the main carers for all children. It is also important to be aware that for Aboriginal and/or Torres Strait Islander people, living together, caring and sharing are a way of life.

Aboriginal and/or Torres Strait Islander people still have close ties with the land and, along with their spiritual beliefs, this impacts further on their health and wellbeing. Do not be offended or hurt if they are not willing to share information related to cultural beliefs or spirituality, as there are certain types of information that can only be known and shared among Aboriginal and/or Torres Strait Islander people (RACGP, 2012).

There are very specific guidelines for caring for Aboriginal and/or Torres Strait Islander people through death and dying, and everything in between. Queensland Health has an excellent resource that would be of benefit for your placement: *Sad news sorry business:*

CASE STUDY 23.1

'23 year old female with abdo pain'

You have just received handover and are commencing an afternoon shift. You have been allocated six patients and you are working with a buddy RN. Belinda Whitby is a 23-year-old female who has been admitted for observations and analgesia. You enter the room which is dark. Belinda is laying curled up on the bed, and her partner Andrew is sitting, fidgeting in the chair. You ask Belinda how she is feeling and assess her pain. Andrew is muttering something under his

>>

breath, but you can't quite make it out. Belinda is not answering your questions. It is not until you review the admission paperwork that you ascertain Belinda is an Aboriginal and/or Torres Strait Islander person. Belinda has been diagnosed with polycystic ovaries and has a large cyst that seems to be causing her pain.

You discuss Belinda's case with the Aboriginal and Torres Strait Islander liaison officer and learn that Andrew is not comfortable with 'women's business'. You go back to Belinda's bedside and ask Andrew if he would like to go and update the family and arrange for aunty

to visit. Andrew looks relieved and leaves you to provide assistance and care for Belinda, who turns over in the bed and engages you in conversation enabling you to provide nursing care and interventions and assist her.

1   Your handover was obviously not sufficient in explaining Belinda's situation. Do you think it is necessary to handover the cultural aspects of patient care?

2   How can you ensure that Belinda's cultural needs are met while she is an inpatient?

3   What aspects will you handover and document regarding Belinda's care?

Guidelines for caring for Aboriginal and Torres Strait Islander people through death and dying, https://www.health.qld.gov.au/__data/assets/pdf_file/0023/151736/sorry_business.pdf.

Aboriginal and/or Torres Strait Islander health workers are unique and hold a special position within their communities. They are community role models, peers, mentors and guides. The main role of the Aboriginal and/or Torres Strait Islander health workers has been described as cultural brokers, acting as cultural mediators between Aboriginal and/or Torres Strait Islander communities and health professionals to meet a duty of care. They also work with traditional healers. Due to cultural dynamics it is not always appropriate for Aboriginal and/or Torres Strait Islander health workers to carry out some tasks. Duty of care needs to be viewed in a flexible manner while maintaining privacy and confidentiality. For example, it may be shameful for a female health worker to discuss health issues with a man. It is common to find liaison officers in hospital-type settings who offer interpretation services including communication education to both staff and clients.

The loss of culture through historical events has caused a further loss in Aboriginal and/or Torres Strait Islander languages. Through ongoing programs, Aboriginal and/or Torres Strait Islander languages are being revived, which will assist in the cultural safety of Aboriginal and/or Torres Strait Islander people through better communication.

Effective communication with Aboriginal and/or Torres Strait Islander people involves respect, dignity and cultural awareness gained through understanding, acceptance and effective interpersonal relationships. Attempting to communicate with any patient by yelling down the corridor at them will not succeed! Ensuring cultural respect and privacy can be maintained is essential in the care of Aboriginal and/or Torres Strait Islander people.

Activity 23.2

Supporting the health-care needs of Aboriginal and/or Torres Strait Islander peoples

Grace is a 38-year-old Aboriginal woman who has presented to the emergency department with high blood sugar levels. Grace is unable to stay in hospital, she states she must return home after you 'fix her up'. Her BGL is 21.7 mmoLs. She has all other vital signs within normal limits, but her urinalysis shows a urinary

tract infection. Grace needs to return home (which is 50 km out of town) to assist with childcare and family routines for the evening.

1   What interventions could you undertake to ensure Grace receives required care?

2   Is there a connection between the UTI and BGL? If so, how could you discuss this with Grace?

3   How can you ensure that you maintain cultural respect for Grace?

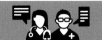

Reflective practice 23.2

Smile

My final placement was in a rural community in New South Wales. I was fortunate enough to gain the placement and was totally out of my comfort zone as 40-degree heat and flies everywhere, as well as dust, were all new concepts to me. Dogs wandered through the hospital and no one shooed them away. I had to stop myself from asking if they were 'allowed' to be there. Clearly they were!

I was working on the only ward in the hospital and the patients varied in terms of what was wrong with them – it was the only ward so everything you could think of was there! There was so much to learn in that regard alone and 70 per cent of my patients were Aboriginal and/or Torres Strait Islander people. For the first few days I was conscious of communicating clearly and that eye contact might not always be maintained. These were the two things I had thought were important. I gained a 'serious' face. I did not smile. I did not look comfortable – of course, hindsight is 20/20! I was so focused on making sure I was respectful I essentially forgot to communicate effectively.

After about two weeks of my placement, many of the 'regulars' started warming to me. They were quick to tell me I needed to smile more and relax. One patient in particular, Mavis, would have me sit with her in the afternoon while she was having dialysis and she would tell me stories of her life and her experiences. She would explain to me that sometimes no words needed to be said. Silence was okay. A smile, a nod, a shrug of the shoulder – these were all meaningful communicating factors. 'Words don't always need to exist nursey', she would say with a big smile. I learnt so much in those few weeks, not just about Aboriginal and/or Torres Strait Islander people, but about communicating, about reading situations, and that sometimes you don't have to talk all the time. 'Just smile nursey', is a saying that I will remember throughout my career.

Hayden Edward, 26, Enrolled Nurse

1   Body language is a powerful communicator. What are your views on 'just smiling' and being more silent in a conversation?
2   How do you think you could gather information about the culture of the Aboriginal and/or Torres Strait Islander people at a placement like this?

Health strategies

Health to Aboriginal and/or Torres Strait Islander people is more than merely the absence of disease. It encompasses the social, emotional and cultural wellbeing of the community as a whole. The National Aboriginal Community Controlled Health Organisation (NACCHO) supports this notion of health (NACCHO, 2017). It can be difficult for Western health professionals to understand some concepts and bush medicine treatments, as both cultures have a different approach to health and disease. Some of these differences are outlined in **Table 23.1**.

TABLE 23.1 Some differences in Aboriginal and/or Torres Strait Islander people and biomedical approaches to disease

Aboriginal and/or Torres Strait Islander people approach	Biomedical approach
Causation	
Serious disease is a result of what is often labelled as magic supernatural influences or breaking of food and social taboo.	The body is seen as a machine that may malfunction.
Context of sick individual	
When in the public eye, the individual is seen in the context of their social and spiritual world.	Diagnosis and therapy centre on individual.
Therapy	
Bush medicines are used unless illness is serious or chronic which then involves intervention of a social or spiritual nature.	Medical or surgical intervention.
Context of belief	
Part of a wider set of ideas from which it is very difficult to separate.	Medicine is a branch of Western knowledge with its own language and culture.

>>

Aboriginal and/or Torres Strait Islander people approach	Biomedical approach
Control	
Minimise the degree of special knowledge accessible to all. One or two individuals have a special understanding of spiritual/social factors of illness.	Doctor-centred and controlled Professional hierarchies with refined knowledge and power at higher levels.

Source: Clarke, P. (2008). `Aboriginal healing practices and Australian bush medicine', *Journal of the Anthropological Society of South Australian*, 33: 17; RACGP (2012). *An introduction to Aboriginal and Torres Strait Islander health cultural protocols and perspectives*; Australian Indigenous Health InfoNet (2013). *Overview of the health of Indigenous people in Western Australia 2013.*

Bush medicine remedies include:

- heated eucalyptus leaves and native honey for severe cold and dysentery
- blue gum poultices for backaches
- steamed and heated gum leaves for headaches
- bed of green leaves on which people would lie for rheumatic problems
- old man weed, a plant common in Victoria's Murray Valley and used as a tonic, also for rheumatism and arthritis, the plant being warmed and wrapped around the affected joint (Clarke, 2008; Australian Indigenous HealthInfoNet, 2013).

Traditional healing practices are specific to individual communities and family groups. They may include traditional song and dance, food and medicine. In some communities the use of traditional healing is predominantly regarded as essential for cultural and spiritual wellbeing. Health-service providers should acknowledge the fact that Aboriginal and/or Torres Strait Islander people choose to use traditional healers. Where Aboriginal and/or Torres Strait Islander people choose to access mainstream services, health professionals need to take into account the individual's cultural and spiritual wellbeing in diagnosis and treatment, and this may involve liaising with traditional healers. There will be contact methods in place at all facilities to ensure this process is as smooth as possible. Again, finding your Aboriginal liaison officer will be essential to understanding these processes.

Strategies to increase participation in health service delivery may include consultation with community representatives and community participation in decision-making processes at all levels. To adequately be able to develop and implement strategies for participation of health services for Aboriginal and/or Torres Strait Islander people you need to be aware of the factors that contribute and predispose these people to ill health.

Geographical remoteness

Geographical remoteness can be difficult when delivering health services in remote areas. In many areas there is a lack of mental health and primary health services leading to inappropriate or premature hospital admission. For Aboriginal and/or Torres Strait Islander people living in remote communities, hospitalisation means leaving their community to receive treatment and some facilities don't allow partners or their family to stay leaving the client estranged from their support network. There is a strong belief in Aboriginal and/or Torres Strait Islander communities that treatment away from home should be the last resort.

Employment

Employment is closely linked with poverty. Until 1966, Aboriginal and/or Torres Strait Islander people were sent to employers on an agreement basis between the employer and Protector of Aboriginal Affairs, in other words they were indentured labour. People worked for minimal wages, were given pocket money and the rest was sent to the Protector. Presently the unemployment rate for Aboriginal and/or Torres Strait Islander people is more than three times that of non-Aboriginal and/or Torres Strait Islander people (ABS, 2013).

Smoking, alcohol and substance abuse

Substance abuse is a real issue in Aboriginal and/or Torres Strait Islander communities. Cigarette smoking is another significant issue. Alcohol is banned in some communities and some states and territories have passed laws and have arrangements with local liquor suppliers regarding limiting purchasing amounts. Strategies such as 'Thirsty Thursday' have been introduced in Tennant Creek to prevent the purchase of large amounts of alcohol on 'pay day'. This was a process pushed by the local elders due to the high incidence of alcohol-related violence and illness on Thursdays (Henderson, 2010).

Mental illness

Aboriginal and/or Torres Strait Islander people have higher rates of suicide, self-harm, substance-induced psychosis and schizoid disorders as compared to non-Aboriginal and/or Torres Strait Islander people. Despite this, Aboriginal and/or Torres Strait Islander people report a high level of life satisfaction, which highlights the strong link between social and psychological wellbeing (Australian Indigenous HealthInfoNet, 2016).

The *Queensland Health Aboriginal and Torres Strait Islander Mental Health Strategy 2016–2021* highlights the increased incidence of mental health conditions among Aboriginal and/or Torres Strait Islander people. The strategy also identifies how the Aboriginal and/or Torres Strait Islander community views mental health and stresses the interrelationship between mind and person. The strategy can be found here: https://www.health.qld.gov.au/__data/assets/pdf_file/0030/460893/qhatsi-mental-health-strategy.pdf.

Key points to consider with Aboriginal and/or Torres Strait Islander mental health are:

- Self-determination – the emphasis is on skilling Aboriginal and/or Torres Strait Islander people to become health workers. This process will enable Aboriginal and/or Torres Strait Islander communities to really be involved in their future health care and address the issues facing them collaboratively. Self-determination enables Aboriginal and/or Torres Strait Islander people to decide what is relevant and what is required for themselves and their community (Eckermann et al., 2005).
- Holistic approach – for Aboriginal and/or Torres Strait Islander people there is a focus on connection to culture, land, spirituality, physical wellbeing, mental wellbeing, family and community. This encompasses their social and emotional wellbeing (Queensland Health, 2016).
- Recognition of the need for services that recognise gender issues in care delivery. In Aboriginal and/or Torres Strait Islander health care, there is 'women's business' for instance, which is health care relating to menstruation or female-specific illness. This is not normally discussed with males present, unless he is an elder (Australian Indigenous HealthInfoNet, 2016).
- Trauma and grief – recognise the historical links to grief and loss and the mental health implications. An example would be the removal from one's family, or having had a family member or significant other forcibly removed (Australian Indigenous HealthInfoNet, 2016).
- Suicide and self-harm – acknowledging links between substance misuse and self-harm, and the increased incidence of mental health issues (Australian Indigenous HealthInfoNet, 2016).

Common medical conditions

Aboriginal and/or Torres Strait Islander peoples are predisposed to and suffer from various health issues. These include:

- There are disturbingly high levels of dental disease in the Aboriginal and/or Torres Strait Islander communities.
- Debilitation due to childhood illnesses is common. Poor health during childhood can create a legacy of health problems in adulthood.

- Trachoma is still prevalent in the Aboriginal and/or Torres Strait Islander communities. Over a third of the population reports trachoma.
- Aboriginal women tend to have more complications during pregnancy related to anaemia, urinary tract infections, cardiac disorders and diabetes. Post-partum haemorrhages, retained placentas and genital tract infections are common post-delivery.
- Respiratory infections with a nasal discharge are common. Possibly exacerbated by lactose intolerance.
- Cases of tuberculosis are still documented with higher prevalence in Aboriginal and/or Torres Strait Islander communities.
- Middle-ear infections such as otitis media have a close relationship with respiratory infections. Clinically this disease from initial episode at infancy can recur with associated rhinitis and rapid progression to perforation. For Aboriginal and/or Torres Strait Islander people there is a distinct difference in the clinical nature of the illness, i.e., tympanic scarring and hearing impairment. There is a link between hearing loss and language development.
- There is a high prevalence of Hepatitis B surface antigen carriers in the Aboriginal and/or Torres Strait Islander communities.
- Gastrointestinal infections are high with Aboriginal and/or Torres Strait Islander children.
- Diabetes is a central health issue. A high number of people still remain undiagnosed and mismanaged.
- Retinopathy is common.
- There are high levels of renal disease.
- Ischaemic heart disease and diseases of the circulatory system account for a substantial proportion of Aboriginal and/or Torres Strait Islander deaths, especially in younger populations.
- Hypertension is a significant problem.
- Hyperlipidaemia was noted to be more common with both genders in Aboriginal and/or Torres Strait Islander communities (Australian Indigenous HealthInfoNet, 2016).

It is clear that much of Aboriginal and/or Torres Strait Islander culture, health and welfare has suffered due to colonisation. The impact of the Stolen Generations, for example, is still not fully understood. There still exists a gross disproportion of increased risk of death in custody, early or premature death, and social inequality in today's society among Aboriginal and/or Torres Strait Islander people compared to non Aboriginal and/or Torres Strait Islander people (Australian Indigenous HealthInfoNet, 2016).

23.4 Evaluating cultural safety strategies

Self-determination

Mainstream health services such as hospitals and primary health-care centres have often been criticised for being inadequate in catering to the needs of Aboriginal and/or Torres Strait Islander people. Poor access to these services has been due to a number of factors; some economic, some geographic. There also are a variety of sociocultural factors involved including the failure of Western health systems to utilise strong kinship networks, which are essential in Aboriginal and/or Torres Strait Islander communities (Australian Indigenous HealthInfoNet, 2016).

The 1970s saw the opening of the first community-controlled Aboriginal medical service. Initially it was supported by volunteers, but is now funded by the Department of Prime Minister and Cabinet. The centres have increased in number and size since this time and focus on the needs of the community (Marlow, 2016).

The 1980s saw the introduction of the Aboriginal and/or Torres Strait Islander Hospital Liaison Officer Scheme. The objective of this scheme was to place Aboriginal and/or Torres Strait Islander people in hospitals to assess and contribute to supporting the health care of

Aboriginal and/or Torres Strait Islander patients. The local Aboriginal and/or Torres Strait Islander community often selected the officers. Since then the role has proven to be incredibly successful – make sure when you are on placement you look up the Aboriginal liaison officer and have a chat with them. You will learn a great deal from them in a mere 10 minutes!

Collaboration

Working as a nurse, it is important to support development of effective partnerships between staff, Aboriginal and/or Torres Strait Islander people and their communities. This collaboration ensures:

- accessibility to service
- affordability
- consideration of socioeconomic status
- accountability
- culturally safe and appropriate health care
- a holistic approach – with community participation and ownership (Australian Indigenous HealthInfoNet, 2016).

Evaluation

As with any nursing intervention, care for the Aboriginal and/or Torres Strait Islander Australian requires evaluation and review. Evaluation needs to incorporate social, spiritual, psychological and physical needs – in other words a holistic approach. Remember that Aboriginal and/or Torres Strait Islander people have strong connections to:

- land
- culture
- spirituality and ancestors
- physical wellbeing
- mental wellbeing
- family/kinship
- community (Queensland Health, 2016).

Providing care for all patients regardless of where they are from or what their culture is must be based on respect, dignity and a holistic approach. Care of Aboriginal and/or Torres Strait Islander people requires a true and unbiased understanding of the history and events that have occurred in Australia. Positive, respectful and dignified nursing care and communication will go a long way in overcoming any potential concerns you may have (Australian Indigenous HealthInfoNet, 2016).

In conclusion

Aboriginal and/or Torres Strait Islander health workers are unique and hold a special position within their communities. They are community role models, peers, mentors and guides to their community. The Aboriginal and/or Torres Strait Islander health workers have been described as cultural brokers, acting as cultural mediators between Aboriginal and/or Torres Strait Islander people and health professionals in order to meet a duty of care. They also work with traditional healers. It is not always culturally appropriate for nursing staff to carry out some tasks, due to cultural dynamics. Men's and women's business needs to be acknowledged as it is not appropriate for a female to discuss male health issues with a man (Eckermann et al., 2005).

Ensuring cultural respect and privacy can be maintained is essential in the care of Aboriginal and/or Torres Strait Islander people. Contacting an Aboriginal and/or Torres Strait Islander interpreter or Aboriginal health/liaison officer in the first instance will also ensure more positive health outcomes. Make sure you review the availability of liaison officers when you are on placement.

SUMMARY

- To develop a therapeutic relationship with Aboriginal and/or Torres Strait islander clients it is important to identify and address cultural factors to ensure cultural safety for clients.
- Nurses need to model cultural safety in their own work practices by engaging in respectful work practices.
- Encouraging self-determination and community control in services and programs is essential to developing effective partnerships between nurses and clients.
- Evaluation of interventions should be undertaken by both nursing staff and clients.

SELF-TEST QUESTIONS

1   What cultural safety issues may arise in the workplace when delivering care to Aboriginal and/or Torres Strait Islander clients?
2   How can a nurse model cultural safety in their work practices?
3   What resources are required to develop strategies for cultural safety in the workplace?
4   Who should be involved in the evaluation of cultural safety strategies?
5   What communication techniques will assist in the provision of culturally safe work practices?

BIBLIOGRAPHY

Aboriginal and Torres Strait Islander people (2000). *Submission to the House of Representatives Standing Committee into the needs of urban dwelling Aboriginal and Torres Strait Islander peoples*. Commonwealth of Australia: Canberra.

Aboriginal Liaison Unit: Women's and Children's Hospital South Australia (n.d.). *Fact sheet*. Retrieved from http://www.wch.sa.gov.au/services/az/other/allied/aboriginal/documents/alu_services_factsheet.pdf.

Australian Bureau of Statistics (ABS) (2013). *4102.0 – Australian Social Trends, Nov 2013*. Retrieved from http://www.abs.gov.au/ausstats/abs@.nsf/Lookup/4102.0Main+Features20Nov+2013. Accessed 4 September 2017.

Australian Human Rights Commission (1997). *Bringing them Home: Report of the National Inquiry into the Separation of Aboriginal and Torres Strait Islander Children from Their Families*. Retrieved from https://www.humanrights.gov.au/publications/bringing-them-home-report-1997.

Australian Indigenous HealthInfoNet (2013). *Overview of the health of Indigenous people in Western Australia 2013*. Retrieved from https://www.healthinfonet.ecu.edu.au/uploads/docs/wa-overview-2013.pdf. Accessed 4 September 2017.

Australian Indigenous HealthInfoNet (2016). *Social and emotional wellbeing: An overview of Aboriginal and Torres Strait Islander health status, 2016*. Retrieved from http://www.healthinfonet.ecu.edu.au/health-facts/summary. Accessed 14 July 2017.

Australian Indigenous HealthInfoNet (2017). *The context of Aboriginal and Torres Strait Islander health*. Retrieved from http://www.healthinfonet.ecu.edu.au/health-facts/overviews/the-context-of-aboriginal-and-torres-strait-islander-health. Accessed 4 September 2017.

Australian Institute of Health and Welfare (2014). *Mortality and Life Expectancy of Aboriginal and Torres Strait Islander People: 2008–2012*. Cat. No. IHW 140. AIHW: Canberra.

Australian Institute of Health and Welfare (AIHW) (2015). *Cultural competency in the delivery of health services for Indigenous people*. Retrieved from http://www.aihw.gov.au/uploadedFiles/ClosingTheGap/Content/Our_publications/2015/ctgc-ip13.pdf. Accessed 21 November 2017.

Australian Institute of Health and Welfare (AIHW) (n.d). *Reports & statistics*. Retrieved from http://www.aihw.gov.au/WorkArea/DownloadAsset.aspx?id=60129548468.

Australian Parliament. House of Representatives. Standing Committee on Aboriginal and Torres Strait Islander Affairs (1992). *Language and Culture: A Matter of Survival. Report of the Inquiry into Aboriginal and Torres Strait Islander Language Maintenance*. Australian Government Publishing Service: Canberra.

Bainbridge, R., McCalman, J., Clifford, A. & Tsey, K. (2015). *Cultural competency in the delivery of the health services for Indigenous people*. AIHW: Canberra.

Berndt, R. & Berndt, C. (1988). *The World of the First Australians: Aboriginal Traditional Life, Past and Present*. Australian Institute of Aboriginal Studies, Aboriginal Studies Press: Canberra.

Berndt, R. & Berndt, C. (1997). *Bringing them home report*. Retrieved from https://www.humanrights.gov.au/publications/bringing-them-home-report-1997. Accessed 14 July 2017.

Brown, A. & Blashk, G. (2006). 'Indigenous male health disadvantage – linking the heart and mind', *Australian Family Physician*, 34(10): 805–96, http://www.racgp.org.au/afp/200510/29470.

Clarke, L., Gray, S., White, L., Duncan, G. & Baumle, W. (2016). *Foundations of Nursing: Enrolled Division 2 Nurses*. ANZ Edition. Cengage Learning: South Melbourne.

Clarke, P. (2008). 'Aboriginal healing practices and Australian bush medicine', *Journal of the Anthropological Society of South Australian*, 33: 17.

Cunneen, C. & Libesman, T. (1995). *Indigenous People and the Law in Australia*. Butterworths Legal Studies Series: Sydney.

Eckermann, A., Dowd, T., Martin, M., Nixon, L., Gray, R. & Chong, E. (2005). *Binanj Goonj: Bridging Cultures in Aboriginal Health* (2nd edition). University of New England Press: Armidale, NSW.

Gray, D. (2006). *Health Sociology: An Australian Perspective*. Pearson/Prentice Hill: Frenchs Forest, NSW.

Henderson, A. (2010). *Push to reinstate 'Thirsty Thursday' grog ban*, http://www.abc.net.au/news/2010-10-22/push-to-reinstate-thirsty-thursday-grog-ban/2308276. Accessed 31 January 2018.

Henderson, G., Robson, C., Cox, L., Dukes, C., Tsey, K. & Haswell, M. (2007). 'Social and emotional wellbeing of Aboriginal and Torres Strait Islander people within the broader context of the Social Determinants of Health', in *Beyond Bandaids: Exploring the Underlying Social Determinants of Aboriginal Health*. Retrieved from http://www.lowitja.org. au/sites/default/files/docs/Beyond-Bandaids-CH8.pdf.

http://www.health.gov.au/internet/wcms/Publishing.nsf/Contemt/mentalpubs/$FILE/wayfor.pdf. Accessed 21 November 2017.

http://www.healthinfonet.ecu.edu.au/health-facts/overviews/selected-health-conditions/mental-health. Accessed 10 October 2017.

Jackson, L.R. & Ward, J.E. (1999), 'Aboriginal health: Why is reconciliation necessary?', *The Medical Journal of Australia*, 170(9): 437–40.

King, I. & Brown, N. (2002). 'Indigenous health: Chronically inadequate responses to damning statistics', *The Medical Journal of Australia*, 177(11): 629–31.

Lowell, A., Brown, I., Marrnayin, B., Flack, M.C. & Snelling, P. (2005). *Sharing the true stories: Improving communication in Indigenous health care*. Retrieved from http://www.healthinfonet.ecu.edu.au/key-resources/promotion-resources?lid=15229. Accessed 17 November 2017.

National Aboriginal Controlled Health Organisation (NACCHO) (2017). Retrieved from http://www.naccho.org.au/. Accessed 9 October 2017.

National Indigenous Health Equality Targets (2008). *Outcomes from the National Indigenous Health Equality Summit*, Canberra, March 18–20.

Marlow, K. (2016). The Redfern Aboriginal Medical Service celebrates 45 years, *NITV*, 6 July. Retrieved from http://www.sbs.com.au/nitv/article/2016/07/06/redfern-aboriginal-medical-service-celebrates-45-years. Accessed 21 November 2017.

O'Brien, G. & Plooij, D. (2006). *Cultural Training Manual for Medical Workers in Aboriginal Communities* (adapted by the Northern Rivers Division of General Practice). School of Social Sciences, Flinders University: Adelaide.

Office of Children and Young People (2002). *Aboriginal Child, Youth and Family Strategy Resource Kit*. NSW Office of Children and Young People: Sydney.

Queensland Health (2015). *Sad news Sorry Business: Guidelines for caring for Aboriginal and Torres Strait Islander people through death and dying*. Retrieved from https://www.health.qld.gov.au/__data/assets/pdf_file/0023/151736/sorry_business.pdf.

Queensland Health (2016). *Queensland Health Aboriginal and Torres Strait Islander Mental Health Strategy 2016–2021*. Retrieved from https://www.health.qld.gov.au/__data/assets/pdf_file/0030/460893/qhatsi-mental-health-strategy.pdf. Accessed 4 September 2017.

Royal Australian College of General Practitioners (2012). *An introduction to Aboriginal and Torres Strait Islander health cultural protocols and perspectives*. Retrieved from http://www.racgp.org.au/download/Documents/AHU/2012culturalprotocols.pdf. Accessed 4 September 2017.

Swan, P. & Raphael, B. (1995). *Ways Forward: National Consultancy Report on Aboriginal and Torres Strait Islander Mental Health*, Australian Government Publishing Service: Canberra, p. 14.

Williams, R. (1999). *Cultural safety – What does it mean for our work practice?* Retrieved from http://www.utas.edu.au/__data/assets/pdf_file/0010/246943/RevisedCulturalSafetyPaper-pha.pdf. Accessed 4 September 2017.

Maternal and infant health care

LEARNING OUTCOMES

After reading this chapter, you should have an understanding of:

24.1 Caring for a mother and her newborn infant as part of the health-care team

24.2 Supporting mother and newborn infant towards identified goals

Special delivery!

The maternity placement I was looking forward to especially seeing a newborn being delivered. I found that it was amazing how this process occurred.

The first week of my placement I was assigned to the prenatal department and was involved in providing prenatal care for women who were coming to the unit for delivery. I was pleased that I could assist here and the skills I had learnt in client assessment were put to good use. I was aware of the different conditions that could arise in pregnancy and was careful to ensure that I checked these assessments carefully.

After the initial week I was then assigned to the delivery ward and the nursery area. I was surprised to find that newborns were very quiet. Every other baby I had spent time with seemed to cry quite loudly. These newborns looked like dolls all swaddled up in their checked bunny rugs. The only time they seemed to stir was around feeding time.

I was able to watch a caesarian delivery in the theatre complex and was fascinated to see the baby squirm and cry on delivery. The midwife showed me how they assessed the baby using the APGAR scoring system. The baby was perfect. Mum and dad were overjoyed and it was very emotional, and I felt quite emotional myself.

I enjoyed my time in this area and looked forward to completing my studies. Who knows? Perhaps this is an area that I will revisit as a registered nurse.

24.1 Caring for a mother and newborn infant as part of the health-care team

Pregnancy is a phenomenal thing. Physiological changes occur from implantation, and for some mothers last until delivery. Nursing care of the pregnant woman is a highly specialised area, with a focus on successful antenatal care. Antenatal care can take place in a hospital or a clinic environment and provides an opportunity for the nurse to provide holistic nursing care, education, support and ongoing assessment. Caring for the expectant mother covers both antenatal and postnatal care.

There are a number of specialised staff involved in the care of the mother and newborn infant. See **Table 24.1** for an overview of some (but not all) of the major health-care team staff involved.

antenatal
Before delivery of the newborn

postnatal
After delivery of the newborn

TABLE 24.1 Team involved in the care of the mother and newborn infant

Staff member	Role
General practitioner	Usually the first health-care team member that the mother makes contact with. They will provide a referral to an obstetrician and link the expectant mother to prenatal services.
Midwife	A registered nurse or midwife who will provide care for the expectant mother throughout pregnancy and delivery.
Registered nurses	Nurses who will assist in the prenatal checks and work in partnership with midwives.
Obstetricians	A doctor with specialised training in the medical care of expectant mothers during pregnancy, labour and after delivery.
Anaesthetists	A doctor who provides anaesthetic services during labour if required.
Radiographer	Will take ultrasounds of baby during pregnancy.
Physiotherapist	A physiotherapist who specialises in the care of the mother before and after pregnancy.
Paediatrician	A doctor who specialises in the care of babies and children.
Neonatal nurses	A nurse who specialises in caring for babies born prematurely or babies who are unwell.
Maternal and child health nurse	A specially trained nurse who will assess children's growth and development from birth to three and a half years.

Pregnancy and foetal development

Working in a specialised area requires the nurse to have a solid foundation of knowledge regarding the conditions in which they will be providing care. This is no different in the maternity area. **Tables 24.2** and **24.3** provide an overview of the changes that occur for both mother and baby during **gestation**. A review of anatomy and physiology prior to a placement in maternity is recommended (see Chapter 7).

The joy of childbirth and pregnancy is not without complication, and nursing management and assessment exists to ensure that high-risk pregnancies are managed differently. Midwifery in itself also identifies that all pregnancies are different and assesses each and every expectant mother as a new case.

Physiological changes that occur in the woman can be categorised as *local* (confined to the reproductive organs) or *systemic* (affecting the entire body). Both the signs and symptoms of pregnancy differ from female to female (see **Table 24.2**), with some women reporting symptoms as early as five weeks pregnancy.

gestation
Development of the foetus during pregnancy

Explore the theory in *Foundations of Nursing* text Chapter 25: Maternal and newborn care

TABLE 24.2 Maternal changes with associated signs and symptoms

Body system	Maternal changes	Associated signs and/or symptoms
Reproductive system	• Uterus becomes progressively larger • Placenta develops and blood flow to uterus is increased • The cervix develops from a rigid to a soft stretchy structure • The cervix produces a mucus plug to stop ascending infection • Increased blood flow to the vagina • Placenta – an organ developed through pregnancy that attaches mother and baby and provides blood circulation from mother and baby • Cervix – the lower part of the uterus that has the opening to the uterus	• Abdominal stretching and enlargement • Nausea and vomiting • Abdominal discomfort • Bluish appearance of labia
Cardiovascular system	• Increase in cardiac output, stroke volume and heart rate • Decrease in systemic vascular resistance from five weeks • The heart is displaced upwards to the left	• Increased pulse rate • Decrease in blood pressure
Haematological system	• Increase in blood and plasma volumes and red cell mass • Increase in clotting factors and fibrinogen	• Anaemia and tiredness • Increased risk for deep vein thrombosis
Respiratory system	• Increase in oxygen consumption • The diaphragm is raised and the ribs flare • The subcostal angle increases • Tidal volume increases and functional residual capacity decreases	• Increased respiratory rate, shortness of breath and poor exercise tolerance
Gastrointestinal system	• Gums become more vascular and oedematous • Intestines are compacted and bowl motility decreases • Stomach capacity decreases and the muscle is relaxed	• Bleeding, tender gums and periodontal disease • Abdominal pain and constipation, haemorrhoids • Heartburn, gastric reflux, nausea and vomiting
Musculoskeletal system	• Relaxation of the pelvic joints and ligaments • Anterior shift in centre of gravity and increased spinal curvature	• Discomfort in the pelvic area • Waddling type gait • Lower back pain
Endocrine system	• Increase in basal metabolic rate • Increase in prolactin production, a hormone responsible for milk production	• Increased temperature • Breast enlargement, tenderness and milk production
Integumentary system	• Increase in melanocyte production and hyperpigmentation	• Darkening over areas of skin, particularly the face and abdomen.

Source: White, L., Duncan, G., Baumle, W., Gray, S. & Ferris, L. (2018). *Foundations of Nursing*, Australian and New Zealand edition, 2nd Edition. Cengage: Melbourne.

Pregnancy is generally 40 weeks. Of course this time can alter due to varying factors, such as prematurity, drug abuse, placenta previa or multiple births. **Table 24.3** outlines the foetal development during gestation.

TABLE 24.3 Foetal development by gestation in weeks

Stage of development	Gestation	Developmental progress
Embryo	0–4 weeks	• Placenta develops and functions to sustain embryo • Primitive central nervous system develops • Primitive heart develops and starts beating • A layer of skin and limb buds form
	4–8 weeks	• Rapid cell division • Spinal nerves, kidneys and lower respiratory system begin to develop • Blood is pumped around vessels • Ossification of the skeleton begins • Head and facial features develop
Foetus	8–16 weeks	• Rapid weight gain and skeletal development • Urine passed, meconium present in the gut • Eyelids meet and fuse • Nasal septum and palate fuse • Primitive reflexes present • Lanugo appears • External genitalia can be differentiated • Foetus can suck its thumb
	16–24 weeks	• Constant weight gain • Vernix appears • Brown fat develops • Sleep and active periods • Ear developing • Skin is red and wrinkled • Surfactant secreted in lungs from 20 weeks
	24–32 weeks	• Legally viable at 24 weeks • Eyelids open • Respiratory movements • Testes descend into scrotum • Skin paler and less wrinkled • Fat and iron are stored
	32–40 weeks	• Weight gain approximately 25 g per day • Lanugo disappears • Hair on head lengthens • Body round and plump • Skull formed but soft and flexible • Can coordinate sucking and swallowing

Source: White, L., Duncan, G., Baumle, W., Gray, S. & Ferris, L. (2018). *Foundations of Nursing*, Australian and New Zealand edition, 2nd Edition. Cengage: Melbourne.

Table 24.4 lists two common complications of pregnancy that are routinely screened for during pregnancy.

TABLE 24.4 Common complications of pregnancy

Condition	Symptoms
Hypertension	High blood pressure brought on by the stress of pregnancy. • proteinuria • oedema • headaches

>>

Condition	Symptoms
Eclampsia	Uncontrolled hypertension that leads to seizures and endangers the life of mother and baby
Gestational diabetes	Pregnancy-induced diabetes It often reverses after delivery but may cause Type II diabetes to occur Refer to Chapter 18 on diabetes

For more information on types of conditions that may occur during pregnancy, visit the following website: https://www.ncbi.nlm.nih.gov/books/NBK326674/.

Labour and birth

Labour occurs in three stages and no two labours are alike. Signs and symptoms of labour include contractions or a 'show' – which is a mucous discharge that is either blood-stained or pink coloured. This is the plug that has been sealing the cervix, so it means that the cervix is starting to stretch. A show can occur hours or even days prior to contractions commencing.

The most common occurrence is 'waters breaking' – the amniotic sac holding the foetus breaks and amniotic fluid leaks or gushes out.

Birth of the infant obviously occurs at the completion of labour. The length of labour differs for each and every woman, and is dependent on many factors such as age, pregnancy complications and previous deliveries. Your role in the birth process will depend upon local policies and procedures. Generally, a midwife is present with the assistance of other nursing staff – enrolled nurses, registered nurses or assistants in nursing, which is your role!

Emergencies can occur during birth. It is important to be aware of where emergency equipment is stored and what your role is during an emergency. Again, this will differ depending on your placement location. Maternal emergencies can also occur in any location (Pillitteri, 2013; NSW Health, 2012; Dempsey et al., 2009, Rizzo, 2015).

Nursing care – assisting the midwife

Childbirth does not complete the nursing care required for both mother and baby. It is merely the beginning of new needs for both patients. Nursing care in this important post-partum period includes assistance and education concerning care of the baby – umbilical cord cleaning, bathing, nappy changing, feeding (breast or formula), and also the care of the mother.

Care of the mother

There is specific care for the mother and baby with each stage of pregnancy. In the prenatal stage care is focused on assessment and early detection of any abnormal health states. See **Table 24.4** for specific health concerns that may develop for the mother as a result of pregnancy. Accurate assessment is critical to pick up health problems and the establishment of a therapeutic relationship will help elicit any further health concerns the mother may have.

During labour, assessment of both mother and baby are conducted. There is specialised equipment used to monitor the infant during the stages of labour. Midwives will also undertake specialised physical checks during the stages of labour, such as assessment of the cervical opening.

In postnatal care we now have two clients – mother and baby. Both are now assessed as individuals. Care of the postnatal mother is as important as antenatal care during labour and delivery. The mother is assessed for any complications that may arise as a result of childbirth.

Some of the common assessments undertaken post-delivery include the following:

- amount of **lochia** post-delivery.
- temperature – indicating fever
- constipation
- special checks if any antenatal complications were present.

The first six weeks post birth is referred to as the **post-partum period**. This is a period of change for the new mother. There are changes in the cervix, vagina, perineum, breasts and hormone levels as the body adjusts to no longer being pregnant.

All interventions in the post-partum period should be family centred so that the family can bond (**Figure 24.1**). Nursing interventions should also be focused on increasing self-esteem for the mother by allowing her to view herself as a new mother (whether it is the first or fourth child!) and bond with her new baby.

lochia
Vaginal discharge after birth

post-partum period
The first six weeks after giving birth

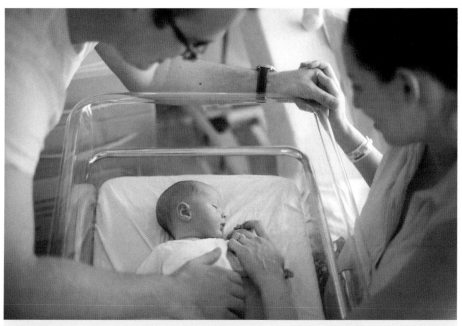

FIGURE 24.1 Psychological impact of birth

Getty Images/Catherine Delahaye.

There are not only physiological changes in the post-partum period, but also psychological changes. Postnatal depression is not uncommon, particularly in first-time mothers. Postnatal depression is a term used to describe mood disorders occurring in women in the first year after the birth of a child. There are three different postnatal disorders that can appear – postnatal blues, depression and psychosis.

Postnatal depression is a true physical illness that affects over 10% of Australian mothers. The depression generally starts after the mother leaves hospital. Generalised signs and symptoms include:

- feelings of inadequacy and irritability
- sleep disturbance
- overly concerned about lack of sleep
- appetite disturbance – poor appetite or overeating
- poor concentration
- memory loss
- inability to do household tasks
- confusion – unable to think clearly
- tearfulness, mood changes
- loss of sexual interest

- feelings of panic, fear of social contact
- fear of harming the baby
- changes in maternal feelings (Pillitteri, 2013; Dempsey et al., 2009; NSW Health, 2012).

Activity 24.1

Postnatal assessment

Locate the policy and procedure for the routine postnatal checks that are performed for the care of the mother following delivery.

1   What is each assessment focusing on?
2   What are the normal parameters for each assessment task?
3   What are some complications that a mother might experience following childbirth?

Care of the newborn

The nurse involved with the care of the newborn baby is in a unique situation. You are providing care for a new life – one that has changed dramatically in such a short period of time. A being that was dependant for much of its growth or gestation now draws its own breath and responds to stimuli out of utero.

The newborn will require routine checks while in hospital. All babies will receive:

- an examination by a doctor or a midwife (usually both) – this is called the newborn examination (see **Figure 24.2**), and is not the exam performed at birth. This examination is always documented in the baby's personal health record.
- a blood test – usually a heal prick test to check for congenital hypothyroidism, phenylketonuria, glactosaemia and cystic fibrosis.
- a hearing test – but this is not in all states in Australia so you will need to ascertain if this is completed in your placement location.

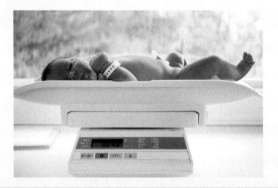

1   A normal full-term infant weighs approximately 3.5 kg and measures about 50 cm when fully extended.
2   Occipitofrontal circumference of the newborn's head is 34–35 cms and the head comprises ¼ of the infant's size.
3   The newborn has two fontanelles. The anterior fontanelle closes at about 18 months and the posterior fontanelle closes at about three months.
4   Vernix caseosa is a whitish sticky substance present on the newborn's skin which has a protective function in utero.
5   The general colour of the skin is pink and may be pigmented with milia, storkmarks, mongolian spots and birthmarks.
6   Meconium is the first stool that the newborn passes and should be checked for in the first 24 hours of life.
7   Observe for bleeding at umbilical site, small spotting when cord falls off, cleaning.
8   The umbilical cord should have two arteries and one vein.
9   Range of movements at hip checked to detect congenital dislocation of the hips.
10 The normal spine for the newborn is 'C'-shaped.

FIGURE 24.2 Examination of the newborn baby

Science Photo Library/Mauro Fermariello.

Each and every newborn is inherently different but similarities do exist! Unfortunately, death occurs even in childbirth. All hospitals will have a specific protocol to follow if the child dies during birth/in utero/or shortly thereafter (Pillitteri, 2013, NSW Health, 2012, Dempsey et al. 2009, Rizzo, 2015).

Reflective practice 24.1

A new beginning

On my second semester placement I went to a regional hospital, just outside of a city. I was walking back from the canteen to return to shift and I was asked for help. I turned around and a woman who was visiting someone was lying on the floor of the main walkway and presumably her waters had broken. There was fluid everywhere; I never thought there would be so much fluid. She was lying on her back and looked frightened. I felt so overwhelmed and unsure of what to do. I decided to just start talking and asking her how she was feeling, how pregnant she was and if this was her first baby. An orderly had passed us also and had called a medical emergency, so I knew that help was coming.

I stayed with this lady right through, my clinical facilitator was amazing about ensuring I could see this unique situation through. Turns out it was Eliza's fourth baby, so she knew pretty much what was ahead. Her labour was well established (I was listening to all the discussions taking place) and she gave birth to a perfect baby boy three hours later. I will never, ever, forget the first little cry he made. It was an amazing sound. The room seemed to echo a big sigh of relief when the cry was audible. Seeing the baby (who was named Mason two days later) was surreal. This little human was totally reliant on Eliza for 39 weeks, and now was breathing and crying and doing all the right things for himself. This experience really opened my eyes to the abundance of areas that nursing can take you. Maternity is definitely one I would like to specialise in.

Holly, 25, EN, 1 year post graduate

1   Would you feel comfortable assisting the visitor in this situation?
2   Why do you think there was a 'sigh of relief' when the baby cried?
3   What, if any, complications could occur for Eliza?

Using correct terminology

As with all nursing communication it is important to use the correct terminology when communicating verbally and documenting. There are specialised terms used as seen in **Tables 24.1** and **24.2** that relate to specific areas of pregnancy, labour and newborns.

When communicating with mothers and fathers it is important to use these terms but also provide a clear explanation of what they mean. You will need to relate these to the words that the parents are familiar with and avoid using jargon without explanation.

Activity 24.2

Communicating effectively

It is essential that you understand the technical terms used in the area of midwifery in order to communicate effectively with other members of the health-care team.
1   Using your handover sheet, work through the terms that relate to three of the clients present in the midwifery unit.

2   Share your definitions with your classmates till all terms have been explained.

Now that you know what the terms mean relate this to your clients. Perhaps you can give a verbal handover of your clients at debrief using the terms that you have defined.

Assisting with lactation

One of the tasks that you will be required to undertake is assisting the mother to breastfeed her new infant. Infants are born with a 'rooting' reflex but the actual latching onto the nipple can be difficult at the start. At times mothers may feel that there is no milk supply, which is normal as *colostrum* is the first fluid that is given to newborns. It usually takes three to four days post-delivery for the milk supply to be present. When the mother's milk does come the breasts can be very hard and full which also makes it difficult for infants to attach to the breast. The mother can be assisted with positioning techniques to enable safe feeding for the infant.

Additional information on infant feeding can be found here: https://www.thewomens.org.au/health-professionals/clinical-resources/clinical-guidelines-gps/.

Activity 24.3

Assisting with breastfeeding

A lot of people feel that breastfeeding is a natural activity that is easily undertaken. This is not the case. Many mothers find it difficult to feed infants for a variety of reasons. Locate the policy and procedure in the workplace relating to lactation.

1   Who is the person that needs to be notified if difficulties are experienced?

Assisting the mother with safe practices in infant care

Providing nursing care to the neonate and their family allows the family to provide care for their child with support – which is an amazing role. Imagine bathing a baby for the first time with no-one to help or show you what to do! Babies are seen as fragile creatures partly because they are so helpless, and new parents can be overwhelmed and incredibly scared with the responsibility of providing total care for their child. Newborn infants are totally dependent on others to meet their needs. Some education may have been delivered during the prenatal period but completing the care on a new infant can be very frightening for some parents. Infants need to have their temperature monitored and controlled through clothing, regular changing of nappies, feeding, sleeping positions, and contact and bonding opportunities.

Your role of the student nurse in this situation is to provide support and education to better arm the parents for the provision of care for their child.

Figure 24.3 outlines a bathing guide for newborns.

Ongoing care of mother

Each new mother requires differing levels of care. For instance, a first-time mother may require much more assistance with breastfeeding, or providing care for their newborn. On the other hand, a mother of five may rely on her life experiences and may not require as much intervention. However, by no means does this allow nursing staff to judge 'who needs what' but requires constant and current assessment of each situation, an assessment skill you will develop as your experience and exposure to this area of nursing develops.

Assessment of the woman during pre- and postnatal periods is undertaken through health interviews, physical examinations, and analysis of laboratory findings. Assessment of her psychological adjustment should begin with her reaction to the birth: Is she happy that the child is a girl or boy? Is she happy to be through with the pregnancy or still longing to be pregnant again? When assessing the quality and quantity of the mother's interaction with the child ask: Does she hold the infant and talk to him/her? Again, it must be stressed that holistic care is required for the mother and the family, in order to promote and facilitate bonding.

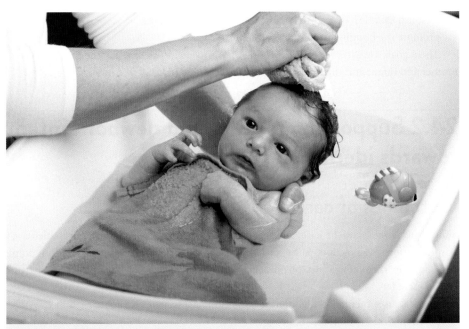

FIGURE 24.3 Bathing guide for newborns

Shutterstock.com/Jandrie Lombard.

It is also important that physiological changes such as uterine involution and lochia flow/amount are assessed.

Documenting and recording observations of the mother and newborn infant

Knowing how to carry out an accurate health assessment – from taking the health history through to performing a physical examination – will help you uncover any significant problems and assist in planning care appropriately. In the maternity area of nursing specialised charts are used for both mother and baby. Like all other areas of clinical care these provide the health-care team with an overview of the mother's and baby's progress. They form part of the client file and are a legal document. For more detailed information on assessment of mother and baby the following websites provide a good introduction:

- World Health Organization (2015). 'Childbirth: Labour, delivery and immediate postpartum care' in *Pregnancy, Childbirth, Postpartum and Newborn Care: A Guide for Essential Practice* (3rd edition), https://www.ncbi.nlm.nih.gov/books/NBK326674/. WHO: Geneva.
- Queensland Department of Health, *Routine newborn assessment*, https://www.health.qld.gov.au/__data/assets/pdf_file/0029/141689/g-newexam.pdf.

Providing holistic care

Holistic nursing covers all components of nursing practice that have healing or caring for the *whole* patient as their goal. Holistic nursing addresses spiritual, psychological, psychosocial, emotional, environmental and physical needs in patients. In the maternity area the goals of nursing care are to:

- ensure the health of the mother
- ensure the health and wellbeing of the newborn

TIP 24.1

Documentation
Ensure that you observe a trained member of staff completing the documentation. The documents are often complicated and it is better to assist with the assessment tasks than trying to guess how to complete the documentation.

Review the skill in Tollefson *Essential Clinical Skills* 2.1 Head-to-toe assessment; 2.3 Temperature, pulse and respiration (TPR) measurement; 2.4 Blood pressure measurement & 7.5 Health teaching

- establish lactation or feeding regime for the newborn infant
- promote the bonding of mother and infant.

These goals are achieved with assessing and implementing care for the individuals, the mother and infant and the family unit (Clarke et al., 2016; Tollefson et al., 2016).

24.2 Supporting mother and newborn infant towards identified goals

Outcomes of care

Simply put, outcomes of care are endpoints or goals that we set for our patients on hospitalisation. Many care paths or care plans have endpoints or explanation points embedded in them. Examples of outcomes of care for a woman during the post-partum period include:

- physical assessment – lochia, uterine condition, assessment of stitches
- psychological assessment – ongoing
- bonding with child and family
- ability to feed and clean child
- ability to change nappy
- education specific to immunisations, health care etc.

Achieving patient goals can be as simple as drawing them up and mapping out 'how to get there'. Collaboration with other members of the multidisciplinary health-care team is also an essential component of achieving patient goals through holistic patient care. Inclusion of the patient's family or significant other is essential – they will be your patient's support person when they are no longer in hospital, a constant source of support and comfort, and more importantly the child's parent. Each patient will have some very personal goals and these need to be respected. Having a newborn can be a very daunting experience initially – because you cannot be certain of any behaviour or habits until you have been able to establish a routine.

Taking time to set goals with your patient enables you to assess their level of understanding. Not all patients will leave hospital fully self-managing – that is why we have domiciliary nursing care and other support mechanisms for the ongoing assessment, support and education in relation to the care of mother, baby and family. (Pillitteri, 2013; NSW Health, 2012; Dempsey et al., 2009; Clarke et al., 2016).

In the care of mothers and babies, discharge planning focuses on holistic care – and referrals to domiciliary or community-based midwifery programs or child and maternal health programs. These programs and the availability of them differ from area to area and state to state. Many hospitals have referrals to 'mother's groups' which slots mothers together with similarly aged children for six to eight weeks of post-partum education and ongoing assessment. This education is delivered by either a midwife or a child and maternal expert (Clarke et al., 2016; Dempsey et al., 2009).

Reflective practice 24.2

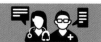

A lesson learnt

When I had my first child, I was 17-years-old. I had no real support mechanisms and I felt like I was always doing the wrong thing. I did not want to breastfeed – a choice that I had many 'lectures' about from some midwives. I now have three children aged 20, five and two. A big age gap, I know. I started my training to be an enrolled nurse when I was 36-years-old. On my second placement I went to a rural hospital and worked in the emergency department. It was the most frightening and amazing placement all in one. A young woman presented, pregnant, alone and very scared. I felt that I could talk to her about my experiences and maybe help her. I started comparing our situations, trying to find common ground – trying to urge her to breastfeed. Turns out I was not supporting her or her needs – I was chasing my own agenda about something profoundly personal. It was an eye-opening experience in many ways and showed me just how easy it is to judge – albeit in the most non-malicious manner – and how much influence we have as a nurse with patients who need our help and advocacy.

This happened a few years ago and now I work in a primary health clinic that offers antenatal and chronic disease management. I have seen the difference it makes to patients to be supported from the outset and listened to. I use my example to any student that will listen as it is invaluable. Just because you are a nurse does not mean you have the right to compare situations or impose your thoughts on a patient.

Kathy, 43, Advanced Practice Enrolled Nurse

Planning care and care goals

Care planning for the maternal patient is unique in that you need to provide care for both the mother and the neonate. As with any care plan, you need to work collaboratively with the midwife to ensure holistic care is being maintained.

In maternal health care, the care required will be heavily reliant upon the client. If this is her first child, for instance, she may require assistance with breastfeeding, feeding, changing or bathing. Even if it is her fourth child, you cannot assume she has all the relevant information to establish feeding or a routine.

CASE STUDY 24.1

Supporting the new mother

Jodie Hynes is a 16-year-old who has just given birth to a boy. Jodie has not had any visitors and has not identified the father of her child. Jodie is having difficulty in bathing her son as she is 'scared' of drowning him.

1   What nursing interventions would be appropriate for the care of Jodie and her son?

2   What other interventions would you consider appropriate for a young mother who does not appear to have any support networks?

3   Is Jodie's age of any significance? How could it impact upon her discharge and ongoing care of her child?

Education

Educational needs for the postnatal client will depend greatly upon identified needs. A large component of care planning and care goals will highlight the educational needs of the client. Each client is unique as is each birth, leaving some women who have already had children confused and overwhelmed by the new arrival. Working closely with the midwife and the client will enable you to establish educational needs – through observation of feeding, bathing, or sleeping safety aspects.

SUMMARY

- It is essential to work as part of the health-care team to ensure that holistic care is provided to ensure best practice in the care of mother and newborns.
- Specialised members of the health-care team are available to assist mothers achieve goals, such as breastfeeding.
- Education may vary depending on the needs of the mother and baby. Nursing staff can model appropriate interactions with newborns to assist mothers with caring for them.

SELF-TEST QUESTIONS

1   What is the required nursing care for postnatal mothers and newborn infants?
2   What are the assessments that are undertaken during antenatal, labour and postnatal times for mother and baby?
3   How can nurses assist the mother in the process of lactation?
4   What education needs to be given to ensure safe practice in caring for newborn infants?
5   How does a holistic approach assist maternal and infant health?

BIBLIOGRAPHY

Clarke, L., Gray, S., White, L., Duncan, G. & Baumle, W. (2016). *Foundations of Nursing: Enrolled Division 2 Nurses* (ANZ Edition). Cengage Learning: Melbourne.

Dempsey, J., French, J., Hillege, S. & Wilson, V. (2009). *Fundamentals of Nursing & Midwifery: A Person-Centred Approach to Care*. ANZ edition. Wolters Kluwer/Lippincott Williams & Wilkins: Sydney.

Diabetes Australia (2015). *Gestational diabetes*. Retrieved from http://www.diabetesaustralia.com.au/Living-with-Diabetes/Gestational-Diabetes/. Accessed 12 March 2017.

Marieb, E. (2014). *Essentials of Human Anatomy and Physiology* (11th edition) Pearson Benjamin Cummings: San Francisco.

NSW Health (2012). *Having a Baby*. Office of Kids and Families: North Sydney. Retrieved from http://www.health.nsw.gov.au/kidsfamilies/MCFhealth/Publications/having-a-baby.pdf.

Pieris-Caldwell, I., Templeton, M., Ryan, C. & Moon, L. (2008). *Diabetes: Australian Facts 2008*. Australian Institute of Health and Welfare: Canberra.

Pillitteri, A. (2013). *Maternal and Child Health Nursing: Care of the Childbearing and Childrearing Family* (7th edition). Lippincott Williams & Wilkins: USA.

Queensland Department of Health (2014). *Routine newborn assessment*. Retrieved from https://www.health.qld.gov.au/__data/assets/pdf_file/0029/141689/g-newexam.pdf.

Queensland Health, Queensland Public Hospitals Health Report (2012). *Patient safety, from learning to action 2012*. Retrieved from https://www.health.qld.gov.au/__data/assets/pdf_file/0022/423472/lta5.pdf. Accessed 12 March 2017.

Raising Children Network (n.d.). *Preparing a newborn bath*. Retrieved from http://raisingchildren.net.au/articles/pip_bathing_newborn.html.

Rizzo, D. (2015). *Fundamentals of Anatomy and Physiology* (4th edition). Delmar Cengage Learning: USA.

The Royal Women's Hospital, Victoria (n.d.). *Clinical Guidelines*. Retrieved from https://www.thewomens.org.au/health-professionals/clinical-resources/clinical-guidelines-gps/.

Tollefson, J., Watson, G., Jelly, E. & Tambree, K. (2016). *Essential Clinical Skills: Enrolled Division 2 Nurses* (3rd edition). Cengage Learning: Melbourne.

Waugh, A. & Grant, A. (2010). *Anatomy & Physiology in Health and Illness* (11th edition). Mosby Elsevier: St Louis.

World Health Organization (2015). 'Childbirth: Labour, delivery and immediate postpartum care' in *Pregnancy, Childbirth, Postpartum and Newborn Care: A Guide for Essential Practice* (3rd edition), https://www.ncbi.nlm.nih.gov/books/NBK326674/. Geneva, CH: WHO.

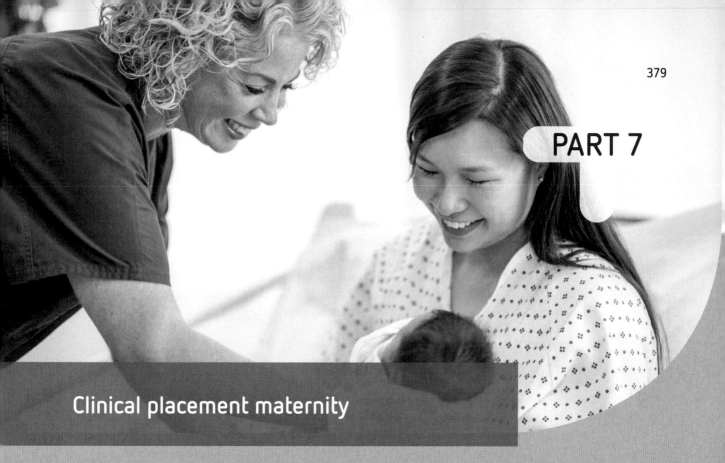

PART 7

Clinical placement maternity

Chapter 25: Improving clinical practice

The maternity experience

I was very lucky to gain a placement in maternity. It was a great insight into the management of such a common condition – pregnancy! The days of the week correlated to clinics and education for expectant mothers, and also postnatal care for those who had already delivered. I soon learnt that pregnancy was different for every woman, and also that there is a great deal of socioeconomic factors that can contribute to antenatal care. Some people had no transport, money or ability to get to appointments. Some people continued to smoke, drink or take illicit drugs while pregnant – without a care in the world – while others had their hearts broken and delivered stillborn infants, miscarried or just could not fall pregnant. I thought maternity would be a happy placement – all about birth and new beginnings. But it was not all happy. Some shifts were so sad. Not because a baby died or anything that horrible, but because it was not always fair. Babies were born with conditions that needed urgent attention, or lifelong care while some mothers faced post-birth complications. It is definitely an area that interests me, but I realise that it is more than just the happy birth! There is antenatal care and education, postnatal care, and the care of the neonate – so many different aspects of maternal care.

The maternity placement will generally be towards the end of your diploma. It will enable you to consolidate your learning from many subjects, such as acute care, anatomy and physiology and, of course, care of the mother and baby.

What kind of patients are in maternity?

Maternity is for care of the mother and her baby or babies. Maternity nursing encompasses the care of the mother pre- and post-delivery, and the care of the newborn. Education, assessment and ongoing review are required for you to be effective in maternity nursing.

In this placement you could be in a hospital environment or in the community setting. The patients you will come across will vary in age and life experiences and may also have health conditions that affect their pregnancy.

Common experiences of student nurses in maternity

Maternity is not just about the birth of a baby. Maternity nursing requires a great deal of education, support and care for both the mother and her baby. Maternal nursing can involve care in the community visiting women and their child for postnatal review and neonatal check-ups, clinic work for antenatal women and acute care in the hospital setting in the birth suite. As enrolled nursing students, you may be allocated to the maternity ward where you will be caring for the mother and her newborn, performing observations on both patients and assisting with delivery of education and health teaching. Establishing feeding and assisting with lactation will also be components of this placement.

Objectives

The objectives that are to be set for this placement need to be contextualised to the maternity setting. Here are some examples of objectives:

* dressing the newborn infant and changing newborn infant nappies
* preparation of feeding formulas
* common obstetric emergencies
* anatomy, physiology and associated terminology related to pregnancy, birth, postnatal period, lactation and care of the newborn infant
* umbilical cord care
* safe practice for bathing, holding, settling and positioning the newborn infant for sleeping
* care of the mother's nipples.

Work allocation

In maternity nursing, often a patient workload is allocated to a team of midwives and nurses. Team nursing is commonly used as it follows the mother from antenatal to postnatal care. Allocation also takes into consideration the needs of the mother and her child. As a student you may administer medications if the unit HLTENN007 has been completed and you are supervised. For more complex management there will be a registered nurse who will undertake specialised activities – such as administration of medications to the neonate. All enrolled nurses and support staff work under the supervision of a registered Division 1 nurse.

Enjoy your placement and ensure you make good use of the valuable time you have in this specialty area.

Improving clinical practice

LEARNING OUTCOMES

After reading this chapter, you should have an understanding of:

25.1 Modelling high standards of performance

25.2 Reflecting on clinical work practices and potential improvements

25.3 Participating in processes for systemic improvement

Clinical practice

I was very interested in learning how the different practices undertaken as part of nursing evolved. After doing the research unit I learnt about evidence-based nursing and how to locate resources that were reputable. I was determined that I would be the best nurse I could be and provide the best care to clients.

I found that applying the knowledge and skills learnt at school to clinical practice was an eye opener. I thought everyone would do things the same way, but this was not the case. On my first placement I thought the registered nurse I was buddied with knew everything. I soon found that this did not always steer me in the right direction and I picked up practices that were not best practice. My clinical supervisor told me to always perform tasks that followed the policies and procedures, even if they took longer, and I found that this did assist in completing my work in the best accepted way.

25.1 Modelling high standards of performance

The key components of modelling high standards of performance are achieved through **collaboration**, communication and **consultation** with all health-care professionals. You will observe the ongoing need for effective communication and how this is a clear pathway to safe and quality patient-care delivery. Health care is an ongoing review process of **continuous improvement** and clinical guidelines are managed through clinical governance or by patient safety and quality officers. Each facility will likely have different methods of review and identification of clinical practices for improvement. A large component of your role as an enrolled nurse will be working out processes for dissemination of information, and for ongoing development and review of clinical practices.

The Nursing and Midwifery Board of Australia has issued the National Enrolled Nurse Standards for Practice (2016), which refers to the scope of practice and the nurse's duties. The frameworks outlined in the Standards for Practice support these duties. The enrolled nurse is responsible for his/her actions at all times and remains accountable in providing delegated nursing care.

collaboration
Working with allied health care and other nursing staff to optimise health care

consultation
Clinical discussion with other health-care team members to enable holistic health care

continuous improvement
An ongoing cycle of improvement to ensure constant review

Organisational vision

Organisational vision and values sound a little non-nursing, that's for sure! Actually they are at the heart of all health-care facilities and in order to provide safe and effective care, health-care facilities need to have clear guidelines as to what their goals are. They need to be measureable to ensure they are actually meeting these goals or targets. In health care, many accountabilities are related directly to clinical care guidelines – things such as medication safety, falls prevention and recognition of the deteriorating patient are some examples.

The vision of the organisation is generally focused on 'better health' for all, or access to health care. Then it is broken down into measurable traits such as commitment to excellence, evidence-based practice, communication strategies or ethical principles, for example.

In working towards improvement of clinical practice, organisational visions and values assist you in the identification of areas for improvement in key accountabilities.

Supporting colleagues

As a nurse, each and every one of us has different life experiences and professional experiences. Imparting knowledge to our peers and colleagues enables ongoing professional development and a level of support. Supporting colleagues can be as simple as listening to an idea for improvement they may have, or assisting them with identified learning needs. Supporting colleagues is entwined with communication and teamwork.

Group work is also another aspect of supporting colleagues. The synergy that results from the interaction between group members is called group dynamics, which influence not only the behaviour of individual members but also the performance of the group as a whole. Effective groups usually have three main characteristics:
- They are formed to accomplish goals.
- They maintain themselves and develop.
- They change/adapt in ways that improve effectiveness.

Another aspect of supporting colleagues is again good and effective communication. Your ability to successfully read a situation and elicit information from your patients, their families and other health-care workers will increase with exposure and practice. Good communication skills are built over time.

Mentoring

Mentoring is a collaborative and reciprocal relationship between two colleagues where there are generally mutual goals and shared accountability which enhances success. Mentoring in nursing is often spontaneous, where an experienced nurse will mentor a newly graduated nurse. In other situations, for example, while you are on placement, you will have a mentor-like relationship with your clinical facilitator (Hnatiuk, 2013).

The role of a mentor is to develop and support clinical and theoretical practice, to bounce ideas off, to answer questions regarding procedures and to offer advice. Mentoring is highly effective, not just in nursing, in establishing workplace safety through supported practice.

Respectful and positive communication

Communication is an ongoing process in all that we do – not just in nursing. Imagine trying to go about your day interacting with goods and service providers and not talking – think about a time when you have had the wrong coffee made because you were misheard, or someone has misunderstood what you are saying and provided something completely different. The same can happen in nursing and health care and this is why communication is ongoing, evolving and needs to be effective.

Wherever you are on placement, take time to review key communication processes – handover is a great example. When does it occur? How does it occur? Is it at the patient's bedside? How are referrals made? Working towards improvement of clinical practice will involve knowing how these processes are undertaken, which will assist your review and analysis for clinical improvement.

Teamwork is not a new concept. Teamwork in health care is essential for effective and safe patient care. Teamwork involves everyone participating actively and positively in the delivery of health care.

Review the skill in Tollefson *Essential Clinical Skills* 3.1 Professional workplace skills – including time management, rounding and personal stress management

Continuous improvement

Continuous improvement is an ongoing process, which is systematic. It is a process that aims to improve the quality of care provided by health-care facilities. It is a cyclical process with four phases that are continually reviewed: plan, do, check and act. They are the cruxes of quality systems for assessing, reviewing and monitoring practice and comparing it to evidence-based practice to ensure care outcomes, innovation and patient safety.

Clinical governance

Clinical governance is closely tied to continuous improvement – it is an ongoing review and is a system that is accountable for quality of care, continuous improvement, minimising risks and fostering excellence in care. Clinical governance is relevant in nursing care due to standards of care and guidelines. The Australian Commission on Safety and Quality in Health Care (2017), has compiled the National Safety and Quality Health Service (NSQHS) Standards – of which there are 10 that are highlighted as areas of concern in patient care delivery.

The standards are as follows:
*   Standard 1 – Governance for Safety and Quality in Health Service Organisations
*   Standard 2 – Partnering with Consumers
*   Standard 3 – Preventing and Controlling Healthcare Associated Infections
*   Standard 4 – Medication Safety
*   Standard 5 – Patient Identification and Procedure Matching
*   Standard 6 – Clinical Handover

- Standard 7 – Blood and Blood Products
- Standard 8 – Preventing and Managing Pressure Injuries
- Standard 9 – Recognising and Responding to Clinical Deterioration in Acute Health Care
- Standard 10 – Preventing Falls and Harm from Falls.

These standards are the cornerstone of patient care and, as such, clinical guidelines and pathways are derived from these standards and clinical reasoning. Medication errors and the repetition of them has led to the development of Standard 4 – Medication Safety, where key identifiers and factors are used to minimise potential harm. See **Figure 25.1** for further explanation of each Standard.

While on placement, particularly in an acute care facility, you will likely see the posters for the NSQHS highlighting the Standards for consumers and all health-care staff. Developing an understanding of improvement in clinical practice is an ongoing process and you can start to identify areas of concern in care delivery just by looking at the 10 standards.

Standard 1 – Governance for Safety and Quality in Health Service Organisations describes the quality framework required for health service organisations to implement safe systems.

Standard 2 – Partnering with Consumers describes the systems and strategies to create a consumer-centred health system by including consumers in the development and design of quality health care.

Standard 3 – Preventing and Controlling Healthcare Associated Infections describes the systems and strategies to prevent infection of patients within the health care system and to manage infections effectively when they occur to minimise the consequences.

Standard 4 – Medication Safety descibes the systems and strategies to ensure clinicians safely prescribe, dispense and administer appropriate medicines to informed patients.

Standard 5 – Patient Identification and Procedure Matching describes the systems and strategies to identify patients and correctly match their identity with the correct treatment.

Standard 6 – Clinical Handover describes the systems and strategies for effective clinical communication whenever accountability and responsibility for a patient's care is transferred.

Standard 7 – Blood and Blood Products describes the systems and strategies for the safe, effective and appropriate management of blood and blood products so the patients receiving blood are safe.

Standard 8 – Preventing and Managing Pressure injuries describes the systems and strategies to prevent patients developing pressure injuries and best practice management when pressure injuries occur.

Standard 9 – Recognising and Responding to Clinical Deterioration In Acute Health Care describes the systems and processes to be implemented by health service organisations to respond effectively to patients when their clinical condition deteriorates.

Standard 10 – Preventing Falls and Harm from Falls describes the systems and strategies to reduce the incidence of patient falls in health service organisations and best practice management when falls do occur.

Australian Commission on Safety and Quality in Health Care

FIGURE 25.1 National Safety and Quality Health Service (NSQH) Standards

25.2 Reflecting on clinical work practices and potential improvements

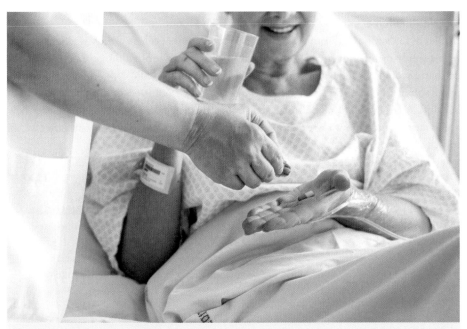

FIGURE 25.2 Medication administration

Getty Images/BURGER.

While on placement, observe who interacts with the patient the most – it is likely that every time, your answer will be the nurse! The nurse is generally the client's first point of contact and spends the most clinical care time with the patients. As a nurse, you will be using clinical guidelines and care plans that have been developed by health-care facilities for the use of all patients. These guidelines are based on the national standards and are an essential component of patient safety.

You will soon observe vast differences in nursing care. One nurse may perform a task in one way and another in a different way. Generally the outcome is the same and there is no patient harm. It is when shortcuts are taken or procedures are not followed correctly that harm can occur. Think of a medication chart – if the identifiers are not present it is not a valid prescription. However, countless times medication has still been administered from an incomplete order.

Practices are audited and reviewed through clinical governance and continuous improvement. The most likely method for identification of potential improvements by the nurse will be through reflection using auditing.

Reflection

Reflection guides us to critically question our actions and practices. It is a great tool for nursing practice – we can always better our practice no matter how experienced we are. Reflection is also a useful tool for students – you will be surprised how much you learn over the duration of a course – and you do not realise it until you reflect upon it! Reflection enables us to view not only our actions but also the actions of others. Think of a fight or feud with a family member or friend – after the dust has settled we often think 'if he/she did not do that, I would not have done this … next time maybe I should …' – this is an example of reflection. In our workplace we reflect upon events or occurrences during the course of our shift. An example would be an arrest or traumatic incident or even something seemingly mundane that turned out to be a 'big deal'. Reflection is a part of our lives – whether we are conscious of it or not!

Reflective practice 25.1

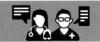

Critical thinking challenge

Reflecting on best practice and quality management, think about areas of your own nursing care that you feel could be improved upon. Then perform an Internet search to see if there are best-practice guidelines in this area.

1   Can you incorporate this into your placement?
2   Or, can you see this occurring in daily practice?

You may not be aware, but reflective practice is something we actively participate in every day. Nurses use evidence-based practice, best-practice guidelines and critical reflection to formulate holistic care plans for our clients. Reflection guides us to critically question our actions and practices. It is a skill highly useful for a student as you will be able to see quite clearly your professional development and growth as a practitioner. You will be surprised how much you learn over the duration of this course, and it is not until you reflect upon it that you are aware of it!

Systemic improvements

Systemic improvements are undertaken through the continuous improvement cycle and clinical governance. As you become more familiar with processes in place for patient safety, and clinical guidelines, it will become easier to recognise potential areas for review or improvement.

Look at how medication charts are being completed. Are allergies documented? Are prescriptions valid and legal? Another significant intervention from systemic review is that of the recognition of the deteriorating patient – the inception of Medical Emergency Teams, the Adult Deterioration Detection Score and clinical alerts are a massive component of this. What system is in place in your current facility?

Best practice

Best practice is a technique or methodology that through experience and research has proven to reliably lead to a desired result. A commitment to using the best practices in any field is a commitment to using all the knowledge and technology at one's disposal to ensure success. Best practice is also referred to as evidence-based practice, which uses guidelines developed through research to replace nursing practices. Examples of this are clinical guidelines that are used for all patient care delivery. Evidence-based practice is objective in its approach, providing the nurse with accurate and accountable information through which the development of guidelines or the review of practice improvement can occur.

As nurses in our daily practice we can identify areas that could be improved upon. These can range from basic nursing skills and techniques, such as hand washing, to time-management skills in care delivery.

Discussing and exploring challenges

Improvements in nursing practice often start from a single event. You may be caring for a patient who had an adverse drug reaction to a medication administered. An effective strategy to ensure this does not occur again would be to document the allergy on the NIMC. This is related directly to the NSQHS Standards – 10 standards which are of considerable concern in health-care delivery in Australia. Another ongoing challenge is the detection of the deteriorating patient. Standard 9 looks at this in great detail, but there are always site-specific occurrences that influence the monitoring and evaluation of inpatients.

Once patient assessment has been completed, you will need to know what information is relevant. Is the patient deteriorating? Are their observations within normal limits? Performing vital signs is useful only if you are reflecting upon the indices and acting upon them.

Clients receive holistic care from a variety of allied health professionals and to enhance patient care your role will be to continually test plans and ideas ordered from these professionals.

Activity 25.1

Applying standards to nursing practice

Review Standard 9 – Detection of the Deteriorating Patient.
1   Why do you think this standard exists?
2   How can you ensure your clinical practice remains vigilant in documenting and reporting observations?

Sourcing information

Other sources of information for review and reflection can be drawn from research and literature reviews. A literature review is a summary of previous research on a topic. Literature reviews can be either a part of a larger report of a research project or a component of a thesis or other research.

Information can also be sourced from and through feedback. There are many types of feedback that can be used, some examples include:
• observation of performance
• testing (drug calculations for example)
• incident reporting
• outcome indicators of care.

Feedback is ongoing and is a component of teamwork. Feedback is a crucial component of information sourcing. Identification of potential improvement in clinical practice takes clinical thinking and reflection. Understanding these concepts and the notion of patient safety and quality processes will enable you to develop potential improvements in clinical care. The more exposure to clinical nursing you gain, the more confident you will be in your reflections, observations and care delivery.

CASE STUDY 25.1

Reflecting on clinical performance

Thomas found that on his next placement, which was the second two weeks of acute placement, he was more prepared and was actually looking forward to spending two weeks in the cardiac medical unit.

Thomas reviewed his clinical journal that he had kept for the first two weeks and identified a few points that he decided to implement in the final two weeks. Thomas had found the planning exercise a good way to organise his time and he also noted that open communication with the clinical supervisor had assisted him in successfully completing his learning objectives.

Thomas decided that he should use some of the time on the weekend before placement reading through his clinical notes on cardiac conditions and what responsibilities and tasks he would likely undertake.

After the initial two days Thomas found that he was enjoying the placement and was managing his workload in a professional manner. One of the clients he was caring for, Paul, was a young man admitted with an arrhythmia for investigation. He had been running and suddenly collapsed and was brought by ambulance to the hospital. Paul had suffered a heart attack as a result of hypertrophic cardiomyopathy (HCM). Paul was withdrawn and appeared very depressed. Reading his notes Thomas noted that Paul was fearful of dying.

Thomas researched the condition and suggested to his buddy that a member of the support group coming in to visit Paul may be helpful. His buddy referred Thomas' ideas to the health-care team at the team meeting and they all agreed that this would be a positive intervention for Paul, if he would accept the proposal.

1   Why is it important to discuss and explore challenges with the registered nurse and the interdisciplinary health team before implementation?

2   How did Thomas comply with this aspect of teamwork?

3   What improvements did Thomas implement for his own area of nursing practice?

Review the skill in Tollefson *Essential Clinical Skills* 7.6 Nursing informatics

25.3 Participating in processes for systemic improvement

Being a part of any improvement process in patient care is not only a positive thing, it is incredibly rewarding. Ensuring patient safety is the epitome of nursing interventions and is generally always reflected in the mission statements of health-care services.

Organisation forums

Once you have completed data collection or reviewed the clinical issue that you wish to improve upon, you will need to ensure that the identified practice has supporting documentation. This will assist dissemination of information.

In order to design your reporting strategy you should consider the following:
*   objectives – what is it you are trying to highlight or review?
*   audience – who are you reporting this too?
*   mode of delivery – report, presentation, delivery at a conference.

Research identifies areas of improvement. Again, the 10 NSQHS Standards were established due to many health-care-related incidents.

A final consideration in disseminating information is to maintain a professional manner. Sometimes, you may come across some issues or problems in the activity you have identified, but remember, these are likely due to your colleagues, and using derogatory terms will not assist betterment in practice.

Activity 25.2

Organisation's forums

While on placement take note of the professional forums that staff can access to report issues or gain information about changes to practice.

1   What forums are available in your clinical area?
2   What type of forums are they, educational or investigative?

Recognising opportunities for systemic improvements to clinical guidelines for nursing practice

On your placement you will notice that there are clinical guidelines and care plans. Once you have identified one to review or improve upon, the process for this proposal needs to be reviewed. How will you gauge the effectiveness of the procedure? Or is it that regardless of the procedure/guideline errors still occur (medication errors are a great example here). There are audit tools for reviewing the 10 NSQHS Standards and these can be used by you to review patients' medication charts, for example, to look for any gaps in prescribing and administering and identify any common consistencies that are potentially causing harm.

Once you have completed the data collection – or auditing or clinical review – you will need to ensure your identified practice has supporting documentation and is clearly outlined for dissemination. Essentially all systemic improvements will follow the continuous improvement cycle – there is no getting around that!

You will need to follow the health-care facility's guidelines. You cannot just audit some charts and determine an outcome if you do not have the support of your colleagues and the approval of your manager or team leader. Information is readily available and you would be incredibly hard pressed to find a team leader or unit manager who did not want their staff to be involved in continuous improvement.

Presenting and arguing ideas for improving clinical practice

Once you have identified and reviewed the clinical process you aim to improve, you will need to ensure that your identified practice has supporting documentation and that you can determine findings (be it from audit or chart review) and report them to your colleagues, or to nursing forums or professional bodies.

The first step in deciding the format of your reporting is to understand the responsibilities you have in reporting the information. This is all reliant upon the reasoning for your review and the process you have undertaken. If, for example, while on placement you reviewed handwashing practices, would you disseminate the information to the ward/department or would you keep it for your learning and reflective practice? All improvement needs to have a reason and an endpoint for reviewing and reflecting.

TIP 25.1

Being a part of the team

When you are on placement, discuss with your facilitator or the nurse educator of the unit you are working on the continuous improvement that is being undertaken in the department. Is there anything that you can assist with? Take the time to review the quality improvement activities and see if you can deduce why they are in place. For instance, in an acute care ward, medication safety and falls would feature highly as ongoing processes.

Identifying and articulating issues and practical processes for implementing change

As your experience and exposure grows, you will notice that you will continually be reflecting, assessing and analysing clinical practice. Whether you use an audit tool or you base your analysis on ongoing errors or systematic gaps, you will soon learn how to ensure that patient safety is paramount because ultimately that is what clinical improvement is all about – the client and their family, and returning them to a state of health that is functional. Our clients are our main focus – their safety, their outcomes and the processes involved that ensure these outcomes marry up.

Activity 25.3

Identify issues that require investigation

All of the interventions that nursing undertakes are based on evidence. Find one of the nursing interventions that you have observed on clinical placement, for example, a particular process for

administration of a medication, and research the background and evidence for how the current practice evolved.

1 Have there been changes to the nursing practice?
2 Why were these changes implemented?
3 What was the outcome of the changes?

Responding to questions with confidence and relevant information

When presenting ways to change accepted practice you need to be able to answer questions relating to how this change will affect both the carer and the client. This will entail having a solid knowledge of what was the accepted practice and why a change is needed.

At times questions may be difficult to answer. If you do not know the answer to any question it is best to respond by saying that you will need to research this area and get back to the questioner.

Engaging with others using professional terminology

As a professional nurse it is important that your communication is structured at the right level for the different types of forums that you may be involved in. During presentations and meetings a more formal type of communication is required. Written material needs to be structured and presented in the correct format so that readers can easily identify the sections, the information being presented and previous findings.

Communicating with others in professional forums also requires a nurse to follow accepted social conventions and practices. It is important to remember that you are representing your workplace and their values and vision.

Feedback

The nature of professional nursing practice is such that competence needs to be evaluated to recognise how the work environment, clients and other staff members impact on the nurse's ability to perform their role.

These elements can cause us to act in a certain way and need to be taken into consideration during assessment and performance management processes. Feedback is crucial for the ongoing processes of continuous improvement, evidence-based practice and systemic review and improvement. Some of the feedback you may encounter includes:

- observation of performance
- audit of documentation (NIMC, for example)
- interview
- peer review
- client feedback.

Feedback is always ongoing, and will be another component of your nursing career – you will receive and give feedback on a daily basis. As your experience and exposure to clinical nursing grows, you will feel more confident in providing feedback. Through mentoring, support and clinical review of practices, your nursing career will strengthen and develop.

CASE STUDY 25.2

Participating in improvements

After the positive feedback Thomas received from the health-care team and Paul, he was keen to develop a network of support groups for clients with cardiac problems to give them additional support both while in the health-care facility and when discharged. Thomas decided to explore how he could implement his ideas for this improvement in the clinical area.

Thomas approached his clinical supervisor and discussed ways in which he could contribute to this improvement. His clinical supervisor suggested that he locate the policy and procedures that related to continuous improvement activities as a starting point. Thomas decided that he would use this experience as a basis for his research activity and gathered clinical research on the effectiveness of support groups for clients with a chronic disease process. Thomas presented his research and literature review to the rest of the class. Thomas also included a register of different types of support groups and services that were available to support individuals with a chronic disease. The class demonstrated their interest by asking a number of questions related to the topic. Thomas was able to answer their queries and direct them to appropriate research papers.

Thomas ended the presentation with a report on how Paul had responded to the intervention and was proud to outline how the unit had decided to implement this intervention and what practical steps were involved in contributing to the implementation of an improvement in the clinical area.

1 Why is it necessary to thoroughly research and prepare for presentations to present an idea for improving clinical practice?
2 What effect does a thorough preparation have on both the presenter and the group it is presented to?

SUMMARY

- A nurse needs to model high standards of performance through communication, sharing information and providing support to colleagues.
- Reflecting on performance enables the nurse to identify areas for improvement in their clinical practice.
- Assisting in the systemic improvement for clinical practice includes engaging in professional communication with colleagues.

SELF-TEST QUESTIONS

1 How can you model high standards of performance in your clinical practice?
2 How can collaboration with other members of the health-care team assist in improving your clinical practice?
3 What methods could you use to identify potential improvements to your clinical work practices?

4   What processes are involved with systematic improvements for clinical placement?

5   How can you contribute to the organisation's processes for systemic improvements to clinical guidelines for nursing practice?

BIBLIOGRAPHY

Borbasi, S., Jackson, D., & Langford, R.W. (2004). *Navigating the Maze of Nursing Research. An Interactive Learning Adventure*. Elsevier Mosby: Marrickville, NSW.

Burns, N. & Grove, S.K. (2007). *Understanding Nursing Research. Building an Evidenced-Based Practice*. Saunders Elsevier: St Louis.

Clarke, L., Gray, S., White, L., Duncan, G. & Baumle, W. (2016). *Foundations of Nursing: Enrolled Division 2 Nurses* (ANZ Edition). Cengage Learning: Melbourne.

DiCenso, A., Guyatt, G. & Ciliska, D. (2005). *Evidence-Based Practice. A Guide to Clinical Practice.*(4th Ed). Elsevier Mosby: St Louis.

Hnatiuk, C. (2013). Mentoring Nurses Toward Success, *Minority Nurse*. Retrieved from http://minoritynurse.com/mentoring-nurses-toward-success/. Accessed 30 March 2013.

Joint Commission on Accreditation of Health Care Organisations. Retrieved from http://www.jointcommission.org/. Accessed 14 July 2017.

National Health & Safety Council, www.nsca.org.au. Accessed 14 July 2017.

National Health and Medical Research Council (2007). *National statement on ethical conduct in human research – updated May 2015*. Retrieved from https://www.nhmrc.gov.au/guidelines-publications/e72. Accessed 14 July 2017.

Nursing and Midwifery Board of Australia (2016). *National Enrolled Nurse Standards for Practice*. Retrieved from http://www.nursingmidwiferyboard.gov.au/Codes-Guidelines-Statements/Professional-standards/enrolled-nurse-standards-for-practice.aspx.

Patton, M.Q. (2002). *Qualitative Research and Evaluation Methods* (3rd edition). Sage: Newbury Park, CA.

Polit, D. & Beck, C. (2010). *Essentials of Nursing Research: Appraising Evidence for Nursing Practice* (7th edition). Lippincott Williams & Wilkins: Philadelphia.

Taylor, B., Kermode, S. & Roberts, K. (2006). *Research in Nursing and Health Care: Evidence for Practice* (3rd edition). Cengage Learning: China.

The Australian Commission on Safety and Quality in Health Care (2017). *National Safety and Quality Health Service Standards*. Retrieved from https://www.safetyandquality.gov.au/our-work/assessment-to-the-nsqhs-standards/nsqhs-standards-second-edition/#NSQHS-Standards-(second-edition).

Tollefson, J., Watson, G., Jelly, E. & Tambree, K. (2016). *Essential Clinical Skills: Enrolled Division 2 Nurses* (3rd edition). Cengage Learning: Melbourne.

Glossary

active listening A technique used to reflect on what a patient has said and can help patients feel more deeply understood

adverse drug reactions (ADRs) Any medication effect other than what is therapeutically intended

adverse event An incident in which harm was done to a person receiving health care, for example from infections, falls resulting in injuries, or problems with medication and medical devices

advocacy The ability to stand up for or represent the interests or rights of another person

advocate A person who speaks up for or acts on behalf of the patient offering support and encouragement to exercise their rights.

advocating To publicly safeguard a person's decisions, wishes and preferences; to ensure the person is treated with respect and that they have the necessary information and support to make an informed choice

Aged Care Assessment Team An interdisciplinary team made up of a doctor, an RN, a social worker and an occupational therapist, assisting the elderly and their carers to determine the care level required to meet the client's needs

Aged Care Funding Instrument (ACFI) A resource allocation instrument that assesses the needs of residents and enables allocation of government funding

allergen A substance that causes an allergic reaction.

alternative therapy Therapies used instead of conventional medical therapy

Alzheimer's disease a progressive disease that leaves a person unable to form new memories and is marked by the loss of other mental functions

anoxic Lack of oxygen

antagonist Drug that blocks receptors, stopping what normally binds to the receptor and as a result inhibits normal response

antenatal Before delivery of the newborn

aseptic non-touch technique (ANNT) Infection control practice used to prevent the transmission of pathogens

atherosclerosis The artery wall narrows due to a build-up of a hard substance that adheres to the surface of the artery wall. Usually consisting of fat, cholesterol and other body substances that bond together

bioethics The application of general ethical principles to health care

biological maturation The process of progressing towards the mature state that occurs in all body systems, organs and tissues

blood glucose level A measurement of the amount of glucose (the principal blood sugar) circulating in the blood

blood pressure A measure of the pressure exerted by the blood on the wall of the artery

blood tests A scientific examination of a blood sample for the diagnosis of illness or detection and measurement of other substances or cells

body cavity An area in the body that contains internal organs

body temperature regulation The internal temperature of the body after the excess heat produced is lost by the body

care plan An individualised document outlining relevant interventions and planned care for the client. It is a communication tool and incorporates the needs of the client

caries Decay of the tooth

chain of infection The circumstances of an infection occurring

Cheyne-Stokes breathing A breathing pattern where the breaths become progressively irregular and shallower followed by periods of strong, deep breathing

clinical hand wash A one-minute hand wash using antimicrobial soap or skin cleanser performed prior to non-surgical procedures requiring aseptic technique

clinical handover The transfer of information, accountability and responsibility for patients from one health-care worker to another

clinical pathways Standardised management plans that are evidence-based and are applicable to the multidisciplinary health-care team

cognitive development The strengthening of the intellect to allow a person to increase ways of learning, thinking, analysing and creativity to enable full interaction with the world and others

collaboration Working with allied health care and other nursing staff to optimise health care

communication The exchange of information, thoughts, and feelings using both verbal and non-verbal methods

co-morbidities The presence of one or more diseases; for example, if a patient has diabetes and hypertension these are co-morbidities when they present with chest pain

complementary therapies Therapies used in conjunction with conventional medical therapy

complex Complicated and intricate – in health care it relates to patients who have multiple conditions or diseases that impact upon the presenting condition

consent Permission or agreement to be allowed to take action or perform some type of care

consultation Clinical discussion with other health-care team members to enable holistic health care

continuous improvement An ongoing cycle of improvement to ensure constant review

cultural safety An environment that is spiritually, socially and emotionally safe as well as physically safe for all people within it

cultural sensitivity Being aware that differences exist between people due to their cultural identity

culturally appropriate care Providing care that is appropriate to the patient's cultural context

culture Dynamic and integrated structures of knowledge, beliefs, behaviours, ideas, attitudes, values, habits, customs, languages, symbols, rituals, ceremonies and practices that are unique to a particular group of people

dementia the irreversible deterioration of intellectual ability accompanied by emotional disturbance

development The growth of the individual from simple to complex functions and skill strengths to enable survival

discrimination Unjust or prejudicial treatment of different categories of people, especially on the grounds of race, age or gender, where the physical, psychosocial, cultural and spiritual environment threatens individuals/group safety and security

duty of care An obligation both moral and legal to ensure the safety of others

electrocardiogram (ECG) Graphical recording of the heart's electrical activity

emergency procedure Outlines an organisation's policies and procedures in response to emergency situations

empathy The ability to understand and share feelings of another person, i.e. 'to stand in their shoes'

ethics Branch of philosophy concerned with determining right from wrong on the basis of a body of knowledge rather than on opinions

evidence-based practice The application of the best available empirical evidence, including recent research findings, to clinical practice in order to aid clinical decision making

exacerbation The time when the symptoms reappear

exudate Fluid that is leaked or drained from a wound. It is a response to the tissue damage in the wound

gestation Development of the foetus during pregnancy

granulation Growth of new tissue in the surfaces of the wound

hazard Anything that has the potential to harm the health and safety of a person

HbA1c A blood test that gives an indication of how well a person's diabetes is being controlled by current lifestyle and treatment

health-care acquired infections (HCAIs) Infections acquired in health-care facilities, or infections that occur as a result of an intervention in a health-care facility

hierarchy of control The process for minimising or controlling risk

holistic Encompassing all aspects of a person, including physical and mental health and wellbeing, spiritual, religious and environmental considerations

homeostasis Balance or equilibrium among the physiological, psychological and spiritual aspects as an integrated whole

implied consent When consent is given implicitly, such as by a person's actions, or lack of actions, rather than expressly (such as verbally or written)

incident report A risk management tool used to describe and report any adverse event that occurs to a client, visitor or staff member

infection Damage to tissue or cells by invading microorganisms

informed consent When the person understands the reason for the proposed intervention, knows the benefits and risks, and agrees to the treatment

interpersonal skills The ability to interact and communicate effectively with other people

law Decisions about conduct that guide the interactions of people. Laws are necessary, binding and enforceable so people can live and work together

life-limiting illness An illness that is expected to cause death

listening Interpreting the sounds heard and attaching meaning to them

lochia Vaginal discharge after birth

manual handling Any activity that requires a person to use force to move, hold or restrain another person or thing

mental health problem Where the person is unable to function to full capacity in society with others due to emotional stresses but is not totally isolated from reality

mental illness When a client is unable to function effectively in society due to emotional stresses that impact on their behaviour and response to others

metabolism The functional activities of cells that result in growth, repair and the release of energy by the cell

mitochondria The energy producing structures in the cells of the body

negligence A general term referring to carless acts on the part of an individual who is not exercising reasonable prudent judgement

non-ambulant Unable to walk

non-weight bearing Unable to support themselves

nutrition All the processes (ingestion, digestion, absorption, metabolism and elimination) involved in consuming and using food for energy

objective data Data that can be seen and measured, and are obtained through both standard assessment techniques performed during the physical examination and laboratory and diagnostic tests

oedema Excessive amount of fluid trapped in the tissue of the body, generally limbs

open disclosure The acknowledgement that harm has occurred to a client while being cared for in a health-care facility

oxygen saturation The percentage of haemoglobin binding sites in the bloodstream occupied by oxygen or the amount of oxygen that has combined with the haemoglobin in the red blood cell and is circulating in the blood

pain Unpleasant sensations perceived by the individual

palliative approach Meeting the needs of the whole person at the end of life – mental, emotional, spiritual relationship and environmental, as well as physical

papillae Small projections on the tongue's surface that allow the person to identify the different tastes of food, for example, the sourness of lemon

pathogen A disease-causing microorganism

pathophysiology The altered functioning of an organ and the resultant symptomology that occurs in a disease state

physical development The changes that occur over the lifespan enabling the person to achieve maturity and increased development of perception and motor skills

postnatal After delivery of the newborn

post-partum period The first six weeks after giving birth

primary health care (PHC) A person's point of entry into the health-care system includes personal care with health promotion, prevention of illness and community development

privacy The right to be left alone, to choose care based on personal beliefs, to govern body integrity, and to choose when and how sensitive information is shared

professional misconduct Poor conduct of a nurse outside their duty as a nurse such as being drunk and disorderly in a public place

psychosocial development The ability to understand emotional responses for both self and others and the ability to interact with others

pulse The number of times the heart beats per minute

remission The period of time that the person does not suffer the symptoms of the disease

respiration Breathing air both in and out of the airways

respite care Care and services that provides a break to caregivers and is used for a few hours a week, for an occasional weekend or for longer periods of time

rigor mortis Stiffening of the joints and muscles of a body a few hours after death

risk assessment Analysis of a hazard in terms of the likelihood of it creating a workplace injury or illness

scope of practice Outlines the procedures, tasks and care permitted under the criteria of the professional licence held by an individual

self-care Learnt behaviour and a deliberate action in response to a need

social hand wash A 10–15 second plain soap hand wash used for daily activities

standard precautions Preventative practice to be used in the care of all clients in hospitals regardless of their diagnosis or presumed infection status

stertorous breathing Noisy breathing

stigma A mark of disgrace associated with a particular quality in which a person is exposed to discriminatory practices by other people based on fear and ignorance

subjective data Include the person's sensations, feelings, values, beliefs, attitudes and perception of personal health status and life situation

surgical hand wash A five-minute hand scrub using antimicrobial soap performed before any invasive surgical procedure

synergy Effect of the use of two or more agents that produces a pharmacological response greater than what would be expected by the individual effects of each agent

TED stockings Elastic stockings that apply pressure to limbs to return fluid back into the circulation system

temperature Measurement of internal body warmth

therapeutic relationship A relationship that encourages the patient to express their feelings, facilitates trust and reduces the anxiety that he or she may be experiencing

thrush Infection of Candida Albicans

unprofessional conduct Poor conduct while undertaking the duties of a nurse. Not providing the agreed level of care

urinalysis Analysis of the urine using an indicator strip

verbal consent When a person expressly grants consent verbally

vicarious liability Where another person or entity, such as the facility, is held responsible for the actions of employees

written consent When a person expressly grants consent via writing

Index

A

Abbey Pain Scale, 142
Abdominopelvic area, 96
Abdominopelvic cavity, 96
ABF. *See* Activity-based funding (ABF)
Aboriginal and Torres Strait Islander health
    care, 352
    communication techniques, 356
    cultural safety guidelines, 355
    cultural safety issue in workplace, 353–355
    cultural safety modelling in work, 355–356
    cultural safety strategies, 356–358, 362–363
    differences in, 359
    health strategies, 359–362
    health-care needs, 358
    issues influencing relationships and
        communication, 353–354
    map, 354
ACAT assessment. *See* Aged Care Assessment
    Team assessment (ACAT assessment)
Accreditation process, 120
Accurate dosage and IV infusion rate
    calculations, 299–301
ACFI. *See* Aged Care Funding Instrument
    (ACFI)
ACHS. *See* Australian Council of Healthcare
    Standards (ACHS)
Acid base balance, 164
Active listening, 83
Active or reflective listening skills, 83
Activities of daily living (ADLs), 158, 190, 206,
    278, 343
    physical impact, 343
Activity theory, 37
Activity-based funding (ABF), 109, 113
Actual or potential health problems, 96–97,
    344
Acute adverse reaction, 310–311
Acute care experience, 290
    kind of patients in acute care facilities, 291
    objectives, 291–292
    of student nurses in acute care, 291
    work allocation, 292
Acute health problems. *See also* Chronic health
    conditions
    emergency department presentations, 320
    impact on person, family or carer, 320
    pathophysiology, 322
    physical and psychological impacts, 321
    planning care for person with, 323–324
    preliminary health assessment and health-
        care team, 320
Acute nursing, 322
    interventions, 325
Acute pain, 141

Acute wounds, 189
ADDS chart. *See* Adult Deterioration Detection
    Score chart (ADDS chart)
ADLs. *See* Activities of daily living (ADLs)
Administering medication
    acute and delayed adverse reactions,
        310–311
    educating person, family or carer, 314
    fluid and electrolyte imbalances, 311
    monitoring and evaluating person's response,
        309, 310
    removing IV cannula, 311–313
Administration routes, 298
Admission(s), 115
    assessments on, 70
    community supports, 75–76
    data for, 74, 75
    issues, 74–75
    preparing for, 70
    procedures, 74
    process for clients, 71
ADRs. *See* Adverse drug reactions (ADRs)
Adult Deterioration Detection Score chart
    (ADDS chart), 291, 328
Advance care
    directives, 45, 147–148, 151
    planning, 147
Advance Care Planning Australia (2017), 147
Advanced life support (ALS), 329
Adverse drug reactions (ADRs), 34, 310–311
Adverse event, 9, 66, 235
Advocacy, 45, 324
Advocate, 236
    for person, 45–46
Advocating, 65
    for clients, 65, 235
    for person, 65
Age-related disorders
    effects of drugs and medications, 34–35
    impacts of, 41–42
    pathophysiological disorders, 35
    physical changes, 32–34
Aged care
    advocate for person, 45–46
    assessment tools, 38–39
    for deceased person, 46
    elder abuse, 45
    funding, 40
    legal requirements and ethical issues, and
        ensuring work practice, 44
    nursing practice, 42–44
    policies and procedures, 45
    reflection about admissions, 41
    requirements and issues, 44
    residential facilities, 43–44
    responding to signs of stress, 46

    standards/accreditation, 40
    support in grief and death, 47
    working in, 31
Aged Care Act 1997, 40, 45
Aged Care Assessment Team assessment (ACAT
    assessment), 39
Aged care environment, nursing practice in, 42
    community services, 43–44
    impact of complex issues on family and
        carers, 42
    promoting health maintenance, 43
Aged Care Funding Instrument (ACFI), 40
Ageing, 32
    myths about, 42
    stereotypes, attitudes, values and beliefs, 42
    theories of, 36, 37
Ageism, 42
Agitation, strategies to relieving, 48–49
AHPRA. *See* Australian Health Practitioner
    Registration Agency (AHPRA)
Airway, compromised, 324
Alcohol, 361
    alcohol-related dementia, 47
Allergens, 92
Allergies, 310
ALS. *See* Advanced life support (ALS)
Alternative therapy, 110–111
Alzheimer's disease, 34, 47
Anaesthetists, 369
Analgesia, 151, 316
Anaphylaxis, 310
Anatomical and medical terminology, 93–95
ANMC. *See* Australian Nursing and Midwifery
    Council (ANMC)
Anoxic injuries, 228, 229
Antenatal care, 369
Anti-embolic aids, 208
ANTT. *See* Aseptic non-touch technique
    (ANTT)
Anxiety, 326
    disorders, 280
Aphasia, 178
APHCRI. *See* Australian Primary Health Care
    Research Institute (APHCRI)
Aprons, 22
Art therapy, 233
Arthritis, 228
Aseptic non-touch technique (ANTT),
    192–193
Assimilation, 93
Asthma inflammatory disease, 228
Atherosclerosis, 226
Attending skills, 83
Audits, 120
Australian Commission on Safety and Quality
    in Health Care, 383

Australian community, 107, 114
  cancer control, 337–338
  cardiovascular health, 338
  diabetes, 339
  effectiveness of community health
    promotion, 116–117
  Emma's story, 117
  emotional and social wellbeing, 117
  environmental and lifestyle factors, 337
  existing health services, 115
  factors affecting health, 114–115
  funding sources for health care in, 113–114
  health education regarding antibiotic use,
    117
  health issues affecting, 336
  health promotion, 116
  injury, 339
  legislation governing drugs in,
    294
  mental health, 339
  musculoskeletal conditions, 339
  obesity, 340
  risk factors for health, 115
  special populations, 337
Australian Council of Healthcare Standards
  (ACHS), 120
Australian Health Practitioner Registration
  Agency (AHPRA), 56, 221
Australian health-care system, nursing within,
  106
  collaborative relationships, 121
  contributing to team, 121, 122
  nurses in health-care system,
    107–112
  reflective practice impacts nursing practice,
    121
  teamwork, 121
  working in professional nursing practice,
    118–120
Australian Nursing and Midwifery Council
  (ANMC), 221
Australian Primary Health Care Research
  Institute (APHCRI), 334
Australian society, 353
  individuals' accessing information, 113–114
  legislation, 109
Autopsy, 152

B

Basic life support (BLS), 329
Bathing, 206
  guide for newborns, 377
Behaviours. *See also* Challenging behaviours
  of concern, 49–50
  conditions and, 280
  dietary change in, 347
  in mental health illnesses, 285
  risk factors, 104
Bereavement care, resources for,
  154

Best practice, 78, 240, 386–387
  outcomes against, 267
BGL. *See* Blood glucose level (BGL)
Bias, 125–126
  identification, 355
  maturation, 91
Bioethics, 62
Biofeedback, 111
Biological
  maturation, 91
  theories, 36
Biomedical risk factors, 104
Biopsychosocial effects, 281
Biopsychosocial health, 281
Bipolar disorder, 280
Birth, 372
  psychological impact, 373
Bleeding, 321
Blood
  handling and storing of, 309
  monitoring and evaluating person's response
    to, 309–314
  pressure, 70
  products, 296–297
  tests, 70, 326
  transfusions, 304–305, 324
Blood glucose level (BGL), 70, 101, 107, 165,
  169–170, 258, 260
BLS. *See* Basic life support (BLS)
BMI. *See* Body mass index (BMI)
Body
  cavities, 96
  interpretation based on structure and
    functioning, 91–94
  interrelatedness of body systems, 322
  language interpretation, 130
  planes of, 94
  relative positions, 94
  structure, 91
  systems, 92–93, 170–172
  temperature regulation, 91
  type of assessment, 101–102
Body mass index (BMI), 261, 340
BPI. *See* Brief Pain Inventory (BPI)
Braden scale, 38
Breast cancer, 337, 338
Breastfeeding, 376
Brief Pain Inventory (BPI), 142

C

CALD communities. *See* Culturally and
  linguistically diverse communities (CALD
  communities)
Cancer, 99, 137, 226
  breast, 337, 338
  cervical, 337, 338
  colorectal, 337, 338
  control, 337–338
  lung, 337, 338

  prostate, 337, 338
  skin, 337, 338
Cannulas, 314
Cardiopulmonary resuscitation, 329
Cardiovascular
  assessment, 184
  health, 338
  system, 32, 92, 181, 370
Care plan(ning), 65, 201, 202, 323, 343
  documentation, 213
  evaluating outcomes and changing care
    plans, 211
  meeting needs of people in, 77
  nursing care process, 212
  of wound, 194–195
Care/caring
  for clients, 8
  comfort, rest and sleep, 208–209
  consent, 202
  dealing with emergencies, 209
  dignity, 204
  documentation, 202–204
  encouraging patient involvement, 178–179
  encouraging person to contributing to own
    independence and mobility, 208
  evaluation, 350
  goals, 379
  implementation to meet identified needs, 205
  of mother, 372–374
  multicultural resources, 205
  of newborn, 374–375
  nutritional needs, 207
  for person from different culture, 109
  for person with diabetes, 236
  personal hygiene, 206
  preparing person for, 202
  respiratory function, 207–208
  skin integrity, 206
Carers, 72
  educating carer on administration of
    medicines, 314
  family and, 347
  impact of complex issues, 42
  using palliative approach, 146–148
  psychosocial impact of palliative care,
    144–145
  support, 235
  understanding of disease process, 229–232,
    261
Caries, 103
Case management, 343
Cerebrovascular accident (CVA), 178
Cervical cancer, 337, 338
Chain of infection, 97–98
Challenging behaviours, 49–50
  impact on person and others, 50
  best practice strategies, 50–51
  determining triggers, 49
  strategies to minimising impact,
    49–51

Challenging wounds, 197–198
Charter of rights and responsibilities, 46
Charting, 100
Chemical incompatibility, 297
Cheyne-Stokes breathing, 150
Chronic health problems, 224, 225. *See also*
    Acute health problems
    body systems, chronic disease states and
        symptoms, 226–229
    care for person with, 224
    community-based care services, 234
    contributing to coordinated service
        approach, 235–237
    identifying impacts, 225–234
    person involvement, 234
    person's and carer's understanding, 229–232
    strategies, techniques and equipment for
        management of, 232
    treatments, 232–234
Chronic pain, 141, 228
Chronic ulcers, 197
Chronic wounds, 189, 197
Cigarette smoking, 361
Circulatory system, 93
Cleaning, 24
Client(s)
    advocacy, 324
    assessing clients' health status, 160
    checking client's physical health status, 99
    clarification of client's physical health status,
        100
    completing charting, 161
    cooperation, 190
    dignity and privacy maintenance, 190
    discharge care and health-care team, 160
    disease, 162–163
    documentation, 173
    example of body systems, 170–172
    health information, 159
    health status, 163
    homeostasis, 163–170
    job role and organisation requirements, 99
    pathophysiology, 161
    physical health status, 99
    planning, 160, 170
    recognising normal readings, 161
    impact of specific interventions, 161
Clinical
    death signs, 151–152
    governance, 383–384
    hand wash, 19
    handover, 86
    investigations and assessments, 100
    judgement, 240
    manifestations of health conditions,
        340–342
    nursing care of wounds, 196
    pathways, 77, 175, 204
    reasoning cycle, 73
    waste management, 26

Clinical assessment, 68
    admission and discharge procedures, 74–76
    analysis of rationale behind decisions, 77
    for clients, 76–77
    collecting and interpreting health data,
        69–74
    confirming nursing interventions, 78
    conflicts, 79
Clinical practice, 381
    applying standards to nursing practice, 387
    discussing and exploring challenges, 387
    modelling high standards of performance,
        382–384
    participating in processes for systemic
        improvement, 388–391
    reflecting on clinical work practices and
        potential improvements, 385–388
CMI. *See* Consumer medication information
    (CMI)
Co-morbidities, 175
Code of ethics, 119
Code Red, 5
Cognitive development, 70
Collaboration, 121, 363, 382
Colorectal cancer, 337, 338
Colostrum, 376
Communication, 50–51, 81, 236, 353
    changes in client's condition, 323
    with clients in health-care facility, 124
    complex, 81–84
    of complex issues to speakers of languages,
        132
    cultural diversity and body language, 131
    cultural diversity and, 130–131
    effective communication in complex
        situations, 81–83
    effective strategies to manage language
        barrier, 131
    with elderly residents, 36
    evaluating effectiveness in complex
        situations, 88
    feedback for performance improvement,
        86–88
    identifying and addressing constraints,
        84
    using information technology, 85
    interpretation of body language, 130
    language barriers, 131
    leading small group discussions, 85
    listening skills, 83
    misunderstandings, 133
    with people from cultures, 132–133
    with people from diverse backgrounds and
        situations, 129
    seeking assistance, 131–133
    skills in nursing practice, 80
    strategies for sensory impairment, 36
    techniques and support services, 146–147,
        356
    verbal and non-verbal, 130–131

Community. *See also* Australian community
    community-based care services, 234
    experience, 331–332
    health promotion effectiveness, 116–117
    health-care service, 335
    liaising with referring agencies and
        community organisations, 256
    placement, 333
    resources and opportunities, 234, 288
    services, 43–44
    supports, 75–76, 350
Companionship, 37
Competence, 57
Complaints, 45, 57
Complementary therapies, 51, 52, 110–111
Complex conditions, nursing care for, 181–184
Complex diseases, 180
Complex interventions, 186
Complex management, 266
Complex needs, nursing care for person with
    critical thinking to improve care quality, 185
    indwelling catheters, 187
    nursing interventions, 175–180, 185–186
    of people with common disorders and
        conditions, 180–184
    quality improvement processes, 186
Complex nursing, 174, 175
    administering prescribed emergency
        medication, 264
    alterations in person's condition,
        266
    complex care needs of person with diabetes,
        262–263
    evaluating and interpreting blood and urine
        test results, 265
    interventions for optimal diabetes health,
        262
    ongoing management of person's condition,
        264
    workload management and re-prioritising
        care activities, 262
Complex wounds, 197–198
Confidentiality, 45, 62
Consent, 45, 190, 202
    form, 203
    informed, 60
    gaining, 204
    written, 202
Constraints on communication, 84
Consultation, 382
Consumer medication information (CMI), 306
Contamination, 29–30
Continuing professional development (CPD),
    221
Controlled Drug Register, 295
Coordinated service approach
    contributing to, 235
    providing education, 237
    role and responsibilities for communication
        and reporting, 236

Coordinated service approach (*Continued*)
  support of family or carer, 235
  variations in person's needs and response of
    health-care team, 237
Cost of treatments, 240
Cough etiquette, 24
CPD. *See* Continuing professional development
  (CPD)
Critical thinking, 73–74, 220, 386
Cultural care, 177
Cultural diversity, 133–134
  and body language, 131
  and communication, 130
  and language barriers, 131
  nursing interventions demonstrating respect,
    176–177
Cultural identity, 125
  caring for person with different, 134–135
  differences in, 126
  food preferences as result of, 278
Cultural safety, 126
  developing strategies for improving,
    356–358
  guidelines, 355
  issue in workplace, 353–355
  modelling in work, 355–356
  process of achieving, 356
  strategies, 356–358, 362–363
Cultural/culture, 125
  appropriate care, 126
  awareness, 355
  backgrounds, 128
  beliefs and practices, 134
  bias and ensuring inclusivity, 129
  considerations, 146
  demographics, 63
  and ethical considerations for research, 243
  influencing feelings and emotions, 126
  issues in open and non-judgemental manner,
    146
  practices, 153
  sensitivity, 126
Culturally and linguistically diverse
  communities (CALD communities), 44
Currency, 248
CVA. *See* Cerebrovascular accident (CVA)

D

Damage or error theories, 37
Data sources, 243
Day Therapy Centres, 43
Death, 141, 151
  caring for person's body after death,
    152–154
  clinical death signs, 151–152
  dignity in, 150
  imminent, 150
  providing support in, 47
  rattle. *See* Noisy respirations
  signs of clinical death, 151–152

Death and Sorry Business, 357
Debriefing, 62
  support and professional, 155
Deceased person, providing care for, 46
Decision-making process, 99, 119, 121
Deep vein thrombosis (DVT), 210, 296
Delayed adverse reaction. *See* Acute adverse
  reaction
Delirium, 48, 280
Dementia, 33, 47, 280
  activities appropriate to person with,
    48
  causes, 47
  frontotemporal, 47
  signs and symptoms, 48
  strategies for, 47–49
Dental caries, 37
Depression, 48, 280, 283
Decision making in PHC, 335–336
Deterioration
  of person, 74
  signs, 148–152
Diabetes, 227, 253, 263, 269, 339, 362
  assessment, 256, 261
  care services, 254
  complex nursing interventions, 262–266
  condition, medications, therapeutic regimes
    and self-management, 268
  determining person's understanding of
    condition, 260
  evaluation and supporting self-management,
    267
  factors impacting person's health, 260
  family or carer's understanding, 261
  holistic nursing assessment, 259
  information on diabetes care and funding
    sources, 254
  liaising with referring agencies and
    community organisations, 256
  management, 268
  medication, 265
  organisations providing services and
    information, 254
  outcomes against evidence-based best
    practice, 267
  pathophysiology, 256–259
  person with, 270
  person's self-management of condition, 269
  reviewing and modifying care plan, 267
  services, 254
  specialist health-care workers, 255
  specialist services and roles of organisations,
    255
  specific health promotion initiatives, 269
Diagnostic Related Groups (DRG), 109, 113
Digestive system, 92–93
Dignity, 204
  in death, 150
  nursing interventions demonstrating respect
    for, 176–177

nursing practice to support dignity and
    privacy, 347
Direct client care, safe work practices for, 4
  Australian codes for emergencies, 5
  hazards in workplace, 6–7
  incidents and injuries, 9
  reducing risk in workplace, 8
  working safely with clients, 7–8
  workplace policies and procedures, 4
Discharge care, 160
Discharge planning, 213–214
Discharge procedures, 74
  community supports, 75–76
  data for, 74, 75
  issues, 74–75
  requirements for, 76
Discrimination, 279
Disease, 162–163
  asthma inflammatory, 228
  complex, 180
  gum, 37
  identification, 103
  infectious, 27
  lewy body, 47
  metabolic, 327
  motor neurone, 228
Disease process
  barriers to education, 231
  education for chronic diseases, 230
  identifying knowledge gaps, 230
  person's and carer's understanding, 229–230
  stage of change and acquisition of new
    behaviours and skills, 232
Disengagement theory, 37
Disposable gloves, 23
Distress
  identifying and responding to signs, 38
  strategies to relieving, 48–49
Diverse groups, promoting understanding
  across, 133
  communication misunderstandings, 133
  cultural beliefs and practices, 134
  dealing with conflict, 133
  difficulties with caring for person with
    different cultural identity, 134–135
  misunderstandings, 133
  resolving differences, 134–135
  impact of social and cultural diversity,
    133–134
Diversity benefits and inclusiveness, 127
  cultural bias and ensuring inclusivity, 129
  identifying cultural backgrounds, 128
  professional relationships, 128
  work practices for safe environment, 129
  working together as team, 129
Documentation, 45, 57–58, 190, 199,
  202–204, 235, 237, 285, 378
  of care plan, 213
Doffing sterile gloves, 24
Donning sterile gloves, 24

Dorsal cavity, 96
Draining systems, closed, 198
DRG. *See* Diagnostic Related Groups (DRG)
Drug
    allergy, 310
    antagonism, 297
    and poisons schedules and classifications, 294–295
    synergy, 297
Duty of care, 59, 60, 64
DVT. *See* Deep vein thrombosis (DVT)
Dying physiology, 148–149
Dying stages, 148
    dignity in death, 150
    ethical issues and concerns, 151
    malignant wound management, 149–150
    management of respiratory and swallowing difficulties, 149
    physiology of dying, 148–149
    signs of clinical death, 151–152
Dysphagia, 178
Dyspnoea, 149

E

Eating disorders, 280
ECG. *See* Electrocardiogram (ECG)
Eclampsia, 372
Economic impacts on health, 109
ECT. *See* Electroconvulsive therapy (ECT)
Education(al), 202, 380
    barriers to, 231
    for chronic diseases, 230
    strategies, 286
Elder abuse, 45
Electrocardiogram (ECG), 70, 161
Electroconvulsive therapy (ECT), 272, 287
Electrolytes, 164
    imbalances, 311
Embryo, 371
Emergency
    medical, 209
    procedures, 5
    response in acute care environment, 328–329
    treatment, 349
    trolleys, 328
Emotional/emotions, 267
    barriers to education, 231
    need, 143–144, 179
    and social wellbeing, 117
    support relating to grief, loss and bereavement, 154
Empathy, 125
Employment, 360
End-of-life decisions, 148
Endocrine system, 33, 92–93, 181, 370
Enrolled Nurse Standards for Practice, 111, 221–222
Enrolled nursing standards, 120
Environment protection authority (EPA), 25

Environmental
    causes, 49
    cleaning, 24
    hazards, 99
    and lifestyle factors, 337
EPA. *See* Environment protection authority (EPA)
Ethical/ethics, 55, 62
    contemporary ethical issues, 63
    dilemmas, 64
    ethical practice, 63
    issues and concerns, 151
    and legal issues, 153
    reporting potential ethical issues, 63
    resolving ethical issues, 63
Evaluation, 267, 363
    component of nursing process, 78
Evidence, 241
    sources, 243
    strength of, 248
Evidence-based practice. *See* Best practice
Exacerbation, 225
Excretion function of body, 93
Exudate, 194
Eye shields/safety glasses, 22

F

Face protection, 22
FACES Scale, 142
Faecal incontinence, 227
Falls risk assessment tools, 39
Falls screening tools, 38
Family, 72
    and carers, 347
    impact of complex issues on, 42
    family/carer support, 235
    family/carer's understanding and involvement in person's diabetes care, 261
Fear, 326
Feasibility, 248
Feedback, 218–219, 387, 390–391
    to colleague, 86
    for performance improvement, 86–88
    professional, 219
    reflecting on, 88
    structured, 86
Fluid imbalance, 311
Foetal development, 369–372
Foetus, 371
Following skills, 83
Food preferences, 278
Frontotemporal dementia, 47
Functional incontinence, 227
Funding sources
    awareness of appropriate, 113
    cost of hospitalisation, 114
    for health care in Australia, 113
    health-care services, 113–114
    information on costs, 114
    for related services, 254

G

Gastrointestinal system, 32, 181, 370
General practitioner, 369
Genitourinary system, 33
Geographical remoteness, 360
Geriatric depression scale, 39
Germs, 28
Gestation, 369
Gestational diabetes, 257, 372
Gibbs reflective cycle, 217
Gingivitis, 37
Gloves, 13, 22–24
Gloving guidelines, 23
Glucose, 256
    storage and conversion in liver, 257
Goggles, 22
Gowns, 22
Granulation, 194
Grey case study, 348
Grief, 361
    providing support in, 47
    stages, 47
Group discussions, leading small, 85
Group dynamics, 382
Group work, 382
Growth function of body, 93
Guardianship, 45
Gum disease, 37

H

Haematological system, 370
Haemorrhage, 194
Hand Hygiene Australia, 18
Hand wash(ing), 18
    with alcohol-based hand rub, 20
    facilities, 20
    frequency, 20
Hazardous manual handling, 7
Hazards, 6
    documentation, 9
    in workplace, 6–7
HbA1c blood test, 268
HCAIs. *See* Health-care acquired infections (HCAIs)
HCM. *See* Hypertrophic cardiomyopathy (HCM)
Head injuries, closed, 229
Health
    employment, 360
    geographical remoteness, 360
    information, 159
    insurances, 113
    maintenance, 43
    medical conditions, 361–362
    mental illness, 361
    smoking, alcohol and substance abuse, 361
    status, 163
    strategies, 359

Health data, 69, 71
    collecting and interpreting, 69–74
    critical thinking, 73–74
    deterioration of person, 74
    developmental stages, 70
    families and carers, 72
    gathering information, 69
    introduction and explanations, 69
    primary health assessment, 69
    vital signs, 70
Health education, 207
    barriers, 345
    effecting change, 346
    and health promotion for illness prevention,
        344
    health promotion programs,
        345–346
    and health-care team role, 237
    regarding antibiotic use, 117
    strategies to support person, 345
Health Practitioner Regulation National Law Act
    (2009), 56
Health problems on person in PHC
    environment, 336
    actual or potential environmental health
        issues, 344
    clinical manifestations of health conditions,
        340–342
    health issues affecting Australian community,
        336–340
    physical, psychological and social impacts on
        activities of daily living, 343
    priorities and potential areas of risk,
        342–343
    sharing information, 343
Health promotion, 116, 286
    and preventative care, 107
    programs, 345–346
    research, 241
Health requirements of older person, 32
    age-related effects of drugs and medications,
        34–35
    age-related pathophysiological disorders and
        preventative care, 35
    age-related physical changes and
        psychosocial needs, 32–34
    assessment of older person, 33
    communicating effectively and making
        adjustments, 36
    companionship and social inclusion, 37
    identifying and responding to signs of
        distress, 38
    oral health problems, 37
    physical changes associated with ageing, 32
    preventative health assessment, 36
    theories of ageing, 36, 37
Health-care. See also Maternal and infant health
    care
    delivery, 112
    environment, 104, 120

facilities, 25, 27, 124, 222
    levels, 108
    person's health-care needs, 346–349
    services, 113–114
    workers in relation to open disclosure, 66
Health-care team, 160–161, 237, 320, 323. See
    also Interdisciplinary health-care team
    gathering information, document and report
        changes, 323–324
Health-care acquired infections (HCAIs), 17,
    210
Health-care system, nurses in, 107
    caring for people from non-Western culture,
        112
    complementary and alternative treatments,
        110–111
    current health issues for health-care delivery,
        112
    medications and PBS, 110
    non-Western approaches, 110
    nurses using strategies to maintain standards
        of care, 111
    political and economic impacts on health,
        109
    positive health outcomes, 107–108
    principles of primary health and wellness,
        107
    sociocultural and social influences affecting
        health, 108
Healthy lifestyle practices, 43
Hearing impairment, 36
Hemiparesis, 178
Hierarchy of risk control, 6
Holistic, 69
    approach, 361
    nursing assessment, 259
Holistic care, 326, 378
    planning, 176
Home care packages, 44
Homeopathy, 111
Homeostasis, 163
    analyse, 169
    BGL, 165
    importance of BGL, 169
    negative feedback controls body
        temperature, 164
    parameters in urinalysis, 166
    tests specific to haemotologic system,
        166–168
HONK. See Hyperglycaemic Hyperosmolar
    Nonketotic Coma (HONK)
Hospitalisation
    cost, 114
    risks associated with, 210–211
Human body, 90, 172
    structural organisation, 91
Hydration, 151
Hydrotherapy, 232
Hyperlipidaemia, 362
Hyperglycaemia, 258

Hyperglycaemic Hyperosmolar Nonketotic
    Coma (HONK), 259
Hypertension, 371
Hypertrophic cardiomyopathy (HCM), 388
Hypnotherapy, 111
Hypoglycaemia, 258, 264

I

Illness prevention, 344–346
Imminent death, 150
Immune system, 92
Immunisations, 27
Immunity function of body, 93
Implied consent, 202
Incident report, 8
    documentation, 9
Incompatibility, 297
Incontinence, 226
Indemnity insurance, 59
Index of Independence in Activities of Daily
    Living (Katz ADL), 38
Indwelling catheters, 187
Infected wound, 191
Infection, 11, 100
    activities to preventing spread, 12
    prevention, 28
Infection control, 24
    hazard management in workplace, 12
    safe work practices for management, 11–12
    and wounds, 196
Infection hazards, 26
    areas of responsibility, 27
    associated with role and work environment,
        26
    control measures to minimising risk in
        accordance, 28
    documenting and reporting activities and
        tasks, 27
    risk assessment, 27
Infection prevention
    hand hygiene, 16
    risk management associating with specific
        hazards, 29–30
    standard and additional precautions for,
        17–26
Infectious diseases, 27
Inflammatory process, 100
Information
    analysing, 247, 249
    comparing and contrasting, 247
    on diabetes care, 254
    feasibility, benefits and risks, 248
    gathering, 244–246
    interpretation based on structure and
        functioning of body, 91–94
    organising, 246
    in practice, 250–251
    prioritising, 247
    relevance of research, 245–246
    requests for, 57

selecting and evaluating, 244–245
sourcing, 387
strength, relevance, reliability and currency, 248
systematic approach, 245
technology to supporting communication, 85
ways to use information in research, 248
Informed consent, 60
Ingestion function of body, 93
Inherited genetic conditions, 98
Injections, 301
Injuries, 9, 339
anoxic, 228, 229
closed head, 229
in Australian community, 339
neurological, 228
penetrating, 228
penetrating, 228
pressure, 197
toxic, 229
Insulin, 256, 264. *See also* Diabetes
Integumentary system, 32, 91–93, 181, 370
Interdisciplinary health-care team, 211, 284, 334
community health-care service, 335
effective decision making in primary health care, 335–336
meetings and service providers, 286
multidisciplinary team, 145
PHC principles and philosophical framework, 334
prioritising needs of individuals, 335
recovery principles with support from, 286
service model and roles of, 334
working with, 144
Internal emergencies, 209
International System of Units (SI units), 299
Internet, 244
Interpersonal skills, 82
Interventions
checking client's physical health status before delivery of, 99
job role and organisation requirements for, 99
Irreversible dementia, 47
Intravenous cannula (IVC), 313
removal, 311–313
Intravenous (IV) solutions, 312
Intravenous fluids, 311
calculating accurate dosages and IV infusion rates, 299–301
considering medication's effect on body, 299
identifying administration route or site for medication, 298–299
legislative and organisational requirements, 301
medication administration and infusion of, 297
monitoring and evaluating person's response to, 309–314

preparing blood and blood products for blood transfusions, 304–305
techniques and precautions specific to person's situation, 301–304
Intravenous therapy, 308–309
administering and storing medication, 305–309
administering medications, 293
assessing effectiveness of pain-relieving therapy, 314–316
minimising potential risk to ensure safe administration, 294–297
standard for schedules of medicines and poisons, 295
IVC. *See* Intravenous cannula (IVC)

J

Journaling, 216, 220

K

Ketoacidosis, 259

L

Labour, 372
Lactation, 375–376
Language barrier management, strategies to, 131
Lasix, 299
Law, 55
Legal and ethical parameters for nursing practice, 54
advocating for person, 65
applying knowledge of legal framework, 59–62
consent, 60
duty of care, 64
ethics, 62–63
interpret referrals or requests for tests on receipt, 62
legal terms, 61
mandatory reporting processes, 61
negligence, duty of care and vicarious liability, 59
open disclosure, 66
privacy and confidentiality, 62
restraint, 60–61
scope of professional nursing practice, 55–58
supporting rights, interests and needs of patients and families, 64–65
writing reports, 61
Legal issues in nursing, 279
Legislation
governing drugs in Australia and New Zealand, 294
legislative and organisational requirements, 301
and policy and procedures, 152

Lewy body disease, 47
Life-limiting illness, 140
Lifestyle choices, impact of, 72
Lifestyle factors, 337
Lifting machines, 7
Linen management, 30
Listening, 83
skills, 83
Lochia, 373
Lung cancer, 337, 338
Lymphatic system, 92, 93

M

Mandatory reporting processes, 61
Manual handling, 240
safe work practices for, 9–10
Masks, 22
Maslow's hierarchy of needs, 336
Massage, 111, 233
Maternal and infant health care, 368
assisting mother with safe practices in infant care, 376
assisting with lactation, 375–376
bathing guide for newborns, 377
complications of pregnancy, 371–372
using correct terminology, 375
education, 380
foetal development by gestation in weeks, 371
holistic care, 378
labour and birth, 372
maternal changes with associated signs and symptoms, 370
nursing care, 372–375
observations of mother and newborn infant, 377–378
ongoing care of mother, 376–377
outcomes of care, 378–379
planning care and care goals, 379
pregnancy and foetal development, 369–372
supporting new mother, 379
team, 369
Meals on Wheels (MOW), 76
Mean, 249
Median, 249
Medical causes, 50
Medical emergency, 209
Medical Emergency Teams (METs), 328
Medications, 110, 287–288, 299, 310
administration, 293, 297, 305, 385
applying 'rights of medication administration', 306–307
applying quality practices and undertaking risk assessment, 308
calculations–conversions, 300–301, 305
and complementary strategies alleviate pain and discomfort, 316

Medications (*Continued*)
drugs and poisons schedules and classifications, 294–295
effects, 34, 299
and elderly, 35
expiry of, 306
handling and storing of medications and blood products, 309
identifying administration route or site for, 298–299
minimising potential risk to ensure safe administration, 294
pharmacology and substance incompatibilities administering, 296–297
preparation for medication administration and infusion, 297–305
purpose and function of prescribing medicine and IV therapy, 296
reporting refusal of medication or IV therapy, 308–309
safe medication administration measures, 308
securing medications in safe manner, 308
suspected incomplete medication ingestion, 308–309
terminology relating to, 299
'Men's business', 357
Mental health, 273, 339
clients, 279
contributing to care planning and conducting initial clinical observations, 282–286
contributing to recovery of person with, 286–288
discharge from mental health facility, 288
legislation and restraint, 277
nursing, 276
placement within mental health environment, 275
problem, 276
responding appropriately to signs of mental illness, 279–282
safe within mental health facility, 282
state/territory mental health legislation requirements, 276–279
Mental Health Act (2014), 277, 287
Mental health experience, 272
kind of patients in mental health facilities, 273
objectives, 273–274
of student nurses in mental health, 273
work allocation, 274
Mental health illnesses, 276, 280, 361
effects on components of individual's life, 281
knowing signs and symptoms, 281
methods of interaction with clients, 282
supporting and valuing person with, 288
Mental illness. *See* Mental health illnesses
Mentoring, 383

Metabolic diseases, 327
Metabolism, 91
Metric system, 299–300
METs. *See* Medical Emergency Teams (METs)
Middle-ear infections, 362
Midwife, 369
MIMS, 297
Mini mental status examination (MMSE), 38
Mitochondria, 98
MMSE. *See* Mini mental status examination (MMSE)
Mobility
devices, 233
equipment, 11
Mode, 249
Modelling high standards of performance, 382
continuous improvement, 383–384
organisational vision, 382
respectful and positive communication, 383
supporting colleagues, 382–383
Monitoring
clients, 100
patient's condition and respecting wishes, 147
person's identified care needs, 210–211
Mood disorders, 280
Morphine, 142, 299
Mother
care of, 372–374
documenting and recording observations, 377–378
Motivation, 160
to change, 231
Motor neurone disease, 228
Movement of body, 93
MOW. *See* Meals on Wheels (MOW)
Multi-resistant staphylococcus aureus (MRSA), 196
Multicultural resources, 205
Multidisciplinary team, 144, 145
Muscle system, 93
Musculoskeletal conditions, 339
Musculoskeletal system, 32, 92, 99, 181, 370
Music therapy, 51, 233
My Aged Care, 44

N

NACAP. *See* National Aged Care Advocacy Program (NACAP)
National Aboriginal Community Controlled Health Organisation (NACCHO), 359
National Aged Care Advocacy Program (NACAP), 45
National Enrolled Nurse Standards for Practice, 382
National Health and Medical Research Council (NHMRC), 17, 243
National Inpatient Medication Chart (NIMC), 301–303, 327
National Palliative Care Strategy (2010), 140

National Safety and Quality Health Service (NSQHS), 327, 383, 384
Naturopathy, 111
Negligence, 59
Negotiation skills, 282
Neonatal nurses, 369
Nervous system, 92, 93
Neurological injury, 228
Neurological system, 33, 181
New Zealand, legislation governing drugs in, 294
Newborns
bathing guide for, 377
care of, 374–375
documenting and recording observations, 377–378
NHMRC. *See* National Health and Medical Research Council (NHMRC)
NIMC. *See* National Inpatient Medication Chart (NIMC)
NMBA. *See* Nursing and Midwifery Board of Australia (NMBA)
Noisy respirations, 149
Non-ambulant bearing, 7
Non-coronial autopsy, 152
Non-disturbance of wounds, 190–191
Non-medication therapies, assessing effectiveness of, 316
Non-pharmacological management, 143
Non-verbal communication, 130–131
Non-weight bearing, 7
Non-Western culture
caring for people from, 112
to health care and nursing practice, 110
Normal ageing, 32
Norton scale, 38
NSQHS. *See* National Safety and Quality Health Service (NSQHS)
Numerical Rating Scales (NRS), 142
Numerical statistics, 249
Nurse/nursing, 236, 241. *See also* Australian health-care system, nursing within
for blood reactions, 304
care process, 212
codes, 56
in health-care system, 107–112
legal issues in, 279
outcomes evaluation in wound care, 198–199
process, 96–97, 185, 189, 204
reason for, 77
research, 241
role, 120, 186
use to maintain standards of care, 111
workload management, 262
Nursing and Midwifery Board of Australia (NMBA), 56, 120, 382
Nursing care
for complex conditions, 181–184
of older person, 42
for person with complex needs, 174–187

Nursing care plan, 267
  admission and discharge procedures, 74–76
  analysis of rationale behind decisions, 77
  care procedures implementation to meet identified needs, 205–209
  for clients, 76–77
  collecting and interpreting health data, 69–74
  confirming nursing interventions, 78
  conflicts, 79
  consulting and collaborating with interdisciplinary health-care team, 211
  contributing to development of, 41
  discharge planning, 213–214
  evaluating outcomes and changing care plans, 211–213
  evaluating outcomes of care providence, 211
  monitoring person's identified care needs, 210–211
  planning care, 201
  preparing person for care procedures, 202–205
Nursing interventions, 185–186, 205, 346
  adjusting nursing interventions, 348
  to assist person with complex needs, 175
  assisting clients to maintain independence, 179
  based on predetermined care plans, 176
  compromised airway, 324
  demonstrating respect for dignity and cultural diversity, 176–177
  dietary change in behaviour, 347
  emergency treatment, 349
  encouraging patient involvement during care interventions, 178–179
  families and carers, 347
  first aid and emergency treatment, 349
  importance of reporting and recording, 179–180
  nursing assessment, 175
  nursing practice to support dignity and privacy, 347
  observing and identifying need for psychological support and care, 325–326
  performance to support health care, 324
  person-centred care, 347
  physical, emotional and psychosocial needs, 179
  planning, prioritising and implementing, 287
  prioritising and modifying nursing interventions, 325
  prioritising nursing interventions according to person's needs, 349
Nursing practice, 55
  acts, guidelines, codes and nursing practice, 55–56
  against ethical and legal requirements, 221
  in aged care environment, 42–44
  analysing information, 247–249

  audits and accreditation processes, 120
  code of ethics and decision-making framework, 119
  documentation, 57, 58
  enhancement, 219–221
  enrolled nursing standards, 120
  gathering information, 244–246
  historical development and current perspectives of nursing, 118
  information in practice, 250–251
  monitoring compliance, 58
  nurse role, 120
  nursing and research, 239
  nursing theorists, 118
  palliative approach to, 140–155
  planning information-gathering activities, 240–244
  in PHC setting, 333–350
  policies and procedures, 56
  principles and parameters of nursing practice, 119
  professional nursing bodies, 119
  requests for information, 57
  responding to complaints, 57
  scope of practice, 56–57, 120
  working in context of, 118
Nutrition, 91, 151
Nutritional needs, 207

O

Obesity, 340
Objective data, 69–70, 91, 211
Obstetricians, 369
Occupational therapy, 232
Oedema, 194
Older person
  aged care assessment tools, 38–39
  aged care requirements and issues, 44–47
  care planning for older person, 38–42
  contributing to development of nursing care plans, 41
  documentation and reporting, 39–40
  health requirements of older person, 32–38
  identifying abilities and limitations for self-care, 40–41
  impacts of age-related disorders, 41–42
  implications of admission, 41
  nursing practice in aged care environment, 42–44
  strategies for dementia, 47–49
  strategies to minimising impact of challenging behaviours, 49–51
  working in aged care, 31
Open disclosure process, 66
Open draining systems, 198
Oral health problems, 37
Oral infections and ulcerations, 37
Organ donation, 152, 153
Organic disorders, 280

Organisation forums, 388, 389
Organisational vision, 382
Oriental medicine, 111
Osteoarthritis, 228
Osteoporosis, 228
Outcomes of care, 211, 378–379
Oxygen saturation, 70

P

Paediatrician, 369
Pain, 228, 314
  assessment, 317
Pain Assessment in Advanced Dementia Scale (PAINAD Scale), 142
Pain management, 141, 143
  non-pharmacological management, 143
  pain assessment tools, 141–142
  pharmacological management, 142
  signs of pain, 141
  strategies, 327
  types, 141
Pain-relieving therapy effectiveness, 314
  clarify location and nature of pain, 315
  identifying signs of pain or discomfort, 314–315
  interpreting observations and evaluating person's pain, 315–316
  medications and complementary strategies, 316
  and non-medication therapies, 316
  recording observations, 316
PAINAD Scale. See Pain Assessment in Advanced Dementia Scale (PAINAD Scale)
Palliative approach, 140, 144
  advance care planning and directives, 147–148
  caring for person's body after death, 152–154
  communication techniques and support services, 146–147
  cultural considerations, 146
  monitoring patient's condition and respecting wishes, 147
  pain management, 141–143
  pathophysiological changes, 141
  person, family or carers using, 146
  person requiring palliative approach to care, 140
  principles, 140
  reflection about loss, 155
  self-care in palliative care role, 155
  signs of deterioration and stages of dying, 148–152
  social, emotional and spiritual needs, 143–144
  spiritual and cultural issues in open and non-judgemental manner, 146
  spiritual support, 144
  working with interdisciplinary team, 144, 145

Palliative care, 140
    experience, 136–138
    principles, 140
    psychosocial impact on family and carers,
        144–145
Palliative sedation, 151
Pancreas, 256
Papillae, 103
Partners in Culturally Appropriate Care
    program (PICAC program), 44
Pathogens, 92
Pathophysiology, 35, 103
    changes, 141
    of diabetes, 256–259
    through observation, 161
Patient identification, 89
Paul's discharge, 75
PBS. See Pharmaceutical Benefits Scheme (PBS)
PE. See Pulmonary embolism (PE)
Penetrating injuries, 228
Performance improvement, feedback for, 86–88
Performance review, 86–87, 222
Periodontitis, 37
Person-centred care, 234, 347
Person's behaviour observation, 285
Person's body after death, caring for, 152
    autopsy, 152
    care of body after death, 153
    cultural and spiritual practices, 153
    emotional support relating to grief, loss and
        bereavement, 154
    ethical and legal issues, 153
    legislation and policy and procedures, 152
    organ donation, 152
    standard precautions, 153
    support needs and resources for bereavement
        care, 154
Person's dignity and uniqueness, respect for,
    287
Person's health-care needs, 346–349
Person's mobility, changes in, 10
Person's needs, variations in, 237
Personal hygiene, 206
Personal protective equipment (PPE), 21, 24,
    209
    aprons and gowns, 22
    eye shields/safety glasses and face protection,
        22
    gloves, 22–24
    masks, 22
Personality disorders, 280
Pharmaceutical Benefits Scheme (PBS), 109,
    110
Pharmacodynamics, 296
Pharmacokinetics, 296
Pharmacological management, 142
PHC. See Primary health care (PHC)
Physical conditions, impact on, 97
    inherited genetic conditions, 98
    pathogens, 97–98

trauma, toxins and environmental hazards,
    99
Physical development, 70
Physical health status
    accurate information about physical health,
        91
    actual or potential health problems, 96–97
    human body, 90
    impact on physical conditions, 97–99
    interpreting information based on structure
        and functioning of body, 91–96
    new language, 96
    physical health status of clients, 99–100
    variations from normal physical health
        status, 100–105
Physical incompatibilities, 297
Physical need, 179
Physical restraint, 279
Physiological incompatibility. See Therapeutic
    incompatibility
Physiotherapist, 369
Physiotherapy, 232
PICAC program. See Partners in Culturally
    Appropriate Care program (PICAC
    program)
Pilates, 233
Planning care, 379
Planning information-gathering activities, 240,
    244
    credible sources of data and evidence, 243
    cultural and ethical considerations for
        research, 243
    current trends, 241
    quality improvement and reflective practice,
        241
    research objectives, 241–242
    research support and improving work
        practice, 240–241
Political impacts on health, 109
Polydipsia, 258
Polyphagia, 258
Polypharmacy, 35
Polyuria, 258
Populations, 337
Post-operative nursing care, 326–327
    promoting post-operative comfort using
        pain management strategies, 327
Post-partum period, 373
Postnatal
    assessment, 374
    care, 369
    depression, 373–374
Power of attorney, 45
PPE. See Personal protective equipment (PPE)
PQRST process, 315
Pre-operative nursing care, 207, 326–327
Predetermined care plans, 176
Pregnancy, 369–372
Preliminary health assessment, 320
Pressure injuries, 197

Preventative care, 35
Preventative health assessment, 36, 38
Primary health
    assessment, 69
    primary health-care environment, 336–344
    and wellness principles, 107
Primary health care (PHC), 334, 335. See also
    Aboriginal and Torres Strait Islander health
    care
    care evaluation, 350
    community placement, 333
    community supports, 350
    documentation, 350
    effective decision making in, 335–336
    health education and health promotion for
        illness prevention, 344–346
    health problems on person in PHC
        environment, 336–344
    interdisciplinary health-care team,
        334–336
    nursing interventions, 346–349
    planned PHC and suitable resources,
        349–350
    principles and philosophical framework,
        334
Prioritising information, 247
Priority of care, 240
Privacy, 45, 62
Professional development, 221
Professional feedback, 219
Professional misconduct, 56
Professional nursing practice. See Nursing
    practice
Professional practice improvement
    facilitating ongoing professional
        development, 221–222
    practice enhancement, 219–221
    reflective practice, 215, 216–219
Professional relationships, 128
Professional terminology, 390
Programmed theories, 37
Prostate cancer, 337, 338
Prosthetics, 233
Protection function of body, 93
Psychological and community intervention,
    145
Psychological barriers to education, 231
Psychological causes, 49
Psychological impact on ADLs, 343
Psychosis, 280
Psychosocial development, 70
Psychosocial need, 179
    of person, 32–34
Pulmonary embolism (PE), 210
Pulse, 70
Pyrexia, 194

Q

Quality improvement processes, 186, 241

R

RACGP. *See* Royal Australian College of
General Practitioners (RACGP)
Radiographer, 369
Re-evaluation of nursing care, 210
Re-prioritising care activities for person, 262
Reality orientation, 51
Recovery principles with support from
interdisciplinary team, 286
Reflection, 216, 220, 386
about aged care admissions, 41
improving practice through, 216
Reflective practice, 215, 216
actively seeking feedback from others,
218–219
barriers to, 217
clinical review, 218
impacts nursing practice, 121
models, 217–218
Registered nurses, 369
Regulation function of body, 93
Rehabilitation, 178–179
centre, 157
experience, 157–158
Relevance, 248
Reliability, 248
Religious care, 177
Reminiscence, 51
Remission, 225
Reporting, 190, 236
and recording, 179–180
Reproduction function of body, 93
Reproductive system, 92 93, 370
Research objectives, 241–242
Respectful and positive communication,
383
Respiratory/respiration, 70, 93
function, 207–208
hygiene, 24
management, 149
new admission of respiratory patient, 73
noisy, 149
system, 32, 92, 93, 181, 370
Respite care, 43
Restraint, 60–61
policy and procedure, 222
Resuscitation trolley, 328
Reversible dementia, 47
Review processes, 222
Rheumatoid arthritis, 228
Rights of medication administration, 306
right client, 306
right documentation, 307
right dose, 306–307
right drug, 306
right form, 307
right response, 307
right route, 307
right time, 307

right to refuse, 307
Rigor mortis, 152
Risk
contamination considerations, 29
management associating with specific
hazards, 29
minimising contamination, 30
protocols for care after exposure to blood
and other bodily fluids, 29
Risk assessment, 6, 10, 27, 39, 282–284, 308
forms, 101
tools, 38–39
Risk factors
for health, 115
with hospitalisation, 210–211
with variations from normal health status,
104
Royal Australian College of General
Practitioners (RACGP), 355–357

S

subcutaneous injection, 265
Safe work practices
for direct client care, 4–9
for managing infection control, 11–12
for manual handling, 9–10
moving people safely, 10
reflecting on, 13–14
working as team to ensuring safe working
environment, 13
Scope of practice, 56–59
Secretion function of body, 93
Seeking assistance, 131, 134
communicating with people from cultures,
132–133
communication of complex issues to
speakers of languages, 132
Self awareness improvement, 126–127
Self harm, 361
Self-administration of insulin, 264
Self-care, 220
identifying abilities and limitations for,
40–41
in palliative care role, 155
Self-determination in mental illness, 361–363
Self-development, recognising need for,
220–221
Self-esteem enhancement, 34
Self-evaluation, 87–88
Self-management, 260
person's understanding of, 268
promoting person's self-management of
condition, 269
specific health promotion initiatives to
support, 269
supporting, 267–269
Self-reflection, journal for, 218
Service model and roles of interdisciplinary
health-care team, 334

Service providers, 286
Short-term care. *See* Respite care
SI units. *See* International System of Units (SI
units)
Skeletal system, 93
Skin, 183, 184, 191, 206
cancer, 337, 338
integrity, 206
SMART format. *See* Specific, measurable,
achievable, realistic and timely format
(SMART format)
Smoking, 361
Social awareness improvement, 126–127
Social hand wash, 19
Social impact
on ADLs, 343
on diverse people, 133–134
Social inclusion, 37
Social need for palliative care, 143–144
Sociocultural and social influences that affect
health, 108
Special senses, 33, 92
Specialist health-care workers for diabetes
management, 255
Specific, measurable, achievable, realistic and
timely format (SMART format), 242
Speech impairment, 36
Spill management, 29
Spiritual
care, 177
issues in open and non-judgemental manner,
146
need, 143–144
practices, 153
support, 144
Standard precautions, 11, 153
colours of bags for waste, 26
environmental cleaning, 24
five moments of hand hygiene, 19
hand washing, 18–20
for infection prevention and control,
17, 18
PPE, 21–24
waste management, 25–26
State/territory mental health legislation
requirements, 276
features of mental health legislation, 277
legal issues in nursing, 279
principles of recovery orientated mental
health practice, 278
rights of person, 278
values and philosophies applying to mental
health care, 277–278
Stereotyping, 42, 281, 353
Sterile gloves, application and removal of,
23
Stertorous breathing, 150
Stigma, 279, 281
Strengths, Weaknesses, Opportunities, Threats
analysis (SWOT analysis), 87–88

Stress
  incontinence, 227
  management, 46
  responding to signs, 46
Student nurses experiences in palliative care, 137
Subacute/rehabilitation setting, 158
Subjective data, 69–70, 91, 211
Substance abuse, 361
Sudden cardiac arrest, 329
Suicide, 361
Support networks, 219–220
Support services, 44, 76
Supporting colleagues, 382–383
Surgical hand wash, 19
Susceptible host, 97
Swallowing difficulties, 149
SWOT analysis. *See* Strengths, Weaknesses, Opportunities, Threats analysis (SWOT analysis)
Syringe driver, 142
Systematic approach, 245
Systemic improvement, 386–387, 388
  engaging with others using professional terminology, 390
  feedback, 390–391
  identifying and articulating issues and practical processes, 390
  organisation forums, 388, 389
  participating in improvements, 391
  participating in processes, 388–391
  presenting and arguing ideas for improving clinical practice, 389
  recognising opportunities for, 389
  responding to questions with confidence and relevant information, 390

T

Team
  approach to safety in workplace, 13
  part of, 389, 390
Teamwork, 121
TED stockings, 7, 208, 327
Temperature, 70
  indicating fever, 373
  pyrexia, 194
  wound, 193
Theatre preparation, 327
Theories of ageing, 36, 37
Therapeutic
  incompatibility, 297
  interventions, 287
  person's understanding of therapeutic regimes, 268
  relationship, 69
  wound, 193

'Thirsty Thursday', 361
Thoracic cavity, 96
Thrush, 103
Time management, 262
Tone of voice, 81
Tooth loss, 37
Toxic injuries, 229
Toxins, 99, 163
Traditional healing practices, 360
Transition Care Programs, 43
Transport function of body, 93
Trauma, 99, 361
Trolleys, 24
Type 1 diabetes, 257
Type 2 diabetes, 257

U

u/a. *See* Urinalysis (u/a)
Ulcers, 197
UN. *See* United Nations (UN)
Unexpected guests, 25
Unfamiliar tasks, 9
United Nations (UN), 276
  principles relating to mental health, 276–277
Unprofessional conduct, 56
Urge incontinence, 227
Urgent responses, 74
Urinalysis (u/a), 70, 161, 165, 266
  parameters in, 166
Urinary system, 92, 93
Urinary/reproductive system, 181

V

Validation therapy, 51
Validity of evidence, 248
Vascular dementia, 47
Ventral cavity, 96
Verbal communication, 130–131, 235, 237
Verbal consent, 202
Vicarious liability, 59
Vision impairment, 36
Visual Infusion Phlebitis Score (VIPS), 313
Vital signs, 70, 74
Voila, 244

W

Waste management, 25–26
Waterlow scale, 39
Wellness, 160
WHO. *See* World Health Organization (WHO)
WHS. *See* Work health and safety (WHS)
Wide qualitative research, 241

Withholding treatment, 151
'Women's business', 357
Wong-Baker FACES pain rating scale, 142
Work health and safety (WHS), 4, 30, 45, 219
Working with diverse people
  benefits of diversity and inclusiveness, 127–129
  communication, 124, 129–133
  culture influences feelings and emotions, 126
  differences in cultural identity, 126
  improving self and social awareness, 126–127
  knowing oneself, 127
  promoting understanding across diverse groups, 133–135
  reflecting on perspectives, 125
  social and cultural perspectives and biases, 125–126
World Health Organization (WHO), 18, 160, 225, 334, 345
Wound
  assessment, 190
  bed presentation, 195
  dehiscence, 194, 195
  dressings, 193, 198, 326
  infection, 194
  malignant wound management, 149–150
  review and reassessment, 199
  swabs, 196
Wound management. *See also* Pain management
  ANTT, 192–193
  applying protocols for, 189–193
  assessing impact of wounds, 193–194
  client cooperation and consent, 190
  clinical nursing care of wounds, 196
  complex or challenging wounds, 197–198
  documentation and reporting, 190
  factors affect wound healing, 192
  maintaining client dignity and privacy, 190
  non-disturbance of wounds, 190–191
  nursing action outcomes evaluation in wound care, 198–199
  planning care, 194–195
  pressure sores, 188
  same wound with different outcomes, 191
  strategies to minimising cross-contamination and spread of infection, 192
Wounds Australia, 189
Writing reports, 61
Written consent, 202

X

Xerostomia, 37